Brains, Behavior, and Robotics

Brains, Behavior, and Robotics

by
James S. Albus

BYTE Books, Subsidiary of McGraw-Hill, 70 Main St., Peterborough, N.H. 03458

The ideas presented in this book represent the
views of the author and not those of the Department of Commerce or the National Bureau of
Standards.

Library of Congress Cataloging in Publication Data
Albus, James Sacra.
  Brains, behavior, and robotics.

  Bibliography: p.
  Includes index.
  1. Artificial intelligence. I. Title.
Q335.A44   001.53′5   81-12310
ISBN 0-07-000975-9   AACR2

3456789 HDHD 89876543

Text set in Times Roman
by BYTE Publications.

Edited by Bruce Roberts and Nicholas Bedworth.

Design and Production Supervision
by Ellen Klempner.

Cover Illustration
by Jonathan Graves.

Production Editing
by Peggy McCauley.

Production by Mike Lonsky.

Typeset by Debi Fredericks.

Printed and Bound by
Halliday Lithograph Corporation,
Arcata Company,
North Quincy, Massachusetts

CREDITS

Chapter 2   **2.1:** from *The Neuroanatomic Basis for Clinical Neurology*, by Talmage L. Peele. © 1961 by McGraw-Hill Book Co. **2.2:** from *Histologia Normal*, by Ramón y Cajal. **2.3:** from *Human Neuroanatomy*, by Raymond C. Truex and Malcolm B. Carpenter. © 1969 by Williams and Wilkins Co. **2.4:** Peele. **2.5:** Ramón y Cajal. **2.6:** from *Bailey's Textbook of Histology*, by Copenhaven *et al.* © 1978 by Williams and Wilkins Co. **2.7:** Truex and Carpenter. **2.8:** Ramón y Cajal. **2.9:** from *Physiology of Behavior*, by Neil R. Carlson. © 1977 by Allyn and Bacon, Inc. **2.10:** from *Organ Physiology, Structure, and Function of the Nervous System*, by Arthur C. Guyton. © 1976 by W. B. Saunders Co. **2.11:** Truex and Carpenter. **2.12, 2.17, 2.19:** Guyton. **2.20:** photo courtesy Drs. M. B. Bunge and R. P. Bunge, College of Physicians and Surgeons, Columbia University.

Chapter 3   **3.1:** from D. Barker, *Quarterly Journal of Microscope Science* 89 (1948): 143-186. **3.2:** Peele. **3.3-3.4:** Guyton. **3.5:** Carlson. **3.6:** from *Submicroscopic Structure of the Inner Ear*, edited by S. Iurato. © 1967 by Pergamon Press. **3.7:** Guyton. **3.8:** Guyton as modified from Skogland, *Acta Physiologica Scandinavica*, Suppl. 124, 36:1 (1956). **3.9:** Carlson. **3.10-3.11:** Guyton. **3.12:** Carlson. **3.13-3.14:** Guyton. **3.15:** from *The Vertebrate Visual System*, by Stephen Polyak. © 1957 by University of Chicago Press. **3.16:** Carlson, redrawn from J. E. Dowling and B. B. Boycott, *Proceedings of the Royal Society (London)* 166 (1966): 80-111. **3.17:** Carlson. **3.18:** Truex and Carpenter. **3.19-3.21:** photos courtesy D. Hubel and T. Wiesel, Professors of Neurobiology, Harvard Medical School. **3.23-3.24:** from *A Textbook of Physiological Psychology*, by S. P. Grossman. © 1967 by William C. Brown Co. **3.25-3.27:** Carlson, **3.28:** from A. R. Tunturi, *American Journal of Physiology* 168 (1952): 712-727. **3.29:** Peele. **3.30-3.22:** Guyton.

Chapter 4   **4.1:** from *Animals Without Backbones*, by Ralph Buchsbaum. © 1948 by University of Chicago Press. **4.3-4.5:** Truex and Carpenter. **4.9:** Guyton. **4.10-4.12:** Truex and Carpenter. **4.13-4.14:** Grossman. **4.16, 4.19:** Peele. **4.22:** Guyton from Warwick and Williams, *Gray's Anatomy*. © 1973 by Longman Group Ltd. **4.23:** Guyton.

Chapter 7   **7.8-7.9:** from "Prospects for Industrial Vision," by Tennenbaum, Barrow, and Bolles. *Computer Vision and Sensor-based Robots*, edited by George G. Dodd and Lothar Rossol. © 1979 by Plenum Publishing Co. **7.20:** from "Attention in Unanesthetized Cats," by Raul Hernandez-Peon, Harald Scherrer, and Michel Jouvet. *Science* 123 (1956): 331-332.

Chapter 8   **8.2-8.5:** photos courtesy Musée d'Art d'Historie, Neuchâtel, Switzerland. **8.6:** photo courtesy Billy Rose Theatre Collection, The New York Public Library at Lincoln Center; Astor, Lenox, and Tilden Foundations. **8.7:** BBC copyright photo. **8.8:** photo courtesy General Electric. **8.9-8.10:** photos courtesy Auto-Place, Inc. **8.11:** photo courtesy Unimation, Inc. **8.12:** photo courtesy PRAB Conveyors, Inc. **8.13:** photo courtesy Unimation, Inc. **8.16-8.17:** photos courtesy Cincinnati Milicron. **8.18:** photo courtesy International Harvester Science and Technology Lab. **8.21-8.22:** photos courtesy Unimation, Inc. **8.23:** photo courtesy Cincinnati Milicron. **8.24:** photo courtesy Astek Engineerng, Inc. **8.25:** Ben Rose photo. **8.27:** photo courtesy Stanford University AI Lab. **8.28:** photo courtesy Cincinnati Milicron. **8.29-8.30:** photos courtesy SRI International. **8.34:** photos courtesy Jet Propulsion Lab.

Chapter 9   **9.5:** photo courtesy Unimation, Inc.

TABLE OF CONTENTS

Opportunities for the Future

Brains, Behavior, and Robotics

CHAPTER **1**

Mind and Matter

What is mind? What is the relationship between mind and brain? What is thought? What are the mechanisms that give rise to imagination? What is perception and how is it related to the object perceived? What are emotions and why do we have them? What is will and how do we choose what we intend to do? How do we convert intention into action? How do we plan and how do we know what to expect from the future?

These questions deal with the innermost secrets of the human brain and have occupied philosophers for centuries. They address the relationship between the environment and the imagination, between reality and belief. These are issues that lie at the very heart of what we know and how we think.

Until recently such questions could only be addressed indirectly by subjective introspection or by psychological experiments in which the majority of the critical variables cannot be measured or controlled. Only in the past three decades, since the invention of the electronic computer and the development of high-level programming, has it become possible to approach these issues directly by building mathematical structures that exhibit some of the mind's essential qualities: the ability to recognize patterns and relationships, to store and use knowledge, to reason and plan, to learn from experience, and to understand what is observed. The appearance of these structures is a critical step in the study of mind, for it is difficult to understand phenomena without a mathematical model. Understanding implies the ability to compare the model's predictions with observed facts and then modify the model until it becomes increasingly accurate in predicting behavior.

Many models of the mind have been constructed in the past. Throughout the ages, philosophers from Aristotle and Descartes to Kant and Bertrand Russell have attempted to formulate models to explain the ability of the mind to reason and wonder, to know and understand. Psychologists from Freud and Pavlov to Skinner and Piaget have attempted to construct theories that explain the phenomena of emotion, learning, perception, and behavior.

Unfortunately, none of these models is able to quantitatively predict or describe the incredible powers and profound capacities of the human mind. Psychological models have been successful to the extent that they generate experiments and produce enormous quantities of experimental data. But no model has yet been able to mathematically predict any significant part of intellectual or emotional experience or to explain how the known anatomy and physiology of the brain generates the cognitive and perceptual properties of the mind.

Many question whether or not it will ever be possible to understand the mind in any significant way. In fact, many believe the mind to be a spiritual entity, separate from the physical body and therefore unknowable within the confines of experimental methods. Mind-body dualism (or separatism) is one of the central tenets of Western thought, founded on the belief that the body is a machine controlled by the brain, while the mind is of the same essence as the soul, separate from the body and therefore from the brain, which is a part of the body.

But the mind influences and controls behavior. How does this influence take effect? A great deal of what we call thinking (a product of the mind) is dedicated to planning for future behavior (a product of the motor system). Where is the interface through which a thought or plan, produced by the spiritual entity of the mind, is communicated to the motor system, a physical entity of the brain?

A tightly coupled interface obviously exists, because many behavioral patterns require a great deal of thinking while they are ongoing. Hunting a dangerous prey or fleeing a tenacious enemy are activities that may fully absorb and challenge both the mind and motor system simultaneously. Where is the division of mind and brain in the midst of a life or death struggle or chase?

In the important battles of life all of the resources of both mind and brain must often be fully utilized. When life itself is at stake or when offspring are threatened, mind and body are united, totally alert, and fully committed. Even in the case of an athlete or musician in the midst of a demanding performance, mind and brain are using every bit of knowledge and skill at their command.

Yet thinking can be, and often is, quite unrelated to ongoing motor behavior. While the body performs a well-known task, the mind can wander. For example, the mind can take flight to distant times and faraway places while we listen to a boring speech. The mind can conceive thoughts that transcend the dreary and often tragic reality of the physical world. The mind can have spiritual and religious experiences that go so far as to deny the existence of the physical world and all its pain and suffering.

How can the mind and motor system be virtually inseparable in one instance and disconnected in another? We have no difficulty understanding how two telephones can be connected at one instant of time and disconnected at another. Perhaps something like this happens in the brain. All that is necessary is for the mind and motor system to reside in geographically, or at least topologically, separate regions of the brain. If we define the mind to be the activity of that portion of the brain where the most sophisticated pattern recognizers, emotional evaluators, and behavioral situation/action rules are stored, and the motor system to be those regions of the brain where the lower-level pattern recognizers and simple behavioral skills are stored, then the mind and motor system are separate physical entities. When these two are electrically or chemically in contact so that they communicate information and command signals, they can act together in concert to perform highly skilled and intellectually clever behavioral patterns. On other occasions, when mind and motor system are functionally disconnected, they can pursue quite separate activities.

The famous split brain experiments of Roger W. Sperry show that when the two sides of the brain are surgically disconnected, they function as two separate brains. Just so, the higher levels of the brain, which produce the activity of mind, can function independently from the lower levels of the motor system when the two are logically disconnected. When nothing demanding is required of the motor system (i.e., when the body is relaxed or engaged in some routine or overlearned task), then the mind can disengage itself from the motor system. The motor system can be given a command to perform a routine task and no further attention is required of the higher levels for long periods of time. During this time the mind is not occupied with supervising the motor system. It is free to "idle" or to otherwise occupy itself with thoughts unrelated to current behavior or sensory experience.

Note the careful distinction between the activity of the mind and the physical structure in which the mind resides. The mind is a process that takes place in the physical structure of the upper levels of the hierarchical control system, the brain. Unfortunately, this leads into a bit of semantic difficulty, for it is common usage to refer to activities such as thinking, wondering, planning, hoping, and dreaming as activities of the mind. Thus, we are confronted with the peculiar notion of an activity of an activity. How can an activity (thinking) be an activity of another activity (mind)? This technical difficulty might best be overcome by an analogy with the computer science concept of a subroutine. A subroutine is a process that evokes another process. It is a process within a process, or, alternatively, a process of a process. Thus, common programming practice provides a good example of an activity of an activity. In short, thinking is a subprocess of mind, as is also imagining, believing, perceiving, and understanding.

The activity of the thinking mind might result in the selection of behavioral goals for intentional action. Alternatively, it could confine itself to the hypothesis of imaginary actions that it had no intention of carrying out. In either case, thinking is the process that generates images and patterns; mind is the process in which the process of thinking takes place.

Thinking allows the mind to generate predictions of the sensory input that would be expected when or if the actions intended or hypothesized by the mind were executed. Predicted input may be generated from memories resulting from past instances of similar actions. Memories may also derive from stories heard or images seen while a similar action was previously being hypothesized. The result is the same. Both hypothetical as well as intended actions generate expectations of sensory experience that are made available to the sensory-processing system. While an intended action is being executed, this internally generated expectation can be compared with the externally generated sensory experience. This makes it possible for behavior to be guided by the difference between observation and expectation. On the other hand, if a hypothesized action is merely imagined, the internally generated expectation can still be analyzed and evaluated as if it had originated from the external world. This gives us the ability to plan, i.e., to think about and evaluate actions before performing them.

If an evaluation modifies a hypothesized action, a new expectation will be generated, leading to a new evaluation, and so on. The looping inherent in this process generates a series of hypotheses, expectations, and evaluations. The result is what we call a thought or idea.

If this simple model of the mind is correct, it suggests that thinking first developed as a means to facilitate behavior. After all, the brain is first and foremost a control system, with a principal purpose of generating and controlling successful goal-seeking behavior in searching for food, avoiding danger, competing for a mate, and caring for offspring. All brains, even those of the tiniest insects, generate and control behavior. Some brains produce only simple behavior, while others produce very complex behavior. Only the most sophisticated and highly developed brains show evidence of abstract thought. Cognitive thought separate from ongoing behavior is a rare and recent phenomenon that occurs only in a tiny fraction of the brains that have ever lived.

In its simplest form, thinking is the "deep structure" of behavior. But in sophisticated brains, it can also generate expectations from hypothesized actions. In its most highly developed form, thinking can be used to hypothesize an entire sequence of actions and analyze the potential consequences of those actions before they are actually performed. It can be used to rehearse future actions or to review past actions. It is thus a mechanism for selecting and optimizing the most advantageous script for behavior in advance. Thinking allows us to analyze the past or to plan for the future; it allows us to select goals and anticipate problems. Thinking provides a means for choosing successful behavioral patterns that confer a clear advantage in the competition for gene propagation.

Of course, once the mechanisms of thinking are developed for selecting and controlling behavior, they can also be used for other purposes. In times of relaxation, thinking can be used to hypothesize actions that yield pleasant memories of the past or joyful anticipation of the future. We can hope and dream and fantasize. Thinking allows us to wonder and calculate and contemplate our place in the universe. It gives us the power to explore the logical consistency of the internal models we use for understanding the environment of the natural elements, the living creation, and the spiritual forces that lie beyond.

If thinking is primarily a high-level mechanism of behavior, then it would seem that any serious attempt to model the cognitive powers of the mind should start with the vastly simpler task of modeling the behavior-generating functions of the lower regions of the brain. Once these are well understood, it could be possible to project our understanding upwards and eventually understand the higher functions of the mind.

For the most part, however, this has not been the approach taken in the study of artificial intelligence. In 1950, Alan M. Turing wrote, "We may hope that machines will eventually compete with men in all purely intellectual fields. But which are the best ones to start with? . . . Many people think that a very abstract activity, like the playing of chess, would be best. It can also be maintained that it is best to provide the machine with the best sense organs that money can buy, and then teach it to understand. . . . This process could follow the normal teaching of a child. Things would be pointed out and named, etc. Again I do not know what the right answer is, but I think both approaches should be tried."

Since that was written, both approaches have been tried. But by far the most effort and commitment of intellectual and financial resources has gone into the first method, the pursuit of abstract reasoning. The entire effort in the field of artificial intelligence has been dedicated to an attempt to model the reasoning power of the thinking mind. This is probably due to the historical fact that most of the brightest pioneers in the field were trained in mathematics, a highly abstract and symbolically orientated science. In a later chapter we will review some of the successes and failures of the artificial intelligence approach to modeling the mind.

In this book we will take Turing's second approach. We will assume that the precursor to intelligence is behavior control; that abstract thought arises out of the sophisticated computing mechanisms designed to generate and control complex behavior; and that first comes the manipulation of objects, then the manipulation of tokens that represent the objects, and, finally, the manipulation of symbols that represent the tokens.

This approach implies that the would-be mind modeler should first attempt to understand and, if possible, reproduce the control functions and behavioral patterns that exist in insects, birds, mammals, and primates. After these systems are successfully modeled, we might expect to understand some aspects of the mechanisms that give rise to intelligence and abstract thought in the human brain.

Even so-called "simple" behavioral tasks are complex. A great deal of intellectual power goes into the most routine of our daily activities. It will be instructive to examine briefly the level of intellectual activity required to perform a typical everyday task.

THE SHOPPING CENTER PROBLEM

Consider the simple task of stopping at a shopping center on the way home from work to buy a record. A detailed examination of your experiences in executing this kind of task will not only illustrate the enormous complexity of the computation and control problems involved, but also demonstrate the range of intellectual capacities needed for such a task.

First, it should be pointed out that every task can be described by a hierarchy of descriptive levels. In the example chosen here, the highest level description is simply < PICK UP RECORD >. The modifier "on the way home from work" describes the time slot in which the task < PICK UP RECORD > is performed.

A second hierarchical level of description is < GO TO SHOPPING CENTER >, < PARK CAR >, < FIND RECORD SHOP >, < BUY RECORD >, < FIND WAY BACK TO CAR >, < LEAVE SHOPPING CENTER >.

A description at a third hierarchical level would break down each of these activities into a sequence of simpler actions. For example, < FIND RECORD SHOP > might decompose into < GET OUT OF CAR >, < LOCK CAR >, < FIND ENTRANCE TO BUILDING >, < WALK DOWN CORRIDOR >, < SEARCH FOR CORRIDOR CONTAINING RECORD SHOP >, < FIND ENTRANCE TO RECORD SHOP >.

A description at a fourth hierarchical level would define each of these activities as a sequence of still more detailed actions: < GET OUT OF CAR > might consist of < REACH FOR DOOR HANDLE >, < PULL HANDLE >, < PUSH DOOR >, < PUT LEFT FOOT OUT >, < TURN BODY LEFT >, < PUT RIGHT FOOT OUT >, < STAND UP >, < STEP FORWARD >.

Each succeeding level would become more refined. A description at a fifth hierarchical level would further break down these activities into a sequence of trajectories of limb movements. At a sixth level each trajectory would decompose into a series of positions and velocities for each of the joints and a sequence of forces in each muscle.

Descriptions at the higher levels are relatively independent of feedback from the environment. < PICK UP RECORD > could apply to virtually any record shop. However, the expansion of this task into the next lower level description depends on the characteristics of the particular record shop in the particular shopping center. At lower hierarchical levels, actions become more and more dependent on detailed conditions in the specific environment and less related to the global purpose under consideration. For example, the third-level task of < WALK DOWN CORRIDOR > requires visual information concerning the position of the walls, the position and trajectory of other persons walking in the same corridor, and the position of obstacles such as benches, potted plants, etc. At the fourth level, the placing of feet and the motions of the body depend on the position of floors, stairs, doors, and windows, etc. Because of the increasing dependence at the lower levels on specific execution-time feedback from the environment, planning is mostly confined to the higher levels.

It is important to understand the sophistication of the high-level perceptual and intellectual capabilities involved in the execution of a simple task such as < PICK UP RECORD >. This can be illustrated by a detailed first person account of the action sequence that actually took place one evening during a stop at the shopping center to buy a record.

On this occasion, I parked my car next to the roofed part of the parking garage as shown in figure 1.1. I got out of the car, with the shopping center building to my back, locked the car door, turned to the right, entered the parking garage shown in figure 1.2, and walked to the shopping center entrance, shown in figure 1.3.

Just this sequence of actions involves a degree of information processing, pattern recognition, and motor-control computations that is well beyond the capabilities of any existing robot system. To make the human body stand up requires a formidable amount of computation involving the coordination of sight, balance, and the tension in hundreds of muscles throughout the body. Inserting the key into the car door lock requires a three-dimensional visual system and a subtle sense of force and touch. Walking erect on two legs over rough surfaces, up and down stairs, and through doorways at a fast pace, avoiding both stationary and moving objects, is a control problem that far exceeds the capacity of any robot-control program. Furthermore, the ability of the vision system to locate and fixate the necessary visual cues to find the shopping center entrance in the confusion of cars, corridors, and lights requires an enormous amount of sophisticated information processing, pattern recognition, and deductive reasoning power.

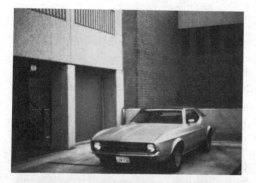

Figure 1.1: *My car parked in the shopping center parking lot next to the edge of the roof of the parking garage. Shopping center building is the brick structure in background.*

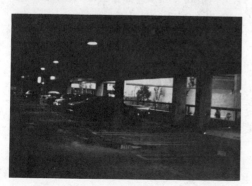

Figure 1.2: *A scene in the parking garage. Directional cues are obtained from the lines painted on the floor, the row of lights in the ceiling, and the row of parked automobiles. Note the wide range of brightness that the visual system must handle.*

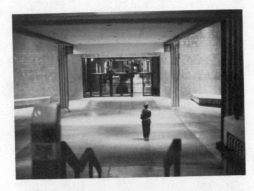

Figure 1.3: *Shopping center entrance. The box in right foreground is a dispenser for tickets to remind customers which door they entered. My failure to take a ticket made the task of finding my way back to my car much more complicated.*

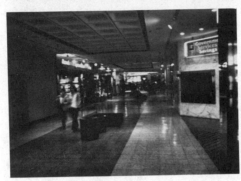

Figure 1.4: *Entrance corridor leading to central hub. The lines formed by floor tiles, walls, and ceiling fixtures assist the visual guidance mechanisms in setting a course. Reflections from shiny surfaces can be distinguished from real objects by the way they move relative to the floor and walls as the eyes move through the environment.*

Upon entering the building, I walked down the corridor shown in figure 1.4. Note that the visual cues in this scene are much simpler than those in the garage. The lines formed by the intersection of the walls, floor, and ceiling apparently converge on the end of the corridor. They are aligned with the flow of motion in the visual field, which always radiates outward from the direction of motion. Any discrepancy between the wall-ceiling lines and the visual flow lines can be interpreted by the vision system as a velocity pointing error. This points out the importance of image motion and visual flow in robot vision, to which we will return.

This particular shopping center consists of a circular building with corridors radiating out like spokes on a wagon wheel. Once I reached the center shown in figure 1.5, the problem then became: "Which way to turn?" Because I did not know where the record shop was, I made an arbitrary choice to follow the flow of the lines counterclockwise. I had been to the record shop once before but did not remember where it was. The only clue that I could recall was that it had an old-fashioned decor. The first corridor was definitely modern in style, so I tried the second, shown in figure 1.6, which had an "old world" appearance. Of course, this required an ability to distinguish old decor from modern.

A search of that corridor turned out to be fruitless. As I returned to the central

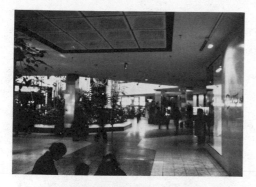

Figure 1.5: *The central hub of the shopping center at the end of the entrance corridor can be seen here. Note the "Gartenhaus" sign on the right, partially obscured by reflected light.*

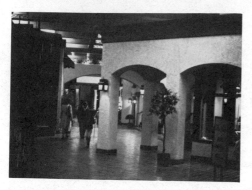

Figure 1.6: *A corridor with an "old world" appearance. Note the brick floor, gas lights, twisting passageways, and arched ceilings. These visual abstractions "match" the wrought iron lamps and bay windows of the record store goal shown in photo 1.7.*

hub, I realized that a linear search of each spoke of the shopping center would require an extensive amount of time, especially since there were three levels to each corridor. At this point, I invoked the strategy "If lost, ask directions." I thus began a subtask, <FIND SOMEONE TO ASK>. The question then became "Who?" I decided to ask one of the nearby shopkeepers and set off to find one who was not busy with a customer. This required the ability to recognize a non-busy shopkeeper.

I finally found such a person in a tobacco shop. He said he wasn't certain, but he thought there was a bookstore that also sold records a few stores down the next corridor. Following this suggestion, I finally came to the record store shown in figure 1.7. This successfully accomplished the <FIND RECORD SHOP> task.

I then executed the <BUY RECORD> task and began the <FIND WAY BACK TO CAR> task. I easily found my way back to the central hub, but now had another right or left decision to make. If I went left and simply retraced my steps, I could surely find my way back, but my previous search had been extensive, and it probably would be shorter and take less effort to continue around to the right. Thus, I continued counterclockwise, attempting to recognize the corridor where I had entered. The first corridor I encountered had a cluttered appearance. I remembered that my entrance corridor had been rather plain. So I rejected this corridor and

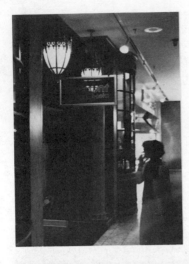

Figure 1.7: *The record store. This was the goal of the <FIND RECORD SHOP> task.*

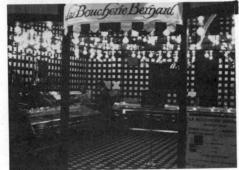

Figure 1.8: *This meat market seen on the way out did not match anything in the memory trace recorded on the trip in.*

moved further to the right. The next corridor appeared plainer, and I decided that this probably was the one. However, after walking halfway down it, I came to a health food store that I did not recall seeing on my way in. But, I wasn't certain—my confidence that I was in the right corridor diminished. Next there was the meat market shown in figure 1.8. Its striking appearance made me almost certain that if I had seen it on the way in, I would have remembered it. Yet just ahead was a door that had a familiar appearance. So, with great misgivings, I pressed onward.

Passing through the door, I encountered the parking garage; because it is a relatively symmetrical structure, I reasoned that it must look the same at every door. How could I be sure whether to go back and search some more—a long walk at best—or go on and risk getting hopelessly lost? I then remembered that I had parked my car at the edge of the roof of the parking garage, and that as I walked from my car to the shopping center entrance, the shopping center building had been on my right. Therefore, if I looked to my left from where I was now, I should see the corner

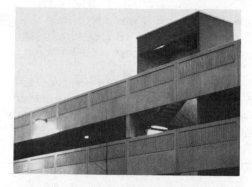

Figure 1.9: *The parking garage seen from the wrong exit. Note that the roof continues to the left as far as the eye can see. If this had been the correct exit, the roof would have ended within sight of this viewpoint.*

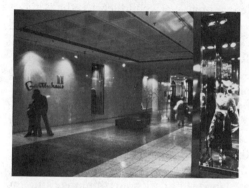

Figure 1.10: *The proper exit corridor seen from the central hub. The Gartenhaus sign triggered a positive recall.*

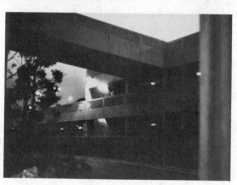

Figure 1.11: *The parking garage seen from the correct exit. The edge of the roof can be seen just where it was predicted by the internal memory model.*

of the parking garage roof. I looked and saw, as shown in figure 1.9, that the roof did not end. I was definitely not at the correct entrance.

Now certain of my error, I retraced my steps to the central hub and continued my search counterclockwise. At the next corridor I saw a sign on the wall, shown in figure 1.10, that said ''Gartenhaus.'' I remembered seeing this sign on my way in. This landmark gave me great confidence. As I progressed down the Gartenhaus corridor, I noticed a window display that I also remembered. I was now certain that I was on the right path. Going out the door, I looked up to the left and, sure enough, there, as shown in figure 1.11, was the edge of the parking garage roof. I had found my way back to the car.

This shopping center experience is interesting from a number of points of view. First, it illustrates the complexity of the so-called simple tasks that we perform every day. If we analyze routine daily activities—getting dressed in the morning, going to school or work, preparing and eating meals, walking through woods or a crowd of people—we will see that these simple activities are composed of intricate and complicated activities of manipulation and locomotion that require many subtle and complex intellectual decisions.

Consider the complexity of the simple task that every child learns, the tying of one's shoe. At a high level we can easily describe the procedure involved: <GRASP THE TWO ENDS, ONE IN EACH HAND>, <FORM A CROSS>, <BRING THE BOTTOM STRING OVER AND AROUND THE TOP>, etc., the type of instructions that might be found in a Boy Scout knot-tying manual. However, try to imagine the instructions required to implement each of these tasks at the lower levels. Imagine the detailed instructions required to describe what to do for every error condition: What if one string slips? What if one is too short to form a loop? How much force should be felt when the task is proceeding correctly? How much is felt, and in which direction, when a mistake has been made? How should a mistake be corrected or would it be easier to start over?

We all perform such tasks every day, apparently without thinking. But the amount of thought involved is considerable, and the amount of computation required to process sensory input (especially visual images) so as to recognize relationships and patterns and to use that information in selecting and executing physical movements is staggering.

Of course, there is nothing terribly mysterious about any of the isolated tasks involved in everyday life. As in the shopping center problem, each task can be broken down into a sequence of simpler subtasks. If there are a sufficient number of levels in the computational hierarchy, each level merely needs to break each task into a few subtasks. If each subtask decomposition is relatively short, it can be learned and can be described by a reasonably compact set of behavioral rules. If the breakdown is predictable, decision points at the various hierarchical levels can each be described by a fairly small set of logical rules involving estimation of the costs and benefits of various alternatives.

Much of the secret of complex behavior lies in structuring the computational task into a hierarchy of computing modules such that each lower level describes the task in only slightly more detail than the level above. This profound principle allows a large number of relatively simple computing modules to be arranged in an integrated system to produce behavior of arbitrary complexity. We will return to this theme many times.

Note that it takes a human being many years to learn the motor skills and intellectual powers needed to perform what adults consider to be routine tasks. A child cannot learn to tie his or her shoes before using the fingers in complex manipulatory tasks for three to five years. Most youths with less than six to eight years experience in finding their way around their neighborhood would not be able to solve the shopping center problem. The apparent ease with which we solve everyday problems is deceptive. Even the enormous computing power of the human brain does not deal with such problems without difficulty.

Of course, once a set of effective procedures and algorithms is learned, the problem appears simple: the many years of learning and practice are behind us. The acquisition of skills and strategies is difficult and tedious, but once learned, their execution comes easily. In many ways, this is analogous to the apparent ease with which performers in an ice skating show execute the most intricate maneuvers. Not evident are the years of practice, the hundreds of failures and falls, the innumerable hours of instruction, and the ruthless competition in which the less talented, less skilled, and less determined performers were weeded out.

This suggests that the truly difficult part of complex behavior is in the learning, or programming, by which the required skills and behavioral rules are acquired. Once effective skills and strategies are mastered, they can be readily applied. It is the discovery of the strategies and the learning of the skills that is difficult. Thus, a person or a robot who comes to some problem with a suitable repertoire of generalized skills will appear very capable and intelligent. A person or robot without these prelearned abilities will appear stupid and clumsy.

The shopping center illustration also gives a number of clues as to how memories are stored in the brain. For example, it suggests that memories are stored in addresses defined by the state of both the body and the brain which existed at the time that the experience originally occurred. The memory of the garage roof's geometrical position was recalled by mentally re-enacting the sequence of states involved in getting out of the car and walking to the shopping center entrance. The mental image of walking with the shopping center building on my right recalled the memory of the edge of the parking garage roof to my back. Similarly, the memory of having seen the "Gartenhaus" sign was triggered by seeing it once again. This implies that the recall of sensory experience can be accomplished by creating the same mental state that was present when the experience was stored. This is what we mean when we say that memory is "context addressable." It is why we are slow to recognize people or objects when we see them out of context in unexpected places. In later chapters we will explore possible mechanisms by which the brain performs this type of memory storage and recall operation. We will also suggest a means by which similar memory mechanisms might be constructed for a robot-control system.

Finally, the shopping center problem demonstrates the amount that can be learned from careful observation and analysis of everyday activities. Nature has provided us with innumerable examples of various degrees of intelligent behavior. Living creatures of every description abound and routinely demonstrate the most amazing feats of manipulation, locomotion, and intellectual decision-making. Many books are available that describe the behavior of various species in great detail. These are valuable in that they relate behavioral patterns and cause-and-effect relationships that are not easily observed. Nevertheless, there is no substitute for direct first-hand observation.

For example, watching an ant climb a tree is enormously instructive in understanding the complexity of legged locomotion. Observation of a beetle walking reveals how such a creature can feel its way along in spite of very poor vision. Or watch a bee move from flower to flower. Imagine the computing power of the visual system that enables it to detect the motion of regions and edges in order to provide the target tracking necessary to maneuver in a field of wild flowers. Watch a duck land on a lake or fly in formation with companions. Consider the computational problems of navigation and flight dynamics. Observe a squirrel jump from limb to limb, a dog bury a bone, or a human play the violin or bake a cake. Consider the problems of visual perception, motor coordination and dexterity, and intellectual decision-making: these are the problems encountered when building a robot. How do bees and ducks and squirrels and humans do what they do? What knowledge is stored internally and how is that internal knowledge used to interpret the sensory input from the external environment?

Without the example of nature, we might easily conclude that intelligent behavior is impossible. But obviously it is not. Even a mosquito can execute an intricate flight pattern, acquire and track a target, avoid getting swatted, execute a precision landing, and perform a complex drilling operation on the skin of its victim. How much computing power is there in the brain of a mosquito? There are but a few thousand neurons in an insect's brain. Surely this is within the capacity of modern computers to duplicate or, at least, simulate.

To learn how creatures of nature do what we would like our robots to do, we'll first examine the computing structure of the brain. To show how the basic elements of perception and behavior are organized in biological organisms, we'll give a brief survey of the structure and function of the sensory-motor system. Then we'll develop a theory of goal-directed behavior and propose a hierarchical structure of computing modules that can produce the elements of such behavior in a robot.

Next, we will construct a neurological model that has the essential properties of the proposed computational modules. We will show how this model can learn, generalize, and recognize patterns. We will then try to show how such a computational hierarchy might recall experiences, solve problems, plan tasks, select goals, answer questions, structure knowledge of the world and events, understand music or natural language, hope, dream, and contemplate the meaning of its own existence.

In the last five chapters, we will return to the subject of robotics and suggest how the proposed hierarchical computing model can be used to build and program robots with significant motor skills and intellectual capacities. Finally, we will offer some speculations on the social and economic consequences of widespread use of robots in the production of goods and services.

CHAPTER **2**

The Basic Elements of the Brain

In order to understand the computational abilities of the brain, it is necessary to understand something of the basic structure and function of the neuronal substrate. This would seem obvious, but many of the so-called brain models that have been proposed in the past bear almost no resemblance to the structure that they claim to model. For example, many early brain models assumed that the brain was a randomly connected network of binary neurons. In fact, the brain is far from randomly connected, and neurons are analog, not digital, computing devices. The neurons in the brain are arranged in quite regular patterns and are grouped in functional divisions. Although the dendrites and axons of the neurons may resemble the random arrays of branches and roots in a forest more than the regular arrays on a semiconductor chip, the interconnections are by no means haphazard. Precise and regular mappings exist from the sensory organs to the sensory-processing regions of the cortex, as well as from the motor centers to the muscles of various parts of the body. Somehow the neurons from one area know how to find and establish contact with neurons in other quite distant areas.

However, the structure of the brain is highly varied from one individual to another, as well as from one neuron to another. There are about as many neurons in the brain as there are trees, bushes, and shrubs in all of the suburban neighborhoods in the United States. And there are about as many different shapes and sizes of neurons as there are different species of woody plants in the American backyard. There are no two neurons exactly alike any more than any two trees are alike. Each neuron is shaped by its surroundings, by the composition of the chemical bath in which it swims, by the hormones it detects, by the electrical and chemical fields and gradients it experiences during its growth and maturing, and by the nature and timing of the electrical impulses and chemical transmitters produced in its vicinity as a result of activity of other neurons. This activity is generated both internally by spontaneous activity such as breathing and heartbeat and externally by events in the environment.

NEURONS

Neurons have four basic parts: a cell body, a set of dendrites, an axon, and a set of terminal buttons. The cell body contains the nucleus and much of the machinery that provides for the life processes of the neuron. Both the dendrites and cell body receive informational input to the neuron. The axon is the output conductor that transmits the neuron's message to its destination. The terminal buttons are located at the ends of the axon and release the transmitter chemicals that pass the neural messages on to the next neuron.

Figure 2.1 shows a typical motor neuron. The cell body of the motor neuron is usually located in the spinal cord, and the axon terminates on a set of muscle cells.

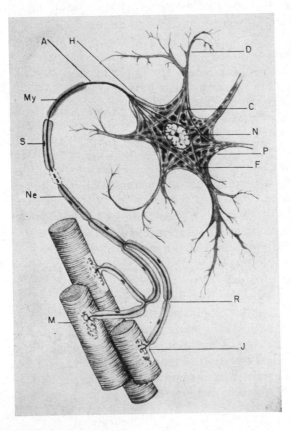

Figure 2.1: *Diagram of a motor neuron. The nerve cell, its axon, and the terminal end-plates on muscle fibers constitute a motor unit. (A) axon, (D) dendrite, (J) motor end-plate, (M) muscle fiber, (My) myelin sheath, (N) nucleus, (R) node of Ranvier, (S) nucleus of Schwann cell. Input arrives via synapses on the dendrites and cell body. Output is carried by the axon. The axon is covered by an insulating sheath of myelin produced by Schwann cells as illustrated in figure 2.19. This drawing is not to scale. The cell body of a motor neuron is typically about a thousandth of an inch in diameter, but its axon may be several feet long. A more detailed diagram of the terminations of the synaptic endings on motor end-plates of muscle tissue is shown in figure 2.12.*

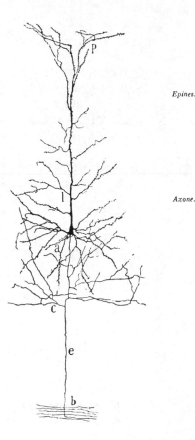

Epines.

Axone.

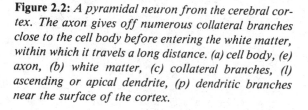

Figure 2.2: *A pyramidal neuron from the cerebral cortex. The axon gives off numerous collateral branches close to the cell body before entering the white matter, within which it travels a long distance. (a) cell body, (e) axon, (b) white matter, (c) collateral branches, (l) ascending or apical dendrite, (p) dendritic branches near the surface of the cortex.*

Long axons like those on motor neurons are encased in an insulating sheath of myelin. Figure 2.2 shows a pyramidal neuron from the cerebral cortex. The axon from this neuron sends out numerous collateral branches close to the cell body before it enters the "white matter"—a layer of millions of myelin-encased axons all bundled together like wires in a telephone cable. It is known as white matter because in a brain preserved in formaldehyde the myelin coating on the axons in the bundle appears whiter than the adjacent regions containing the cell bodies and dendrites. These latter regions comprise the "grey matter." The color of the white and grey matter in photographs, however, depends on the type of stain which is used to prepare the brain tissue. For example, the Weigert-Weil stain turns the white matter black, as in figure 2.3.

Different types of stain can be used to bring out different aspects of a section of neural tissues. Figure 2.3 shows three types of stain used on the same region of cortical tissue. Golgi stain brings out the entire shape of a few selected neurons including the dendrites and axons. Nissl stain brings out 100 percent of the neurons

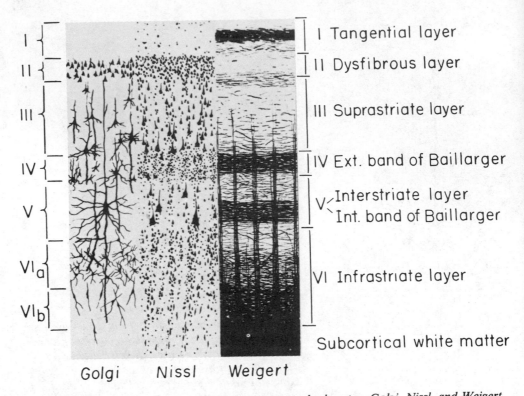

Figure 2.3: *The cell and fiber layers of the human cerebral cortex. Golgi, Nissl, and Weigert refer to the types of stain that bring out various features of neural tissues. See text for further explanation.*

but shows only the cell bodies. Weigert stain brings out the myelinated axon fibers. Figure 2.4 shows the Nissl-stained cell bodies in seven different regions of the cerebral cortex. Note the distributions of cell layers in the different regions. This suggests that different types of computations are being performed in these various regions.

Figure 2.5 shows a variety of neurons in the cerebral cortex. Note that some of the axons descend into the white matter, but that others rise and enter the fiber layer near the surface of the cortex, and still others remain confined to a volume within the grey matter near the neuron of origin. Figure 2.6 illustrates a number of different types of neurons. Note that all except one have the basic form of dendritic inputs, cell body, and axon output. The unipolar sensory neuron (A) shown in figure 2.6 is different. It has free endings that pick up sensory signals and transmit them to the terminal arborizations in the spinal cord. The cell body of the unipolar neuron hangs off to the side.

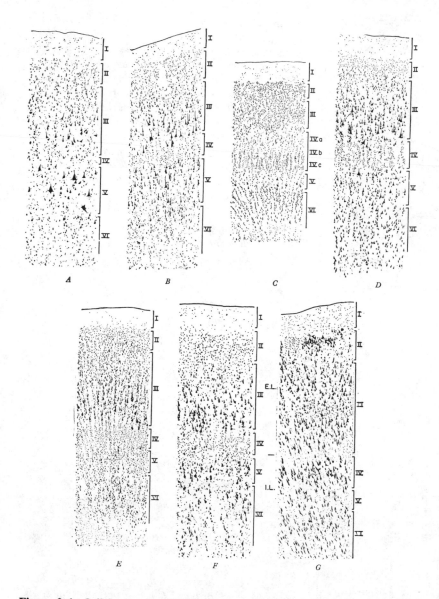

Figure 2.4: *Cell body organization in various cortical regions stained with Nissl stain. (A) Precentral region, Brodmann area 4. (B) Postcentral region, Brodmann area 3. (C) Primary visual cortex, area 17. (D) Superior temporal cortex, areas 41 and 42. (E) Associative visual cortex, area 19. (F) Temporal cortex, area 21. (G) Inner temporal cortex, area 28. The numbered Brodmann areas refer to the map of the cortex shown in figure 4.19.*

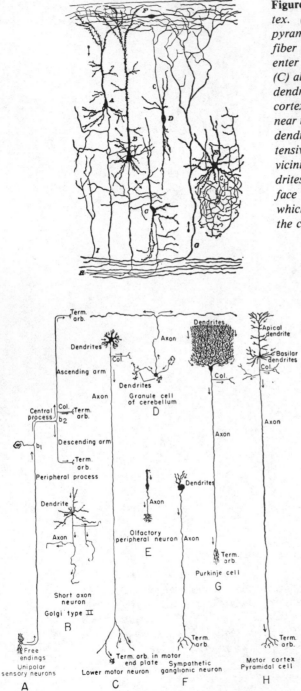

Figure 2.5: *A variety of neurons in the cerebral cortex. (A) and (B) are medium- and large-sized pyramidal cells with dendrites that extend into the fiber layer near the cortical surface and axons that enter the white matter after sending out collaterals. (C) also sends an axon into the white matter, but its dendritic field is confined to the lower layers of the cortex. (D) sends its axon upwards into the fiber layer near the cortical surface. (E) is an interneuron whose dendritic field is small and whose axon branches extensively within a region confined to the immediate vicinity of the neuron. (F) is a neuron whose dendrites and axon lie within the fiber layer near the surface of the cortex. (G) is an incoming axon fiber which terminates on dendrites in the fiber layer near the cortical surface.*

Figure 2.6: *Schematic representations of a variety of neuronal types. (A) shows a unipolar sensory neuron. The free endings pick up sensory information such as touch, cold, or pain. This neuron enters the spinal cord, where it branches, sending ascending and descending collaterals to make synaptic contact with neurons at several different levels of the cord. (B)–(H) are a variety of neurons from different parts of the nervous system. Arrows denote the direction of information flow.*

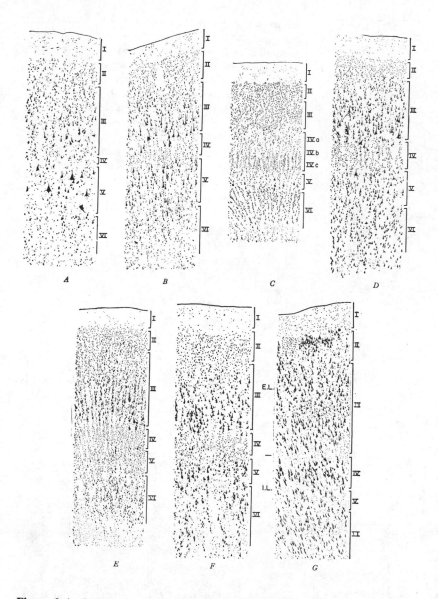

Figure 2.4: *Cell body organization in various cortical regions stained with Nissl stain. (A) Precentral region, Brodmann area 4. (B) Postcentral region, Brodmann area 3. (C) Primary visual cortex, area 17. (D) Superior temporal cortex, areas 41 and 42. (E) Associative visual cortex, area 19. (F) Temporal cortex, area 21. (G) Inner temporal cortex, area 28. The numbered Brodmann areas refer to the map of the cortex shown in figure 4.19.*

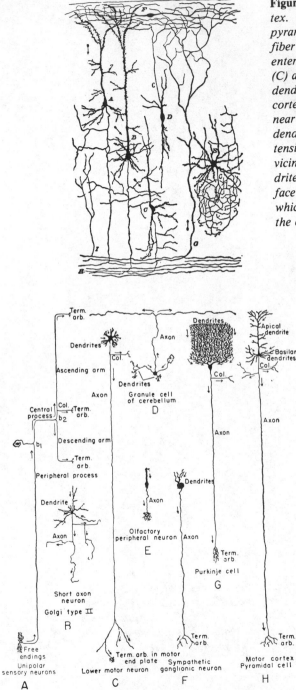

Figure 2.5: *A variety of neurons in the cerebral cortex. (A) and (B) are medium- and large-sized pyramidal cells with dendrites that extend into the fiber layer near the cortical surface and axons that enter the white matter after sending out collaterals. (C) also sends an axon into the white matter, but its dendritic field is confined to the lower layers of the cortex. (D) sends its axon upwards into the fiber layer near the cortical surface. (E) is an interneuron whose dendritic field is small and whose axon branches extensively within a region confined to the immediate vicinity of the neuron. (F) is a neuron whose dendrites and axon lie within the fiber layer near the surface of the cortex. (G) is an incoming axon fiber which terminates on dendrites in the fiber layer near the cortical surface.*

Figure 2.6: *Schematic representations of a variety of neuronal types. (A) shows a unipolar sensory neuron. The free endings pick up sensory information such as touch, cold, or pain. This neuron enters the spinal cord, where it branches, sending ascending and descending collaterals to make synaptic contact with neurons at several different levels of the cord. (B)–(H) are a variety of neurons from different parts of the nervous system. Arrows denote the direction of information flow.*

The size and shape of each neuron depends on the particular computational job it is asked to perform. Some neurons, such as the giant pyramidal cells, are large, with cell bodies up to a tenth of a millimeter in diameter and axons that can reach two feet or more in length. Other neurons are tiny, like the granule or stellate cells, measuring only a few thousandths of a millimeter in diameter with axons that reach less than a millimeter or two.

DENDRITES

The dendrites of a neuron resemble the branches or, in many cases, the roots of a tree. Dendrites are covered with synapses much like the branches of a bush are covered with buds in the spring. See figure 2.7. Synapses are the receptor sites that receive the input signals from the axons of other neurons. Some neurons have dendritic trees that branch extensively and receive inputs from thousands of other neurons. The Purkinje cell, for example, has upwards of 200,000 synaptic inputs. Other neurons have only a few dendrites and receive a small number of inputs. The cerebellar granule cell typically receives from one to eight inputs.

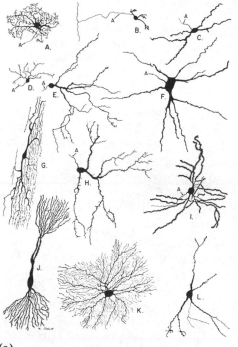

(a)

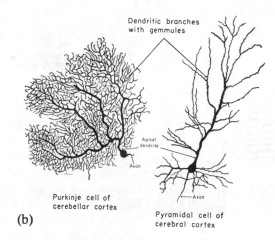

(b)

Figure 2.7: (a) *Some characteristic neurons whose axons (A) and dendrites remain within the central nervous system.* **(b):** *Two principal types of neurons in the cerebellar and cerebral cortex. Dendritic branches are covered with synaptic terminals.*

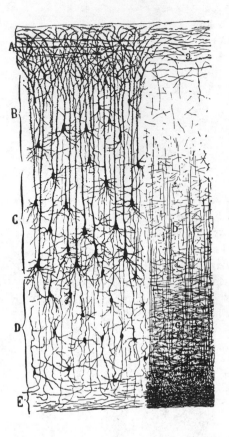

Figure 2.8: *An illustration of the packing density and layered organization of the cerebral cortex. At the left are the cell bodies, dendrites, and outgoing axons shown in Golgi stain. On the right is a Weigert stained section of the same region showing many axon fibers entering and leaving.*

The tree-like structure of the dendrites produces a forest-like structure in a section of neural tissue. This is illustrated in figure 2.8. On the left of this figure is an illustration of the packing density of cell bodies and dendrites in the cerebral cortex. On the right, the axon fibers entering and leaving the same region are illustrated. At the top right is the layer of input fibers that are making synaptic contact with the apical (i.e., top) dendrites. In the middle and bottom right are the axons and collaterals of the axons that are leaving the cell bodies en route to the white matter and thence to distant regions of the brain.

Although the dendritic branches of neighboring neurons intermingle, there is still a lot of empty volume in the brain that is not completely filled with dendrites. Axons pass through this space, occasionally making synaptic contact with dendrites or cell bodies.

The remaining space is filled with glial cells. The name comes from the Latin word for glue. For many years the function of the glial cells was unknown except for their obvious utility in filling space between neurons and holding the brain in one piece. Today we know that the glial cells surround the neurons with a very special

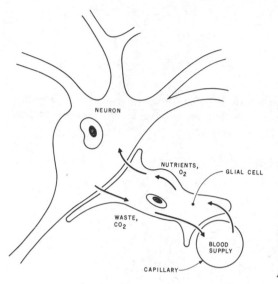

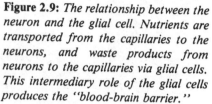

Figure 2.9: *The relationship between the neuron and the glial cell. Nutrients are transported from the capillaries to the neurons, and waste products from neurons to the capillaries via glial cells. This intermediary role of the glial cells produces the "blood-brain barrier."*

enriched and purified fluid environment. They transport substances essential for metabolism from capillaries to the neurons and transport waste products from neurons to the capillaries, as illustrated in figure 2.9. This produces the so-called "blood-brain barrier." Glial cells regulate the chemical composition of the extracellular fluid and even act as housekeepers by digesting and removing neurons that die from injury, disease, or old age. In addition, they insulate neurons from each other so that their electrical messages do not get scrambled.

AXONS

Axons are long tubes that carry the neurons' electrical messages from the cell body to the terminal buttons. The terminal regions of axons typically form branches and attach themselves via buttons to synaptic sites on the dendrites and cell bodies of the receiving neuron as illustrated in figure 2.10. In some cases the axon of the sending neuron will climb over the surface of the dendrites or cell body of the receiving neuron like a vine, making repeated synaptic contacts. This is illustrated by the climbing fibers in figure 2.11. In other cases, the axon of the sending neuron will simply pass through the dendritic tree of a receiving neuron, making contact with the few synaptic sites that happen to lie in its path, as illustrated by the parallel fibers in figure 2.11.

Some neurons send axons to distant places in the brain or spinal cord. Motor neurons leave the brain entirely to terminate on muscle cells and glands in the

Figure 2.10: *A typical motor neuron showing synaptic buttons from other neurons terminating on the cell body and dendrites.*

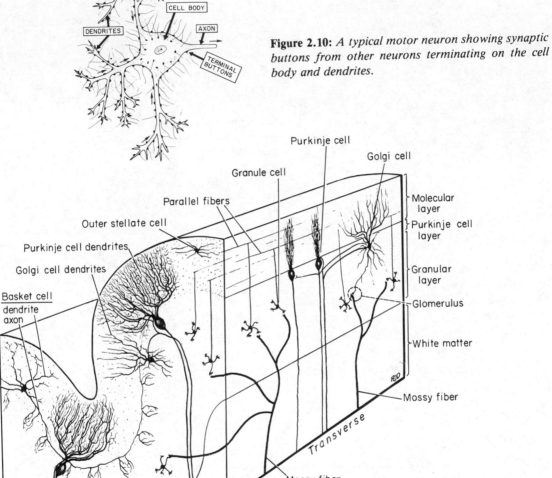

Figure 2.11: *A schematic diagram of the cerebellar cortex showing cell and fiber arrangements. Climbing fibers entwine about the branches of the dendritic trees of the Purkinje cells, making repeated synaptic contact. This is quite different from the passage of the parallel fibers through the dendritic trees of the Purkinje cells. Synaptic contacts here are made only at those dendritic sites that happen to lie directly in the path of the passing fiber.*

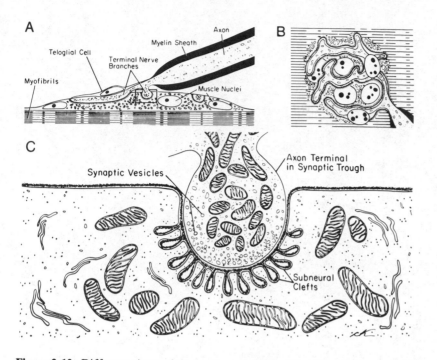

Figure 2.12: *Different views of the motor end-plate. (A) side view, (B) top view, (C) magnified side view showing the axon terminal contact with the motor end-plate.*

peripheral regions of the body. Figure 2.12 shows several views of the neuromuscular junction, sometimes called the motor end-plate. Other neurons send axons only to nearby neurons. Some axons travel long distances, branching only occasionally and ending with terminal buttons on target neurons in very specific regions. Other axons branch extensively, ending in thousands, or even hundreds of thousands, of synapses over a large and diffuse volume.

SYNAPSES

The synapse is an electrical gate, or valve, whose resistance to the flow of current is controlled by the receipt of transmitter chemicals from the axon buttons of other neurons. Three typical synapses are shown in figure 2.13. When an electrical signal reaches the buttons at the terminal ends of the axon, tiny packets, or vesicles, that contain a transmitter chemical are released. This transmitter diffuses across the narrow gap between the button and the synaptic receptor site on a dendrite or cell

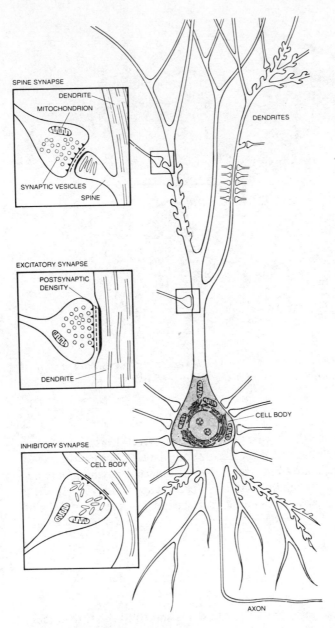

Figure 2.13: *Different types of synapses on a typical neuron in the brain. Excitatory synapses tend to have round vesicles and a continuous dense thickening of the postsynaptic membrane. Inhibitory synapses tend to have flattened vesicles and a discontinuous postsynaptic membrane. [From "The Chemistry of the Brain," by L. L. Iversen. Copyright © 1979 by Scientific American, Inc. All rights reserved.]*

body of the receiving neuron. The presence of the transmitter causes an electrical current to flow in the synapse of the receiving neuron. This current may be either positive or negative, depending on the type of transmitter chemical released.

As a general rule, a particular neuron releases only one type of transmitter chemical. Thus, neurons can be classified as either excitatory (i.e., causing positive current to flow in receiving neurons) or inhibitory (i.e., causing negative current to flow). There is a synaptic receptor for every axon button. Thus, there are two types of synaptic receptor sites: excitatory and inhibitory. A single receiving neuron may have both excitatory and inhibitory inputs. Communication of information across synapses is one-way, flowing from the terminal buttons of one neuron to the dendrites or cell body (and in some cases to the axon) of another neuron.

MEMBRANE POTENTIAL

Neurons have a skin consisting of an electrically insulating membrane of lipid. This membrane is an active living organ that creates an electrical potential across itself by pumping positively charged sodium ions out of the cell and replacing them with positively charged potassium ions. The membrane is quite impermeable to the sodium ion, so most of the sodium pumped out stays out. However, it is relatively permeable to potassium ions, so much of the potassium pumped in leaks back out. This is illustrated in figure 2.14. The result is a net negative charge inside the cell of about −70 millivolts. The neuron thus uses the sodium-potassium pumping action of the cell membrane to turn itself into a tiny electrical battery.

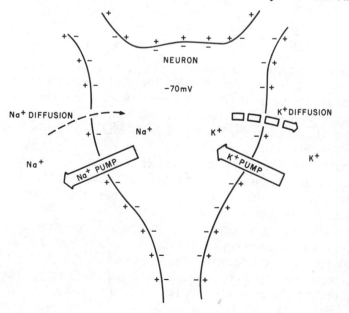

Figure 2.14: *Pumping action of the neural membrane causes an electrical potential to develop between the inside and outside of the neuron. Sodium (Na⁺) ions are pumped out and potassium (K⁺) ions are pumped in. The membrane is normally impermeable to sodium and large negatively charged ions, but partially permeable to potassium. Thus, many of the K⁺ ions pumped in leak back out, but few of the Na⁺ ions pumped out can get back in. The result is that an electrical potential of about −70 millivolts develops across the neural membrane.*

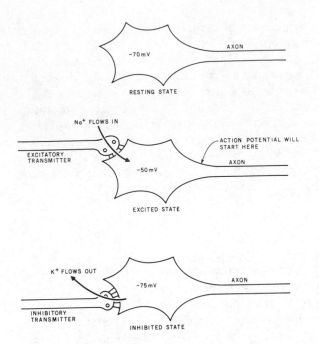

Figure 2.15: *Action of transmitter chemicals causes selective changes in the permeability of the synaptic membrane. Excitatory transmitter increases permeability to sodium (Na⁺) ions. An inflow of Na⁺ ions reduces the negative potential inside the neuron. Inhibitory transmitter increases permeability to potassium (K⁺) ions. An increased outflow of K⁺ ions increases the negative potential inside the neuron.*

The presence of transmitter chemical causes changes to occur in the size or the configuration of tiny pores in the synaptic membrane. The excitatory transmitter opens pores that allow positively charged sodium ions to flow back into the cell. This current flow discharges the electrical voltage of the cell battery. Thus, the excitatory transmitter causes the receiver cell battery to depolarize or decrease its negative voltage. This is illustrated in figure 2.15.

The presence of an inhibitory transmitter at an inhibitory synapse opens other pores that are constructed to allow potassium ions to flow out of the neuron. This current flow increases the charge of the cell battery. An inhibitory input, then, causes the neuron to retain or even increase its normal negative battery voltage.

Using these excitatory and inhibitory transmitters, the neuron is able to receive messages and compute functions. The neuron computes by summing the total of all the positive and negative currents induced in the dendrites and cell body by the transmitter chemicals. In most cases this computation is not just a simple arithmetic sum, because the voltage in the cell body is influenced by the relative strength of the

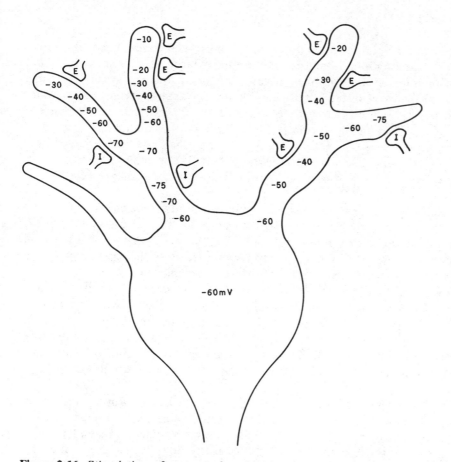

Figure 2.16: *Stimulation of a neuron by synaptic inputs of different types located at many points on dendrites produces a variety of electrical effects depending on the location and time sequencing of the various inputs.*

various synapses, the relative time of arrival of inputs from different sources, and even the relative positions of the various synapses on the dendrites and cell body. Thus, as shown in figure 2.16, the result of the neuronal computation may be a very complex function of the totality of the inputs.

The electrical voltage in the cell body of a neuron at the point where the axon is attached represents the result of its computation. It is its output. This voltage is a piece of information, a scalar variable representing the state of the neuron. It is the value of a parameter that may indicate some condition or event or the presence of some pattern or relationship.

ACTION POTENTIAL

Once the neuron has computed its result, it must then communicate this information to its destination, which can be another neuron, a muscle, or a gland. Transmission is not a simple problem, because the signal voltage is small (less than a tenth of a volt), and the distance may be quite far. The axon that must carry this information is very long compared to its diameter so that its electrical resistance is high. This means that the signal voltage of the neuron will be dissipated in transmission unless some means can be provided for boosting the signal strength along the way. This is the purpose served by the action potential. The action potential allows the signal voltage of the neurons to be transmitted over long distances by encoding it as a string of pulses.

The walls of the axon tube have the ability to produce a dramatic and rapid momentary reversal of the battery voltage in the axon. If the signal voltage of the neuron cell body rises above about -50 millivolts, the membrane walls of the axon that connect to the cell body suddenly drop their resistance to the passage of sodium ions. This allows sodium ions to rush into the axon causing its voltage to completely reverse polarity and go positive to about $+50$ millivolts. However, this is a momentary effect that disappears in about 0.5 millisecond to be replaced by an equally sudden drop in the resistance to potassium. This causes potassium ions to rush out of the axon, which in turn causes the axon to return to a voltage even more negative than before the inrush of sodium. This entire sequence of events, illustrated in figure 2.17, happens in about one millisecond. The result is an electrical impulse that is called an "action potential."

The action potential propagates down the axon like a spark down a fuse, as illustrated in figure 2.18. As each section of the axon generates an action potential, it depolarizes the section next to it so that it also generates an action potential. Thus, no matter how long the axon may be or how many times it branches, an action potential can be transmitted without loss in intensity.

In vertebrates, most axons that travel any significant distance are covered with an insulating sheet of myelin. The role of the myelin is to increase the speed and efficiency of the axon transmission. The myelin is interrupted every tenth of a millimeter or so by a patch of bare axon. These patches, called the nodes of Ranvier, are shown in figure 2.19. The current flow necessary for generating the action potential in the axon wall cannot pass through the myelin insulator as it does while propagating in an uninsulated axon. Instead it must flow around the myelin insulation, which causes the action potential to jump from one node to the next. This greatly increases the speed of propagation from about 30 meters per second in an unmyelinated axon to about 300 meters per second in a myelinated axon. It also decreases the amount of energy expended in each action potential, because the ionic currents of the action potential flow in only a tiny fraction of the axon surface.

The myelin is composed of the insulating membrane of a special type of cell called the Schwann cell that wraps itself around and around the neuron axon, as

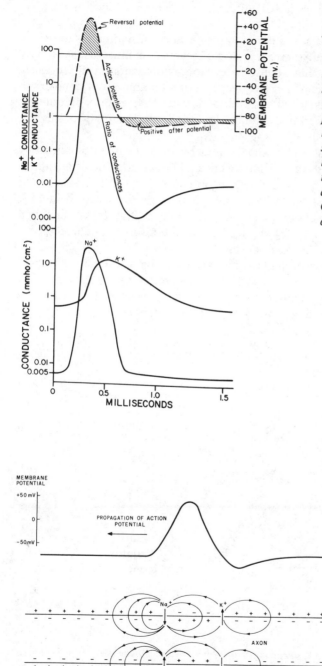

Figure 2.17: *Changes in sodium (Na⁺) and potasium (K⁺) permeability (i.e., conductance) versus time during the course of the action potential. Once the axon membrane potential rises above about −50 millivolts, Na⁺ conductance spontaneously increases several thousand percent. When this happens, Na⁺ ions rush in, causing the potential inside the axon to rise to about +50 millivolts. Then within about 0.5 millisecond, the sodium conductance drops almost as abruptly as it rose. Meanwhile, potassium conductance begins to rise, causing K⁺ ions to rush out and driving the axon potential even more negative than before. Gradually, over about 1.5 milliseconds, the conductances and voltage return to normal.*

Figure 2.18: *The action potential propagates down an axon like fire on a fuse. The presence of a positively polarized action potential at one point on an axon causes currents to flow in adjacent regions. These raise the potential in those regions above the −50 millivolt threshold, triggering a spontaneous increase in Na⁺ permeability. The result is that the leading edge of the action potential sweeps down the axon. The trailing edge of the action potential is produced by the drop in Na⁺ permeability and the simultaneous rise in K⁺ permeability. This quenches the action potential, so that a voltage pulse, or spike, of about one millisecond is propagated down the axon. The propagation speed depends upon the axon diameter and whether it is covered with myelin.*

shown in figure 2.19. A cross-sectional microphotograph of a myelinated axon appears in figure 2.20.

Following an action potential is a period during which the axon is less sensitive to depolarizing stimuli. Gradually, over a period of several milliseconds, sensitivity returns to normal. The result is that a constant level of depolarization will produce a string of action potentials at a constant frequency. A greater amount of depolarization will cause a higher frequency. A lesser amount will cause a lower frequency. Thus, an analog voltage in the cell body can be converted into a series of pulses at a particular frequency.

When each action potential reaches the terminal buttons, it causes the release of a number of vesicles containing transmitter chemical. The rate at which transmitter is released depends on the rate at which action potentials arrive. The amount of transmitter chemical released at the terminal buttons is proportional to the analog voltage in the cell body that generated the string of action potentials at the beginning of the axon. In other words, the analog voltage in the cell body of one neuron is converted into an analog input in the next neuron.

Neurons are *not* binary devices, and the brain is not a digital computer. The all-or-nothing character of the action potential does not mean that the neural signal is a Boolean variable. The action potential is simply an encoding mechanism that the brain uses for transmitting analog variables over long distances. Analog signal

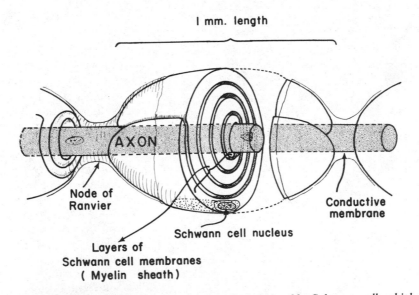

Figure 2.19: *An insulating sheath of myelin is formed by Schwann cells which wrap themselves around the axon. Uninsulated patches between myelinated sections are called nodes of Ranvier.*

values are encoded as pulse frequency, or pulse spacing, or in some instances such as in the localization of audio signals, as the phase, or relative time of arrival of action potentials from two locations.

Signal encoding by action potentials unfortunately introduces quantization noise into the information channel. This is because the action potential is a discrete event, as is the pulse spacing between action potentials. The encoding of a continuous voltage as a string of pulses is a form of quantization. The brain overcomes this noise by redundancy; many neurons transmit the same message, each encoded slightly differently. The average of a large number of neurons produces the accuracy needed for precise control. This redundancy also provides improved reliability, important in a structure in which approximately ten thousand neurons die every day of disease, injury, or old age.

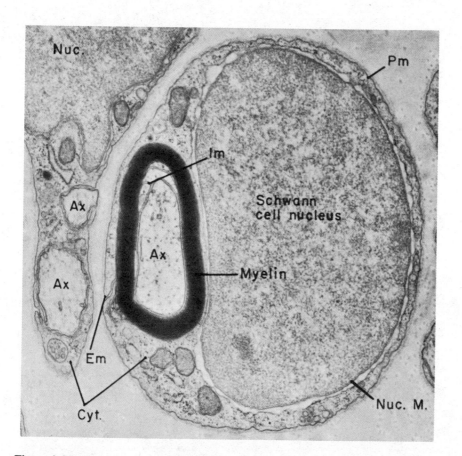

Figure 2.20: *An electron micrograph of a cross-section of a myelinated axon (Ax) magnified 27,000 times.*

Neurons are the transistors, resistors, capacitors, and wires of the brain. Like the individual circuit elements in a computer, neurons need to be interconnected in specific ways to produce the computational power of the brain. In the next two chapters we will briefly discuss the basic structure of the neuronal circuitry and the networks of interconnecting pathways that collect sensory data, analyze information, and generate motor behavior.

CHAPTER **3**

Sensory Input

Input to the brain arrives through a number of different pathways, including through the five senses: sound, sight, smell, taste, and touch. However, these are only the inputs that reach the conscious part of the brain. A number of subconscious senses are also important to the generation and control of behavior. For example, the proprioceptive senses monitor the position, force, and velocity of motion in the muscles and joints. These senses provide feedback to the neural servomechanisms that control the muscles in the production of smooth and dexterous movements of the body, limbs, and digits. Without these senses, skilled movements such as walking, running, jumping, and manipulating objects in the natural environment would be impossible.

One of the most important of the proprioceptive sensor mechanisms is the muscle spindle organ, shown in figure 3.1, that measures the degree of stretch in muscles. Another is the Golgi tendon organ, which measures the tension in tendons. There are also sensing organs in the joints that measure the position and rate of motion of the joints.

Another set of sensing organs that operates primarily below the level of consciousness is the sensors of the vestibular system. These measure the forces of gravity and both linear and angular accelerations and provide the information necessary to maintain balance and stability while the body maneuvers through its environment.

The vestibular sensors are a part of the structure of the inner ear. They are housed in a bony cavity with three interconnecting, fluid-filled semicircular tubes, or canals, shown in figures 3.2 and 3.3. Portions of the vestibular canals widen into chambers called ampullae into which protrude flexible structures called cupulae, shown in figure 3.4. The bases of the cupulae contain hair cells, of which two types appear in figure 3.5, that can detect the smallest bending motion of the cupulae resulting from movement of the fluid. The arrangement of the cupulae in the chambers of the canals is shown in figure 3.3. Whenever the head is rotated, the fluid in one or more of the semicircular canals is set in motion, causing the respective cupulae to be deflected. The hair cells attached to each cupula are deflected, and their neuronal firing rates are a measure of angular acceleration. Two other chambers called the utricle and saccule contain a set of weights called otoconia that is suspended on a gelatinous layer also containing hair cells. These are shown in figure 3.6. If the position of the head changes with respect to gravity or if a linear acceleration occurs, the otoconia are displaced so that the hair cells buried in them can report the direction of tilt or acceleration.

The vestibular system is the inertial guidance reference. Information from the vestibular system is combined with force, velocity, tension, and position information from tendon, stretch, and joint receptors. Together, these form the vestibular reflex that functions like an autopilot to maintain balance during a variety of bodily motions. The neuronal computational mechanisms for the vestibular and stretch reflexes are discussed in the next chapter. Circuit diagrams for the stretch reflex are shown in figure 4.6; diagrams for the vestibular reflex appear in figure 4.13.

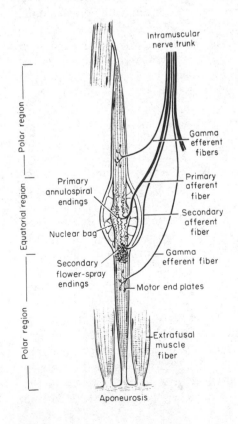

Figure 3.1: *Diagram of a muscle spindle organ that measures the degree of stretch in the muscles. The two ends of the spindle organ attach to motor muscle tissue. Sensory nerve endings in the equatorial region generate action potentials whose frequency is proportional to the amount by which the spindle organ is stretched. The afferent fibers carry this sensory information back to the central nervous system. Gamma efferent fibers excite tiny muscles in the polar regions of the spindle organ itself, shortening it, and hence increasing its sensitivity to stretch of the motor muscle to which it is attached.*

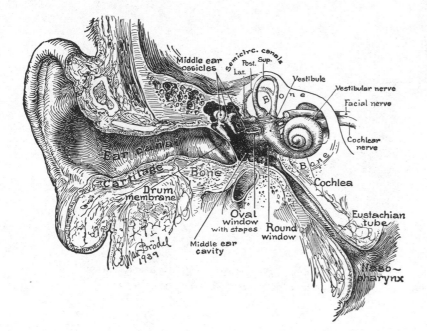

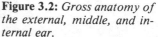

Figure 3.2: *Gross anatomy of the external, middle, and internal ear.*

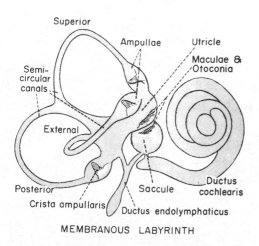

MEMBRANOUS LABYRINTH

Figure 3.3: *Enlarged view of the vestibular apparatus and cochlea illustrating the positions of the ampullae and maculae.*

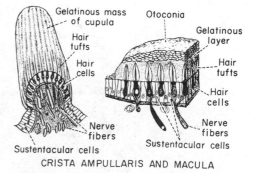

CRISTA AMPULLARIS AND MACULA

Figure 3.4: *Hair tufts from the hair cells are embedded in the gelatinous mass of the cupula that extends into the ampulla of the semicircular canals. Rotary acceleration of the head causes the fluid in the semicircular canals to deflect the cupula and excite the hair cells.*

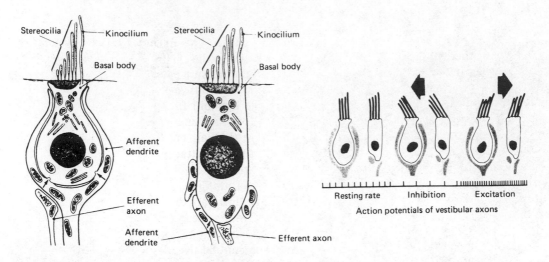

Figure 3.5: *Two types of vestibular hair cells. Deflection of the hairs in one direction slows the normal firing rate of action potentials in the vestibular afferent axons. Deflection of the hairs in the opposite direction increases the firing rate.*

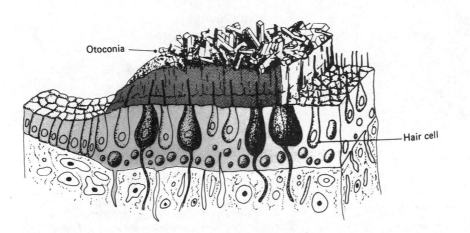

Figure 3.6: *Hair tufts from hair cells are also embedded in the gelatinous layer beneath the calcium carbonate crystals making up the otoconia. Linear acceleration of the head causes a shearing force that deflects the gelatinous layer, exciting the hair cells.*

TOUCH

There are at least seven different types of touch sensors. These are shown in figure 3.7. First, there are free nerve endings that are found in the skin as well as in many other places in the body. These can detect very slight pressure and provide an extremely sensitive sense of touch. Second are Meissner's corpuscles, which have localized pressure-sensing capabilities. Abundant in the lips and fingertips, these provide a high degree of spatial localization of the sense of touch and make it possible to discern the shape of objects by touch. Third are the hair end-organs that detect the mechanical deflection of the hairs to which they are attached. Pacinian corpuscles, fourth, are particularly sensitive to vibration or rapid changes in pressure such as might result from a blow. They are also found in the joints where they are thought to signal the rate of motion of the joints. Fifth are the Ruffini end-organs that signal the continuous deformation of the skin and deep tissues. These are also found in joints where they signal the degree or position of joint rotation. Figure 3.8 illustrates the type of information that is transmitted to the brain from joint angle receptors. Additional types of touch receptors called Merkel's discs and Krause's corpuscles are sixth and seventh, respectively. These are located in various parts of the body and report different kinds of tactile information.

There are also specific sensory nerves for heat, cold, pain, and itch, all of the free nerve ending type. The pain sensors are calibrated so that they begin to signal pain precisely when tissue damage begins to occur.

In addition, there are visceral sensors that measure the condition of the internal organs, the pressure in arteries, the degree of expansion of the lungs, the digestion of food, the operation of the kidneys, the regulation of temperature, etc. An entire subdivision of the nervous system, called the autonomic nervous system, is dedicated to the control of the innumerable regulatory and control functions of the body's life support system. Figure 3.9 illustrates the basic structure of the autonomic nervous system and the type of organs it controls. We will not deal further with this portion of the nervous system as it has little direct connection to the part of the brain that generates and controls intentional behavior.

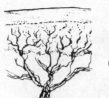
Free nerve
endings

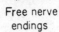
Merkel's
discs

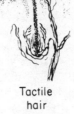
Tactile
hair

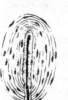
Pacinian
corpuscle

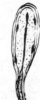
Meissner's
corpuscle

Krause's
corpuscle

Ruffini's
end-organ

Golgi tendon
apparatus

Muscle
spindle

Figure 3.7: *Several types of sensory receptors.*

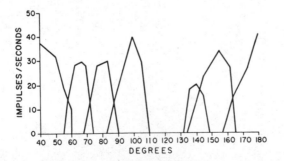

Figure 3.8: *Response of several different nerve fibers from sensory receptors reporting the position of the knee joint in a cat.*

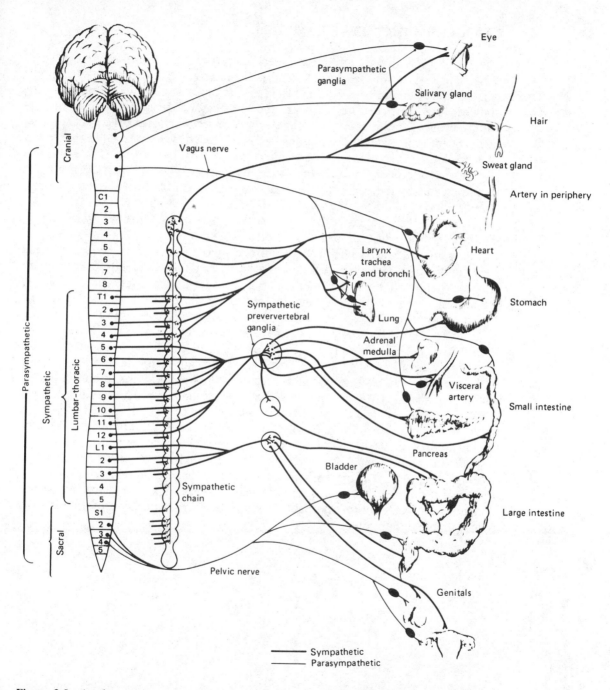

Figure 3.9: *A schematic overview of the autonomic nervous system and the organs it enervates.*

LAW OF SPECIFIC NERVE ENERGIES

For every sensory input there are specific nerves for each of the different sensations. This feature is called the law of specific nerve energies or "place encoding." For example, the brain knows that touch has occurred at a particular point on the body because a particular nerve fiber connected to a touch sensor at that point is carrying a string of action potentials. The strength of the touch is encoded by the firing rate. The location of the touch and the fact that a touch has occurred (as opposed to heat or pain) is encoded in the particular touch fiber that is firing. There are also several specific sets of fibers that report painful stimuli. The location of the pain is communicated by the particular set of active pain fibers, and the intensity is communicated by the number of pain fibers that are firing as well as by their rate of firing. Similarly, there are nerve fibers that are sensitive to heat and cold. Their respective rates are an indication of how hot or how cold it is.

As a general rule, the intensity of sensory input is encoded by the rate of firing such that each increase of stimulus intensity by a certain percent tends to cause an increase in firing rate by a fixed amount. This leads to a logarithmic, or power law, relationship between stimulus intensity and firing rate. This is called the Weber-Fechner Law after the two gentlemen who first carefully measured the effect; see figure 3.10. However, this power law is only a steady-state approximation, considerably modified by the temporal relationships between stimulus and firing rate. The firing rate of a sensory neuron is typically quite high at the onset of the stimulus and then decays rapidly to a much lower value as the stimulus remains constant. The rate of decay varies from one type of sensory cell to another and is effected by an inhibitory influence of the receptor circuits adjacent to the one being stimulated. As shown in figure 3.11, the activity of a Pacinian corpuscle pressure sensor decays to zero in about a tenth of a second; a hair-receptor touch sensor activation also decays to zero in about a second. A muscle spindle or a Golgi tendon organ firing decays more slowly, over five or ten seconds to about 50 percent of its initial value. Pain-receptor input, however, does not decay. In fact, under some conditions, the threshold for excitation of the pain receptors becomes progressively lower as the painful stimulus continues.

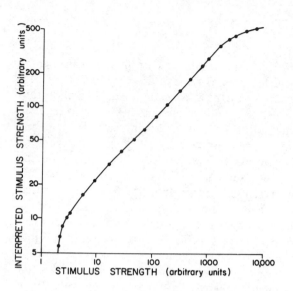

Figure 3.10: *A plot of nerve firing rate versus stimulus strength demonstrating the Weber-Fechner logarithmic or power law. Note that the logarithmic relationship does not hold at either very weak or very strong stimulus strengths.*

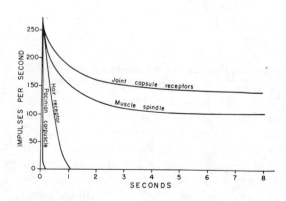

Figure 3.11: *A plot of the firing rate of several types of sensory neurons versus time. Muscle spindle and joint receptors are most sensitive at the onset of a stimulus, and the firing rate decays with time. Hair receptors and Pacinian corpuscles sense only transitory stimuli.*

VISION

One of the most important and widely studied of the senses is vision. As can be seen from figure 3.12, the mechanical features of the eye are very like those of a camera, with a lens that focuses the incoming light to form an image on a photosensitive surface, the retina. There is also an iris that can change the f-stop to regulate the amount of light reaching the retina; adjustment of the iris increases the dynamic range of illumination over which the eye can function by 30 times. However, the largest portion of the eye's dynamic range comes from photochemical changes in the retina that adjust the sensitivity of the rods and cones. This latter process has a time constant of several minutes, whereas the iris can adjust in a fraction of a second as the gaze shifts from bright sunlight to shadow and back again. The muscles of the iris are controlled by a reflex feedback system that is sensitive to the level of illumination on the retina. The neuronal pathway for this reflex is illustrated in figure 3.13.

The muscles that adjust the focus are controlled by a much more complex reflex composed of several components. One component comes from the convergence of the two eyes, i.e., the amount the two eyes are turned inward to point at a target. The second comes from the fact that red and blue light focus at slightly different distances through the same lens. The third is a slight oscillation in the focusing muscles at a rate of one-half to two times per second. This causes the focus to "hunt" around the point of maximum sharpness.

The fact that there are two eyes can be used to advantage in different ways depending on the requirements of the particular species. For creatures of prey, like rabbits and deer, the eyes are located on opposite sides of the head so as to cover the entire hemisphere of the environment and warn of impending predators. For hunting species, the eyes are located in the front of the head so that the visual fields overlap, providing stereo depth vision. Among other things, this enables the brain to continuously compute the distance to objects in the visual field. Stereo depth vision measurements are highly accurate for distances within grasping or jumping range.

The resolution of the eyes is extremely high in the center of the field of view (the fovea) and falls off rapidly in the peripheral regions. In humans the area of high resolution is only one half of one degree in diameter, or roughly the size of the image of the full moon. This is a very small area, but it is exactly in the center of the field of view and is kept pointed at the center of attention at all times by an extraordinarily rapid and precise servo-like system. The photoreceptors in the fovea primarily send signals to shape recognizing circuits in the higher level visual-processing centers of the brain. The photoreceptors in the surrounding regions of the retina primarily send signals to the areas that detect motion and position of objects and which direct the eye muscles to point the fovea at points of interest. The pointing of the eyes is controlled by three pairs of extraocular muscles: the lateral and medial recti, which move the eye from side to side; the superior and inferior recti, which move it up and down; and the superior and inferior oblique, which rotate the eyes, maintaining the visual fields upright and keeping the right and left fields in registration. The circuitry for the control of eye-pointing movements is shown in figure 3.14a and b.

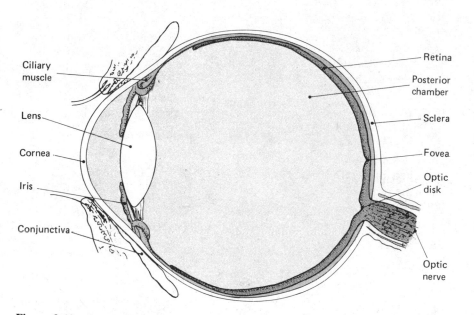

Figure 3.12: *A cross-section of the human eye.*

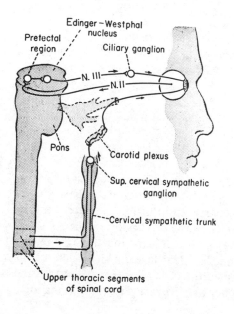

Figure 3.13: *A schematic diagram of the neuronal system that controls the iris. This system controls the intensity of the image formed on the retina.*

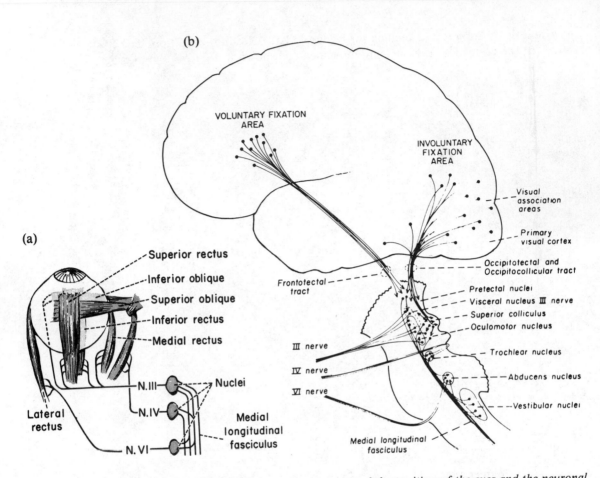

Figure 3.14a: *The extraocular muscles that control the position of the eyes and the neuronal nuclei that control them.* **b:** *The computing centers and neuronal pathways involved in the control of eye position.*

THE RETINA

The retina is composed of several layers as shown in figure 3.15. First is the pigment layer that lies on the inside surface of the eyeball farthest from the lens. Second is the layer of rods and cones, or the photosensors, and third is the outer limiting membrane. The outer nuclear layer, which contains the cell bodies of the rods and cones, is fourth. Fifth is the outer plexiform layer, which is the location of the first synapses in the visual pathway. Sixth is the inner nuclear layer, which contains the cell bodies of the horizontal, bipolar, and amacrine cells. These provide the first layer of processing of the visual image. The inner plexiform layer, which is the loca-

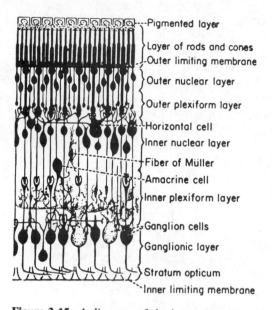

---Pigmented layer

}Layer of rods and cones
}Outer limiting membrane

}Outer nuclear layer

}Outer plexiform layer

--Horizontal cell
}Inner nuclear layer

Fiber of Müller

Amacrine cell

}Inner plexiform layer

Ganglion cells

}Ganglionic layer

}Stratum opticum
Inner limiting membrane

Figure 3.15: *A diagram of the layered architecture of the retina. See text for a description of the function of the different layers.*

tion of the second level of synapses, is seventh. Eighth is the layer of ganglion cells whose axons make up the optic nerve; these axons leave the eyeball and terminate in the lateral geniculate body of the thalamus and in the superior colliculus. The ninth layer is the optic nerve fibers on their way out of the eye. The inner limiting membrane, the tenth layer, separates the retina from the vitreous humor, which fills the interior of the eyeball. A more detailed diagram of the retina illustrating the fine structure of the various cells and synapses is shown in figure 3.16.

It is apparent from this anatomical structure that a great deal of processing of the visual image must take place on the retina itself, a fact that has been confirmed by neurophysiological experiments. The bipolar cells transmit excitatory information directly from the rods and cones to the ganglion cells immediately beneath them. The horizontal cells transmit inhibitory information to ganglion cells from rods and cones in the surrounding neighborhood. This produces the "center-on, surround-off" response of many of the ganglion cells. A model of the circuit connections that produce this response is shown in figure 3.17. A structurally similar but functionally inverse set of interconnections produces the "center-off, surround-on" response. There are about the same number of ganglion cells with the "center-off" response as with "center-on."

The amacrine cells are also inhibitory cells, but their response is transitory in contrast to the continuous response of the bipolar and horizontal cells. When the photoreceptors are first stimulated, the amacrine response is intense, but this signal dies away to almost nothing in a fraction of a second. This transient response produces a sensitivity to changing light intensities, hence serving to detect motion in the visual scene. Many of the ganglion cells that exhibit the on-center or off-center response also have a transient response. Some produce a burst of action potentials when the light stimulus is first turned on. Others produce a burst when the light is turned off. This information is used at higher levels in the visual-processing system to detect an object's direction of motion.

The percentage of ganglion cells that are sensitive to motion is much higher in the peripheral field of view than in the central. This is why moving objects in the peripheral field can be readily detected, whereas stationary objects are not. The survival advantage of this is obvious. Moving objects are much more likely to be of immediate importance than stationary ones: a moving object may be an approaching enemy, or it may be a fleeing prey. When the eye is moving linearly through the environment, the apparent motion of stationary objects is inversely proportional to their distance. An object that appears to be moving rapidly represents a potential collision. The ability of the vision system to detect moving objects over a wide field of view directs the attention to important areas of the environment. This guidance information sets the extraocular muscles to point the high-resolution part of the visual field in that direction. Thus, the eyes tend to be kept pointing at the portion of the visual field where the "action" is.

The recognition of motion is a relatively simple computation compared to the recognition of shapes. Many lower forms can discriminate moving objects quite well, but have virtually no capacity for recognizing stationary objects. For example, motion discrimination is particularly well developed in the retina of the frog. In the famous paper "What the Frog's Eye Tells the Frog's Brain," Lettvin, Matturana, McCulloch, and Pitts first discovered the extensive processing of motion signals that takes place in the retina. The frog retina processes the visual signal to the extent that there are neurons in the optic nerve of the frog that reveal the position and trajectory of flying bugs accurately enough so that the frog can snap them out of the air with one flick of its tongue. Yet a frog will starve to death while looking at dead bugs apparently because it cannot see them.

Higher forms, such as mammals, typically perform more sophisticated analyses of shape and delay the detailed processing of motion data until higher levels in the brain where other information can be integrated into the processing. However, even in humans, the detection of motion begins in the retina itself, and this analysis remains an important component of the visual data-processing system.

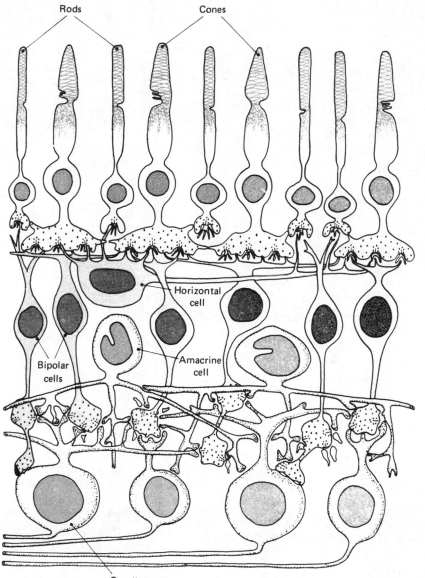

Figure 3.16: *Details of the retinal circuitry.*

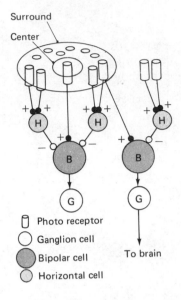

Figure 3.17: *A neural model that can account for the behavior of a ganglion cell with "center-on, surround-off" response.*

COLOR VISION

There are three kinds of cones that have differential sensitivity to red, green, and blue light. The rods are most sensitive to green. When all three types of cones are equally stimulated, the perceived color is white. Different amounts of stimulus of the various cones produce the perception of color. All the different colors, shades, and hues that can be perceived arise from various combinations of stimuli of the three types of cones.

Both rods and cones can change sensitivity to adapt to differing light levels. As the light level decreases, the cones can increase sensitivity by about 60 times. However, the rods can increase sensitivity by more than 25,000 times. Thus, in dim light, vision is primarily generated by the rods that can't discriminate color. In brighter light, vision is mediated primarily by cones, and colors are perceived.

A single ganglion cell may be stimulated by a number of cones or only a very few. When all three types of cones stimulate the same ganglion cell, the signal transmitted is the same for any color. Such a ganglion cell is sensitive only to light intensity, but not to color. Many other ganglion cells are excited by one color cone and inhibited by another. Thus, color discrimination and analysis also begin in the retina.

HIGHER LEVEL PROCESSING

The retinal ganglion cells send most of their axons to the lateral geniculate body of the thalamus. From there the visual information is relayed to the visual cortex through the pathways known as the optic radiations, shown in figure 3.18. In the lateral geniculate, the optic fibers terminate in six layers as shown in figure 3.19.

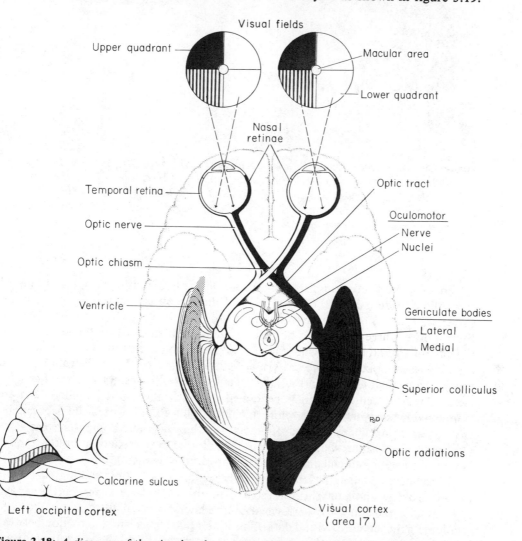

Figure 3.18: *A diagram of the visual pathways viewed from the underside of the brain. Note that input from the left visual field falls on the right half of the retina in both eyes and projects to the visual cortex on the right side of the brain. Input from the right visual field falls on the left half of the retina in both eyes and projects to the visual cortex on the left side of the brain.*

RIGHT EYE

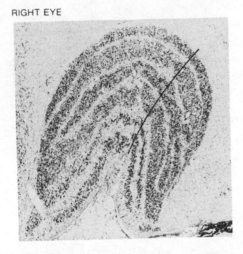

Figure 3.19: *A section through the lateral geniculate nucleus showing the layered structure. Cells in layers 1, 4, and 6 (numbered from the bottom to top) receive input from the eye on the opposite side. Cells in layers 2, 3, and 5 receive input from the eye on the same side. The maps are in register, so that the neurons along any radius (black line) receive signals from the same part of the visual scene.*

Layers 2, 3, and 5 (counting from the surface of the thalamus inward) receive inputs from the outside half of the visual field of the eye on the same side of the head. Layers 1, 4, and 6 receive signals from the inside of the visual field from the eye on the opposite side of the head. Thus, the lateral geniculate body on the left side contains input from the right visual field of both eyes and the lateral geniculate on the right contains input from the left visual field of both eyes. The registration of two images from the two eyes in the lateral geniculate bodies establishes the basis for stereo depth perception. Signals generated by black and white ganglion cells are found mainly in layers 1 and 2, while signals carrying color information occur mainly in layers 3 through 6. The receptive fields in the geniculate bodies have the same on-center or off-center shapes similar to those found in the retina, although a much higher percentage of geniculate cells respond to movement.

The lateral geniculate also receives a large number of fibers coming back from the visual cortex and from the brain stem. This means that the cortex has the capacity to modify the functions performed by the lateral geniculate so as to filter and manipulate the incoming visual data. This looping structure and interaction between incoming data and higher processing levels is characteristic of all the input pathways in the brain.

Axons from cells in the lateral geniculate travel primarily to area 17 of the cortex, the primary visual cortex. Neurons that respond to lines at specific orientations are found here. Some neurons respond to dark lines on light background, others to bright lines on dark background. Still other neurons respond to edges between dark and light regions. Figure 3.20 shows the different kinds of responses for neurons in the lateral geniculate and the cortex. These line and edge detectors were first observed by David Hubel and Torsten Wiesel. These neurons are termed simple if they are sensitive to edges and lines in a particular orientation and position. Neurons that have the same sensitivity to lines and edges at particular orientations but respond if the stimulus is anywhere within a large area of the visual field are termed complex. Still other neurons are sensitive to angles and corners; these are termed hyper-complex.

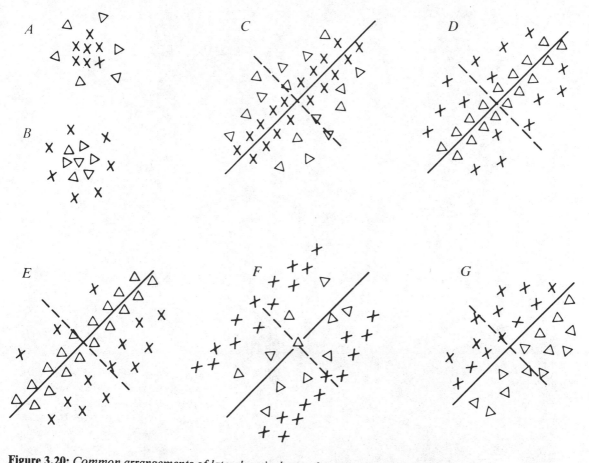

Figure 3.20: *Common arrangements of lateral geniculate and cortical receptive fields. (A) On-center geniculate receptive field. (B) Off-center receptive fields. (C-G) Various arrangements of simple cortical receptive fields. "X" areas are excitatory "on" responses; "△" areas are inhibitory "off" responses. Receptive fields shown here are all at the same angle, but each type occurs in all orientations.*

The visual cortex is markedly layered as can be seen in figure 3.21. Neurons with the center-surround response tend to be located in layer IV. Simple line and edge detectors lie just above them, and complex neurons are located in layers II, III, V, and VI. The complex neurons can be further categorized; the ones found in each layer are very different in a number of ways.

(a)

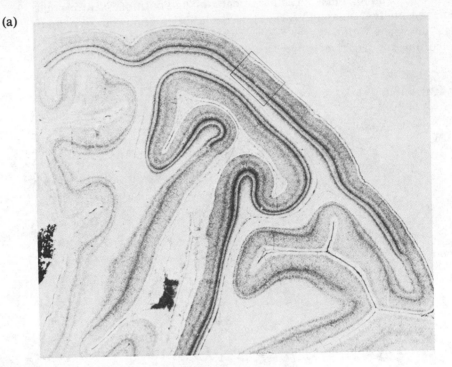

(b)

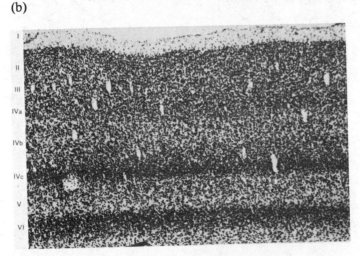

Figure 3.21: *Section of visual cortex stained by the Nissl method, which makes cell bodies, but not fibers, visible. In (a) the visual cortex can be seen to be a layered sheet of neurons about two millimeters thick. The black rectangle outlines a section similar to the one shown in (b). A section (b) of primary visual cortex enlarged about 35 diameters. The white gaps are sectioned blood vessels.*

The neurons in the various layers also transmit their outputs to different destinations. Layer VI projects back to the lateral geniculate; layer V projects to the superior colliculus; layers II and III send their outputs to other parts of the cortex.

The visual cortex is also organized in columns that are arranged perpendicularly to the cortical surface. All the neurons in a particular column are sensitive to lines and edges at a particular orientation. If an electrode is driven through the cortex at an angle so as to successively sample neurons from adjacent columns, the preferred orientation gradually shifts as each new column is encountered. This is illustrated in figure 3.22. Recent experiments, using radioactively labeled cell nutrients that can reveal which neurons have recently been more active than their neighbors, have shown that this pattern of shifting preferred orientation repeats every millimeter or so. Every square millimeter of cortex corresponds to one resolution element of the visual field. The high-resolution region of the fovea thus occupies a relatively large percentage of the visual cortex.

Sensory data from the primary visual cortex go to a number of other regions where they are processed further and integrated with information from other sensory pathways. We will deal with these higher level functions in a later section.

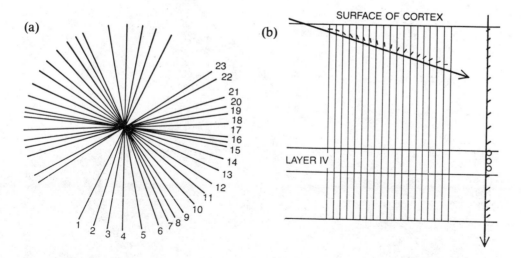

Figure 3.22: *Orientation preferences of 23 neurons encountered as a microelectrode penetrated the cortex obliquely are charted in (a). Adjacent columns of the visual cortex contain neurons with receptive field orientations that are rotated progressively as shown in (b). All neurons within a single column have the same orientation, except for layer IV where circularly symmetrical fields are encountered. This pattern repeats as each receptive field merges with the next. [From "Brain Mechanisms of Vision," by D. H. Hubel and T. N. Wiesel. Copyright © 1979 by Scientific American, Inc. All rights reserved.]*

HEARING

Next to vision, hearing is the most extensively studied sense. The neural input to the audio system begins in the cochlea. Sound enters the ear and the vibrations are coupled from the ear drum into the fluid-filled cochlea by means of a mechanical impedance transformer made up of three tiny bones called the hammer, anvil, and stirrup. The cochlea is a snail-shaped compartment consisting of two- and three-quarter turns of a gradually tapering cylinder as can be seen in figures 3.2 and 3.3. This cylindrical tube is divided along its length into three sections. A cross-sectional view is shown in figure 3.23. Pressure changes caused by sound vibrations enter the oval window and cause the fluid in the *scala vestibuli* to move back and forth. This motion is transmitted through the two membranes to the fluid in the *scala tympani*, which causes the round window to move in and out. The result is that the basilar membrane flexes up and down.

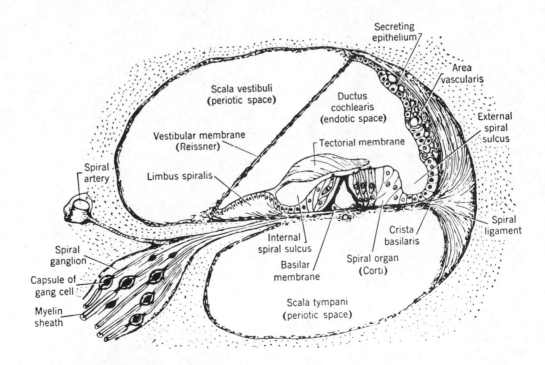

Figure 3.23: *Cross-section of the cochlea. Pressure changes caused by sound vibrations are transmitted through the oval window into the fluid in the* scala vestibuli. *This produces motion of the fluid filling the cochlea and causes the basilar membrane to flex up and down.*

Tiny hairs are stretched between the tectorial membrane and the hair cells on the basilar membrane, as shown in figure 3.24. These are deflected by mechanical motion of the basilar membrane. The hair cells are sensitive to mechanical deflection of the hairs and generate electrical signals as a result of the vibrations produced by sound. The hair cells do not produce action potentials because they do not need to transmit their information over any distance; rather, dendrites from the bipolar neurons of the spiral ganglion make synaptic contact with the hair cells. These bipolar neurons produce action potentials that encode the auditory information for transmission to the cochlear nuclei.

The fluid in the center section, the *ductus cochlearis*, has an electrical potential of $+80$ millivolts relative to the rest of the cochlea. Because the hair cells have a -70 millivolt potential, there exists a -150 millivolt potential across the membrane of the hair cells. The high electrical potential is thought to increase the sensitivity of the cell to small movements of the hairs.

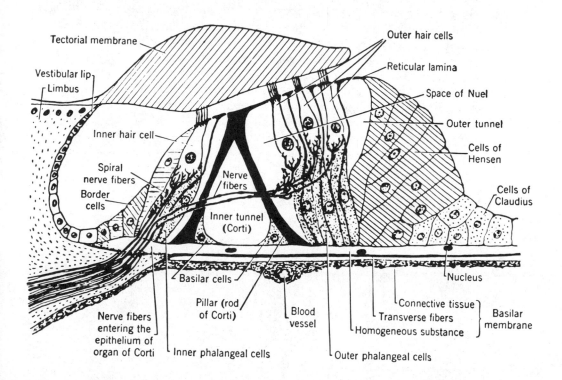

Figure 3.24: *Enlarged cross-section of basilar membrane showing the relationship of the cochlear hair cells to the tectorial membrane. As the basilar membrane flexes up and down in response to the pressure waves of sound, the hairs connected to the tectorial membrane are deflected back and forth. This produces an electrical signal in the hair cells and causes action potentials to be produced on the neurons of the spiral ganglion.*

There are about 20,000 outer and 3500 inner hair cells. Neurons in the spiral ganglion synapse with these outer hair cells on a ten-receptor/one-neuron basis. Though the inner hair cells are less numerous, neurons in the spiral ganglion synapse with these inner hair cells on a one-receptor/one-neuron basis. Thus, the inner hair cells are more heavily represented in the cochlear nerve.

Recordings made from the cochlear nerve indicate that different bipolar neurons are sensitive to sounds with different pitch. Figure 3.25 shows the so-called "tuning curves" for single auditory nerve fibers. The frequency discrimination evidenced in these neurons is much better than would be predicted from the mechanical tuning of the resonant cavity of the cochlea itself. Lateral inhibition of the type which produces the center-surround effect in the visual system may account for this phenomenon.

It may also be that feedback from higher levels in the auditory system can sharpen the frequency sensitivity through some form of a phase lock loop or autocorrelation effect. The cochlear nerve also contains information sent from the superior olivary nuclei to the point of origin of the auditory signal, shown in figure 3.26. These outward-conducting (efferent) axons synapse directly on the cell bodies of the outer hair cells and on the dendrites of the bipolar neurons connected to the inner hair cells. These efferent fibers convey inhibitory signals, but their exact function is unknown. In any case, the cochlear ganglion neurons produce outputs similar to the output of a comb filter. The firing rate on any particular neuron is analogous to the value of a Fourier coefficient in a frequency spectrum.

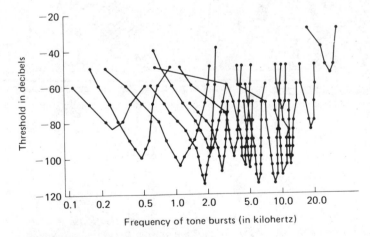

Figure 3.25: *Tuning curves of single auditory nerve fibers. Each individual nerve fiber is maximally sensitive to a single frequency and moderately sensitive to a band of nearby frequencies.*

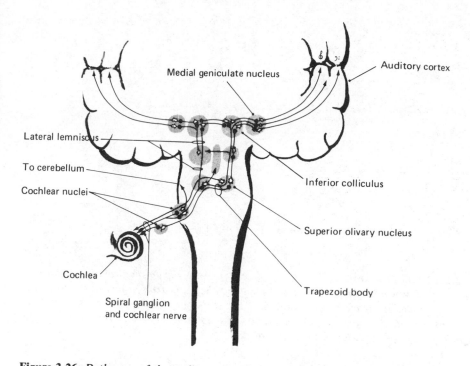

Figure 3.26: *Pathways of the auditory system. Note that signals flow in both directions in the auditory nerve. Sensory information originating in the cochlear hair cells flows to the cochlear nuclei and superior olivary nuclei on the way to the inferior colliculi, the medial geniculate, and the auditory cortex. However, signals originating in the superior olivary nucleus also travel back to the cochlea where they modify the behavior of the hair cell receptors.*

At low frequencies, cochlear neurons tend to fire in synchrony with the displacement of the audio pressure wave. At frequencies above about 500 hertz, cochlear neurons cannot fire fast enough to keep up with every cycle of the vibration. However, they can fire on every other cycle or at integer submultiples of the audio frequency. For example, in figure 3.27 the vibration of the basilar membrane is shown at the top duplicating the pressure fluctuations of the sound wave. Fibers (a) through (e) fire at slower rates, but at integer submultiples of the frequency of the sound wave. Thus the combination of fibers (a) through (e) contains all the information of the original signal. We will suggest in a later section how this combination might be made. The synchrony in the neuron firing patterns means that the cochlear comb filter preserves phase information as well as extracting frequency components.

Loudness is encoded by the number of impulses per cycle of the sound vibration as well as by the number of neurons responding to the sound.

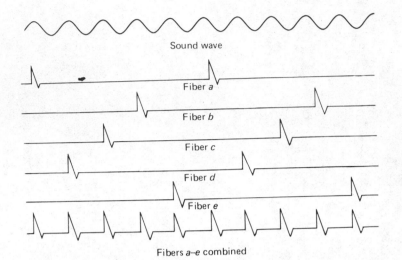

Sound wave

Fiber *a*

Fiber *b*

Fiber *c*

Fiber *d*

Fiber *e*

Fibers *a–e* combined

Figure 3.27: *Cochlear neurons tend to fire in synchrony with the mechanical displacement of the hair cells. However, at frequencies above about 500 hertz, neuron firing rates cannot keep up with every cycle of the mechanical motion. Thus, different neurons fire on different sub-multiples of the sound frequency. A combination of many fibers contains the frequency and phase information of the original sound signal.*

The neuronal pathways of the auditory information are shown in figure 3.26. Nerve fibers from the spiral ganglion enter the cochlear nuclei located in the upper part of the medulla. At this point, all the fibers synapse. From here the signals pass mainly to the opposite side of the brain stem through the trapezoid body to the superior olivary nucleus. Some fibers go to the superior olive on the same side. The superior olive also sends some fibers back into the cochlea to synapse on the hair cells and on the dendrites of the spiral ganglion cells near where they pick up their input from the hair cells. This architecture has many similarities to the design of a phase lock loop or to an autocorrelation mechanism.

From the superior olivary nucleus, the auditory pathway passes upward to the nucleus of the lateral lemniscus. Many fibers pass through this nucleus on their way to the inferior colliculus where most terminate. From here neurons send their axons to the medial geniculate body of the thalamus where all the fibers synapse. From here the auditory tract spreads by way of the audio radiations to the auditory cortex located mainly in the superior temporal lobe.

It should be noted that fibers from both ears are transmitted through auditory pathways on both sides of the brain. Also many fibers enter the reticular system. There are inputs to the cerebellum from several different levels of the auditory system.

The auditory system is complex. The pathway from the cochlea to the cortex

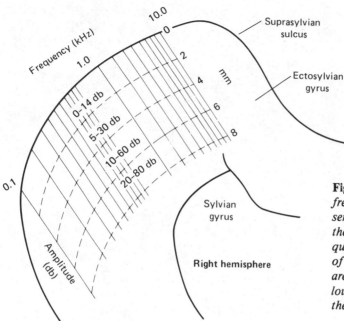

Figure 3.28: *Localization of intensity and frequency in the auditory cortex. Neurons sensitive to lower frequencies are located to the left, and those sensitive to higher frequencies are to the right along the surface of the cortex. Cells sensitive to soft sounds are near the surface, and those sensitive to loud sounds are several millimeters beneath the surface.*

passes through at least four and as many as six neurons. Yet a high degree of tonal organization is maintained. Figure 3.28 shows the representation of frequency and intensity on the surface of the auditory cortex. This type of mapping exists at all levels of the auditory pathway. However, the synchrony of action potentials with sound waves is not preserved beyond the superior olivary nucleus except for sounds below 200 hertz.

TASTE AND SMELL

For primitive creatures, taste and smell are the most important senses. Certainly, from an information processing standpoint, these senses are the simplest. Molecules entering the mouth or nose react directly with chemically sensitive neuronal detectors to create the sensation. Specific chemical reactions with specific incoming molecules create the basis for taste and smell discrimination. Very little additional processing is necessary to relate the neuronal signals to specific objects or events in the external environment.

The tongue, palate, pharynx, and larynx contain approximately 10,000 taste buds. Most of these are located such that they open into tiny trenches that trap saliva. The taste receptors are connected with the free endings of unipolar sensory neurons whose cell bodies are located in the ganglia of the seventh, ninth, and tenth cranial nerves. These are, respectively, the facial, glossopharyngeal, and vagus nerves. These pathways are shown in figure 3.29.

There are four types of taste buds that respond differently to the four types of taste: sour, salty, bitter, and sweet. The response of these four types of cells to the four types of taste are shown in figure 3.30. The various complex tastes that the brain can recognize arise from various combinations of these four sensors. This is analogous to the eye where all the colors result from various combinations of the three-color receptors in the retina.

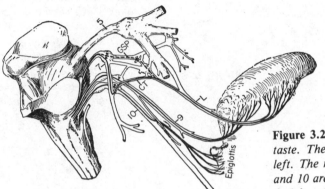

Figure 3.29: *Pathways for the sense of taste. The brain stem is shown on the left. The nerve bundles labeled 5, 7, 9, and 10 are, respectively, the trigeminal, facial, glossopharyngeal, and vagus nerves.*

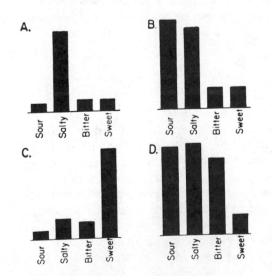

Figure 3.30: *Specific responsiveness of four different types of taste buds. Type A is particularly sensitive to salty tastes. Type B is sensitive to both sour and salty. Type C is sensitive to sweet, type D to sour, salty, and bitter. Tastes other than the four primary tastes are detected by various combinations of the four types of taste buds.*

The nerve fibers from the taste receptors synapse in the nuclei of the *tractus solitarius*. Cells from these nuclei synapse in the thalamus, and from the thalamus taste fibers are transmitted to the opercular-insular area of the cerebral cortex. This is next to the area that receives touch, pressure, and pain sensations from the tongue.

The smell sensors reside within two patches of mucous membrane inside the nasal cavity. Receptor cells have tiny cilia that protrude into the mucus. These receptors are neurons whose axons pass through tiny holes in the bone on the roof of the nasal cavity into the olfactory bulb. The precise details of the chemistry and neurophysiology by which odor-producing molecules interact with the cilia of the olfactory receptors to produce action potentials is unknown.

The senses of smell and taste are often confused. Persons with bad colds often claim they have lost their sense of taste. However, tests have shown that the loss is that of smell rather than taste.

Output from groups of olfactory cells make synaptic contact with mitral cells in synaptic clusters called glomeruli. The mitral cells make up the olfactory bulbs, and their axons give rise to the olfactory tract as shown in figure 3.31. The olfactory tract then enters the limbic lobe of the brain making synaptic contact in several limbic nuclei as shown in figure 3.32.

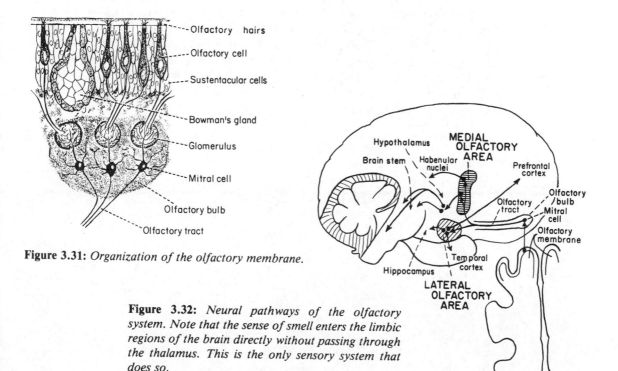

Figure 3.31: *Organization of the olfactory membrane.*

Figure 3.32: *Neural pathways of the olfactory system. Note that the sense of smell enters the limbic regions of the brain directly without passing through the thalamus. This is the only sensory system that does so.*

It is significant that the olfactory tract enters the limbic system. In lower animals the olfactory limbic cortex makes up the bulk of the cortical regions. The limbic system is the seat of the emotions and functions as the evaluation system that distinguishes good from bad. In lower forms the primary good–bad judgments concern whether to eat something or not, a decision based mostly on the sense of smell. In higher forms the good–bad decision mechanisms are much more complex and must deal with a much wider range of sensory inputs and behavioral choices. Hence, the limbic system in higher forms is much larger and receives highly processed input from all the senses.

CONCLUSIONS

This brief survey of the sensory input channels makes it clear that a great deal of information processing goes on in the sensory pathways, starting in the sensory receptor cells themselves. Each sensory pathway has a number of computational modules dedicated to the processing of that particular input. Many, if not most, of these modules receive input from the higher centers of the brain as well as from the sensory input receptors. Outputs from the sensory-processing modules often travel both to low-level, behavior-generating modules as well as to higher levels in the sensory-processing system. Gradually, as the sensory data makes its way toward the higher levels of the brain, it becomes integrated with data from other senses. How does this complex interaction of sensory input and higher level signals generate the phenomenon of perception? How is the perceived sensory information translated into behavioral actions? Before addressing these fundamental questions in the study of the brain, it will be useful to examine the neurological structures where this translation is performed.

CHAPTER **4**

The Central Nervous System

$\mathbf{T}$he human central nervous system, the most complex structure in nature, consists of trillions of neurons connected together in such a way to produce the phenomenon of conscious cognitive behavior and imagination. In the peripheral regions of the sensory and motor systems, specific neurons and clusters of neurons tend to have specific functions. However, at the higher levels in the neuronal hierarchy, the various modalities become intermixed, and it is not possible to relate a specific neuron with a specific muscle or sensory receptor. Areas in the higher regions of the brain tend to be related to specific behavioral actions, such as eating, articulating thoughts, or thinking about spatial relationships.

This transformation from specific effectors and receptors to specific behavioral actions takes place gradually, as the number of synapses from the periphery grows. It is the natural result of a hierarchical goal-directed system. As will be seen later in figure 9.1, the computational modules at each level in a hierarchy have more general concerns than do the modules beneath them. At the very bottom, the computations concern only a single muscle group. At slightly higher levels, computations concern coordination of several muscle groups. At higher levels still, the motion of an entire limb or concerted actions between limbs are computed. Finally, at the highest levels of the brain, the entire body must be coordinated in a single activity directed toward a future goal which may be expressed symbolically or even philosophically. Hierarchical command and control structures which extend beyond the single individual allow groups of individuals or entire societies to be coordinated in the pursuit of family, tribal, or national goals.

We will begin this progression from the bottom up, starting with the motor neurons of the spinal cord. As we go, we will note significant features of the structure of the brain that are pertinent to the computing architecture we'll later propose for robot-control systems.

The most obvious hierarchical partitioning of the central nervous system divides it into three levels. At the lowest level is the spinal cord; above that is the

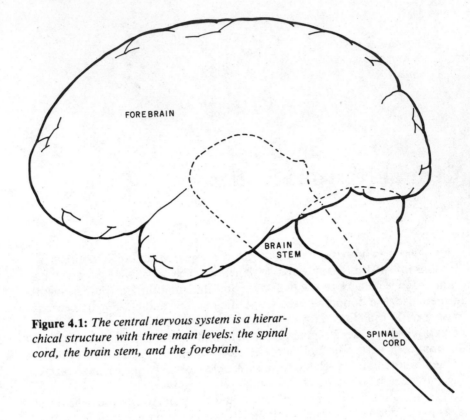

FOREBRAIN

BRAIN STEM

SPINAL CORD

Figure 4.1: *The central nervous system is a hierarchical structure with three main levels: the spinal cord, the brain stem, and the forebrain.*

brain stem, and finally at the top is the forebrain, shown in figure 4.1. Within each of these three main subdivisions, there are many intermediate levels.

THE SPINAL CORD

The spinal cord is much more than a bunch of axons carrying commands from the brain to the muscles and sensory information from the sensor organs to the brain. The cord contains a number of computing centers that coordinate extensor and flexor muscles to facilitate standing, walking, running, and jumping. It generates complex reflexes such as the one that causes a falling cat to land on its feet and those that generate rhythmic stepping motions, reciprocal stepping of opposite limbs, diagonal stepping of all four limbs, and even scratching movements. These computing centers constitute the first and second levels in the sensory-motor hierarchy controlling the limbs, hands, feet, and digits.

The spinal cord also houses command centers for a number of autonomic reflexes including changes in vascular constriction due to heat or cold, localized sweating, and motor functions of the intestines and bladder. These autonomic computational centers need to know the type and amount of physical activity that is ongoing in the muscles in support of intentional behavior so that they can intelligently allocate the body's resources, such as the blood supply, the digestive juices, etc. These computing centers receive their higher level input commands from the place in the intentional motor system where activity is actually being generated. Figure 3.9 shows the physical relationship between the autonomic and the intentional nervous systems.

Large sections of the spinal cord are made up of grey matter: dendrites, cell bodies, and axon buttons. The computations required for generating and controlling the reflexes are performed here. The white matter of the spinal cord consists of axon bundles, wrapped in myelin, carrying sensory and control signals. Some of these bundles carry commands from the brain to the motor neurons. Some carry sensory signals from the skin, muscles, and joints to the brain. Others carry information back and forth between computing centers in the grey matter of the cord itself.

Even in the simplest of creatures the computations in what corresponds to the spinal cord are extensive. For example, in insects the nerve cord that runs the length of the body is the primary, if not the only, computational organ. As can be seen in figure 4.2 the brains of the planaria, the earthworm, and the amphioxus are virtually nonexistent. All muscle coordination is performed in the cord. Even in the bee, the brain is hardly larger than the eyes. It is thus not surprising that the behavior of an insect is stereotyped, i.e., a particular stimulus produces a predictable response. Insect behavior is generated entirely at one, or at most two, hierarchical levels.

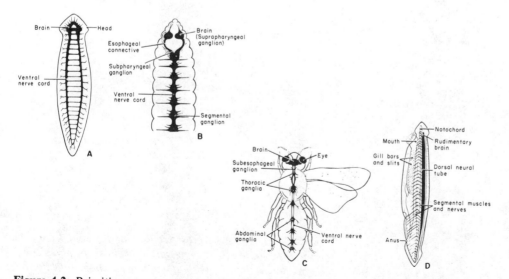

Figure 4.2: *Primitive nervous systems: (a) planaria (b) earthworm (c) bee (d) amphioxus.*

68

This does not mean, however, that the motor patterns of the insects are simple. The muscle coordination required to produce the flight patterns of a bee, dragon fly, or mosquito, or the climbing skills of an ant or beetle are considerable. Even though these types of movements are apparently computed in a one- or two-level computing structure, the amount of multivariable computation that goes on in the insect brain is astonishing. A close examination of the manipulatory dexterity in the leg of an ant reveals a degree of control sophistication not found in any existing laboratory robot. The spinal cord is thus a formidable computational machine and has been so from the beginning. It is, in fact, the basic building block of the brain. It is the first and second level input-output computational module.

If the spinal cord of a higher mammal is cut in two, the exposed face of the cut has a cross-sectional appearance, as illustrated in figure 4.3. The dark regions in the diagrams correspond to the grey matter at different levels in the spinal cord. Notice the resemblance to a pair of horns. The upper part of these figures is toward the back. The upper horns are thus the dorsal or posterior horns. The lower part is toward the front. These are the ventral or anterior horns.

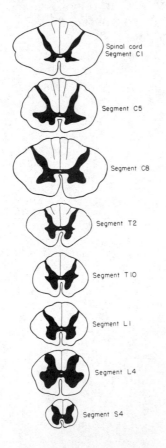

Spinal cord
Segment C1

Segment C5

Segment C8

Segment T2

Segment T10

Segment L1

Segment L4

Segment S4

Figure 4.3: *Diagrams of cross-sections of the spinal cord at several different levels showing variations in shape and size of the grey and white matter. Letters and numbers indicate the spinal vertebrae at the corresponding level.*

The motor neurons are located in the anterior horns as shown in figure 4.4 and the axons of the motor neurons leave the cord in a series of little bundles along both sides of the front of the cord. These bundles gather together to form the ventral roots. A similar series of little bundles, consisting of axons from sensory neurons in the periphery, enter the spinal cord from the rear. These are called the dorsal, or posterior, roots and are shown in figure 4.5.

The sensory neurons are unipolar neurons. One unipolar neuron is shown in figure 2.7a. The cell bodies of the unipolar sensory neurons reside in the bulges called the dorsal root ganglia. The axons from the dorsal roots may synapse on sensory-processing neurons in the posterior horns, or they may travel into the anterior horns to synapse on the motor neurons. The posterior horn neurons send axons up the cord toward the brain.

The dorsal and ventral roots merge into single bundles called spinal nerves before leaving the protection of the bony channel of the spinal vertabrae. The spinal nerves often follow blood vessels and branch repeatedly, as the motor axons trace out pathways to the muscles they control and the sensory axons fan out to the sensory endings by which they are stimulated.

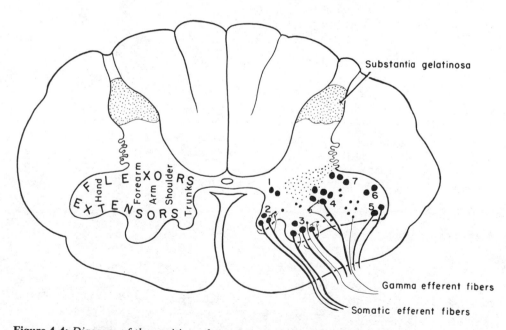

Figure 4.4: *Diagram of the position of motor neurons in the forward grey horn of a lower cervical segment of the spinal cord. On the left is shown the locations of motor neurons controlling specific muscle groups. On the right are the axon pathways leaving the cord. Note that some collaterals from outgoing axons return to synapse on intermediate cells.*

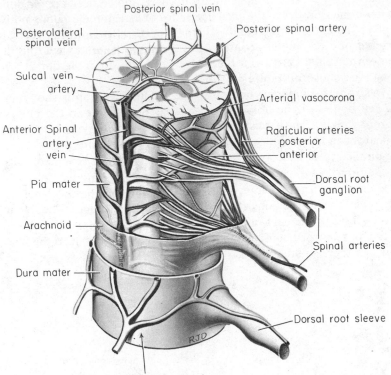

Posterior spinal vein

Posterolateral spinal vein

Posterior spinal artery

Sulcal vein artery

Arterial vasocorona

Anterior Spinal artery vein

Radicular arteries posterior anterior

Pia mater

Dorsal root ganglion

Arachnoid

Dura mater

Spinal arteries

Dorsal root sleeve

Internal vertebral venous plexus

Figure 4.5: *The axons of motor neurons leave the front of the cord in a series of small nerve bundles that gather together to form the anterior roots. Sensory neurons enter the cord from the rear through the dorsal roots, which split into similar bundles. The anterior and dorsal roots join to form the spinal nerves, which leave the protection of the spinal column and travel to the muscles and sensory receptors in the periphery. All neural tissue in the central nervous system is covered by two membranes: the arachnoid and the dura.*

THE STRETCH REFLEX

It is perhaps not surprising that the first computational level in the sensory-motor system is the best understood. The servo level control system in the vertebrate motor system is primarily composed of the stretch reflex. Figure 4.6 illustrates the essential components of the stretch reflex. The muscle spindle attached to a muscle bundle contains a sensory ending that sends out a stream of action potentials whenever it is stretched. The rate of the pulses is proportional to the amount of stretching. The axon carrying this signal from the muscle spindle enters the spinal cord through the dorsal root. There it terminates with an excitatory synapse on the motor neuron which controls the muscle bundle to which the spindle is attached. When the muscle is stretched, the spindle increases its firing rate. This excites the motor neuron, which commands the muscle to contract, thereby counteracting the stretch. The net result tends to keep the muscle at a constant length despite variations in external load.

The advantages of this system are clear: the stretch reflex in the muscles of the legs tends to hold the body upright. If the body starts to fall forward, the muscles in the back of the legs are stretched; this activates the stretch reflex to contract these same muscles and pull the body back erect.

The spindle also has a tiny auxiliary muscle of its own that can be used to contract and hence shorten the tissue by which it is attached to the much larger muscle bundle. The relationship between the muscle spindle and the larger muscle bundle is shown in figure 3.1. When the tiny attachment muscles contract, they shorten the overall length of the spindle, and the spindle then fires at a shorter length. The neurons that control these shortening muscles, called gamma neurons, essentially set

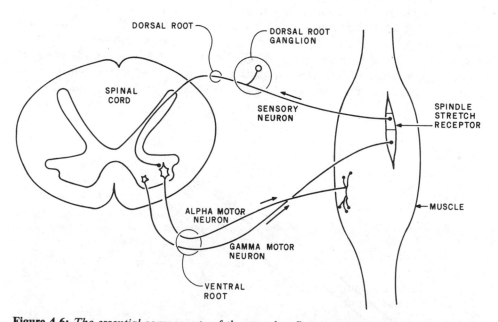

Figure 4.6: *The essential components of the stretch reflex. A sensory neuron from a spindle stretch receptor enters the cord through a dorsal root and makes excitatory synapses on an alpha motor neuron. When the muscle to which the spindle is attached is stretched, the resulting activity on the sensory neurons excites the motor neuron to counteract the stretch. The gamma motor neuron can shorten the spindle organ to increase the sensitivity of the stretch receptor.*

the length of the spindle at which a certain firing rate will occur. If the gamma neurons fire rapidly, the spindle will start firing when the muscle bundle to which it is attached is stretched only a little. If the gamma neuron is firing slowly or not at all, the spindle will not respond until the muscle bundle is stretched to a much longer length. Figure 4.7 is a set of curves illustrating the input–output of the spindle at various firing rates on the gamma neuron.

The output of the spindle sensor travels to the spinal cord where it enters through the dorsal roots and terminates with excitatory synapses on the dendrites of the alpha motor neurons as shown in figure 4.6. When the gamma neuron fires at a rate g_1, it shortens the ends of the spindle to a length $l(g_1)$. If the muscle bundle attached to the spindle is stretched by more than an amount $L(g_1)$, the spindle will fire, sending a signal to the motor neuron that controls the muscle bundle commanding it to resist further stretching. Thus, the gamma neuron can set the point at which the stretch reflex resists further movement. The effect is that the limb moves to a position set by the firing rate on the gamma motor neuron. The gamma neuron, muscle spindle, and motor neuron thus comprise a position servo. A particular firing rate on the gamma neuron tends to produce a particular length of a muscle and hence a particular position in the joint angle.

Figure 4.8 shows a schematic diagram of the computing modules involved in the gamma position servo. The position command enters the motor-output module and generates a particular firing rate on a gamma neuron. The gamma neuron sends its indication of what the spindle length should be to the sensory spindle where it becomes an expected position. The spindle compares the actual position with the expected and puts out an error signal, which comes back to the motor output module

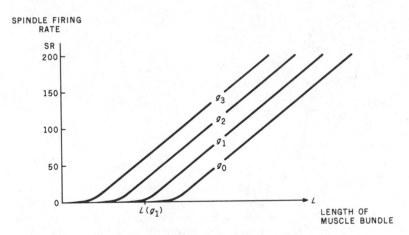

Figure 4.7: *A plot of spindle firing rate vs. length of motor muscle for various levels of gamma neuron activity g_0, g_1, g_2, and g_3.*

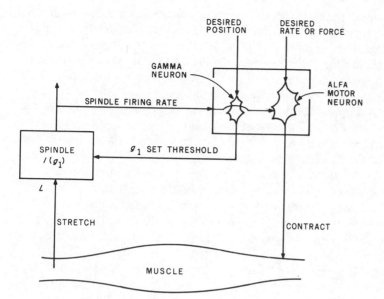

Figure 4.8: *A schematic diagram of the relationship between the motor neurons, muscles, stretch sensors, and input commands from higher motor centers.*

as an excitatory feedback signal. The motor-output module, whose output is the alpha motor neuron, then uses this feedback together with input from other motor centers to compute its output signal, which it encodes as a firing rate to the muscles.

Some of the other motor center inputs come from commands to and feedback from other limbs. The rest of the other inputs come from higher motor centers: pyramidal fibers come directly from the motor cortex; extrapyramidal fibers come from the red nucleus, the *substantia nigra*, the subthalamic nucleus, and the vestibular nucleus. These all synapse directly on the motor neurons. These inputs essentially command the motor neurons to fire at a particular rate and so produce a particular force or rate of contraction of the muscles. This is represented in figure 4.8 as a rate or force command input to the motor module.

In addition to the muscle spindles that measure the amount of stretch in the muscles, there are the Golgi tendon organs that measure the tension in the tendons. Axon fibers from the Golgi tendon organs enter the dorsal roots and make excitatory synapses on interneurons. These interneurons then make inhibitory synapses on the motor neurons. The overall effect is to limit the force exerted by the muscle to prevent excessive stress from tearing the muscles or tendons. When tension in the tendon organs approaches the danger level, the tendon organ fires vigorously, causing a relaxation of the muscle. Signals from the tendon organs thus provide the motor output module with the information necessary for servoing the force in the tendons. It is thought that force commands from higher in the motor system modulate the gain in the inhibitory portion of the tendon organ loop. If the inhibitory signal is equal to the difference between the commanded and the observed tension, the motor neuron will increase its firing rate whenever the tension falls below the commanded value. Correspondingly, the motor neuron will reduce its firing rate when the tension rises above the commanded value. The result is that the force in the muscle is servoed to the commanded value.

Animals with severed spinal cords can still produce a number of coordinated reflex actions. Almost any kind of tactile stimulus will produce the flexor reflex that withdraws the limb from a noxious stimulus. The basic neuronal circuitry involved in the flexor reflex is illustrated in the left side of figure 4.9. A large number of neurons are involved in any coordinated action, even of this simple kind. If the stimulus is weak and localized, it may not activate enough neurons to elicit the withdrawal. However, if it is intense or widespread, the resultant signal will produce the reflex action.

There are three basic types of neuronal circuits in the reflex system: (1) diverging circuits to spread the signal to the necessary muscles for withdrawal, (2) reciprocal inhibitory circuits to relax the antagonist muscles, and (3) oscillatory circuits to prolong the withdrawal action after the stimulus is removed.

In addition, as shown in figure 4.9, an axon pathway crosses over to the opposite side of the cord, carrying the signals necessary for the crossed extensor reflex. Approximately 0.2 to 0.5 seconds after a stimulus elicits a flexor reflex to withdraw the one limb, the opposite limb begins to extend, pushing the body away from the stimulus.

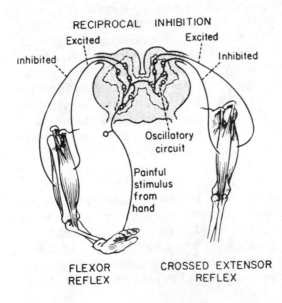

Figure 4.9: *The flexor reflex, the crossed extensor reflex, and reciprocal inhibition. These work together to produce coordinated activity that moves the body away from a noxious stimulus.*

There are also reflex pathways that travel up and down the cord on both sides. These are the mechanisms that produce the righting reflexes and the diagonal stepping of all four limbs.

The spinal cord possesses a large computing capacity just related to motor reflexes. It also contains a number of sensory-processing modules, or nuclei: the nucleus dorsalis, sometimes called Clark's column, the intermediomedial nucleus and several others. The neurons in these nuclei receive input from the sensory neurons of the dorsal roots, as well as collaterals from the motor-command neurons of the pyramidal and extrapyramidal tracts. They send their axons upward to the cerebellum, the thalamus, and other spinal cord neurons. These nuclei are certainly involved in some of the spinal reflexes as well as in other sensory-processing computations which are not as well understood as those of the spinal reflexes.

SPINAL TRACTS

In addition to the computing centers located in the grey matter of the horns of the spinal cord, there are also a great number of axon pathways in the spinal cord that carry motor command signals from the brain and sensory signals to the brain. Figure 4.10 illustrates some of the sensory pathways to the cerebral cortex from the touch and pressure sensors and from the joint receptors for position and movement. Data carried by these pathways is processed through two sets of computing centers: one set in the medulla consists of the nucleus gracilis and the nucleus cuneatus, and the other in the thalamus is the ventral posterolateral nucleus. However, there is another pathway for touch sensors that goes directly to the thalamus and from there to the cortex. A third pathway for heat, cold, and pain receptors also travels directly to the thalamus and on to the cortex. Finally, there is a pathway for data from muscle spindle and tendon organ information that travels to the cerebellum. Most of these fiber bundles give off collaterals to various nuclei in the spinal cord and brain stem as they pass by.

An equally diverse set of axon pathways travels downward. For example, figure 4.11 shows the pyramidal motor pathways that travel directly from the motor cortex to the motor neurons in the ventral horns. These fibers, named pyramidal fibers, pass through the triangular-shaped regions called the pyramids in the medulla. There also exists a second set of motor-command fiber pathways from the vestibular system to the motor neurons, and a third set from the red nucleus and the tectum to the motor neurons.

Each of these pathways contains many hundreds of thousands of individual axons, far more than necessary simply to move the limbs and report the results. The purpose of such large numbers is twofold. Redundancy is the first: large numbers of nerve fibers can be rendered inoperative through injury, yet the system can still function, or at least can recover its function. The second is precision: an individual neuron is a noisy and unreliable information channel; if the same information is encoded by many neurons, the statistical average of all the signals is much more precise than any one signal by itself. A large number of motor neurons makes possible very precise movements, and a large number of sensory neurons makes possible a very fine degree of sensory discrimination.

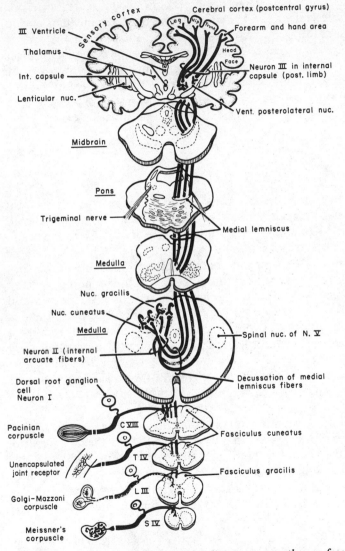

Figure 4.10: *Some of the upward traveling sensory pathways from touch and pressure sensors and joint receptors to the cerebral cortex. Data carried by these pathways is processed through the nuclei gracilis and cuneatus and then through ventral posterolateral nucleus of the thalamus. There are three other sensory pathways: for touch sensors; for heat, cold, and pain sensors; and for stretch and tension sensors.*

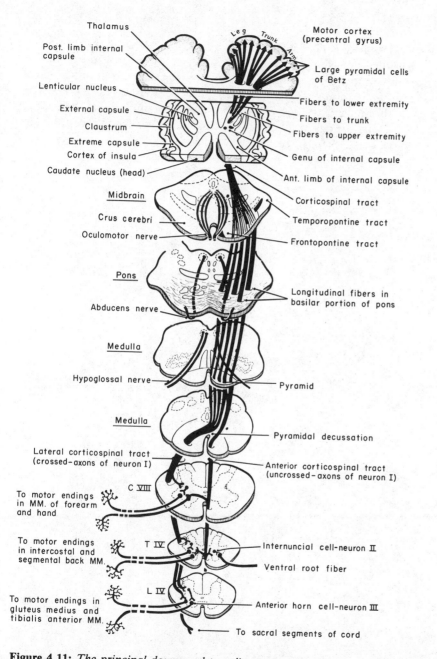

Thalamus

Post. limb internal
capsule

Lenticular nucleus

External capsule

Claustrum

Extreme capsule

Cortex of insula

Caudate nucleus (head)

Leg   Trunk   Arm

Motor cortex
(precentral gyrus)

Large pyramidal cells
of Betz

Fibers to lower extremity

Fibers to trunk

Fibers to upper extremity

Genu of internal capsule

Ant. limb of internal capsule

Corticospinal tract

Temporopontine tract

Frontopontine tract

Midbrain

Crus cerebri

Oculomotor nerve

Pons

Abducens nerve

Longitudinal fibers in
basilar portion of pons

Medulla

Hypoglossal nerve

Pyramid

Medulla

Pyramidal decussation

Lateral corticospinal tract
(crossed–axons of neuron I)

Anterior corticospinal tract
(uncrossed–axons of neuron I)

C VIII

To motor endings
in MM. of forearm
and hand

To motor endings
in intercostal and
segmental back MM.

T IV

Internuncial cell–neuron II

Ventral root fiber

To motor endings in
gluteus medius and
tibialis anterior MM.

L IV

Anterior horn cell–neuron III

To sacral segments of cord

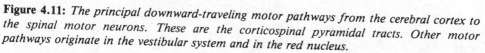

Figure 4.11: *The principal downward-traveling motor pathways from the cerebral cortex to the spinal motor neurons. These are the corticospinal pyramidal tracts. Other motor pathways originate in the vestibular system and in the red nucleus.*

THE BRAIN STEM

At the top of the spinal cord just above where the cord enters the skull is the imposing structure of the brain stem shown in figure 4.12. In lower forms the computational centers of the brain stem are the highest levels that exist. But in humans, the brain stem is subordinate to many layers of higher level computational centers. The relationship of the brain stem to the rest of the brain in the human can be seen in figure 4.1. The bulges of the cuneate and gracilis nuclei can be seen in figure 4.12 at the top of the spinal cord where it joins the medulla oblongata.

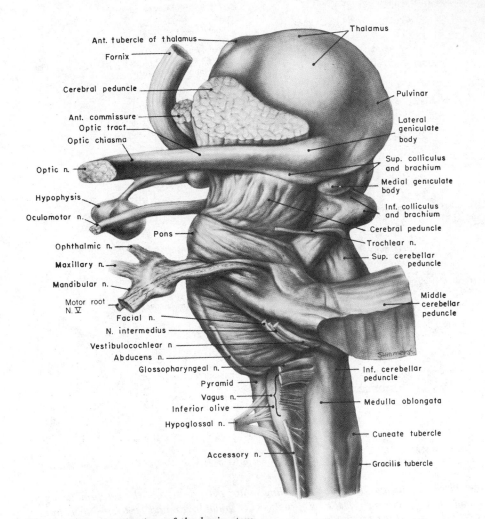

Figure 4.12: *A side view of the brain stem.*

A number of nerve bundles enter and leave the brain stem. The accessory nerves receive from and transmit to the neck and upper torso musculature. The hypoglossal nerve carries taste information and controls the tongue muscles. The vagus and glossopharyngeal nerves send and receive from the larynx, trachea, esophagus, heart, and chest and abdominal viscera. The abducens, trochlear, and oculomotor nerves control the muscles that position the eyes. The vestibulocochlear nerve conveys information from the ears and vestibular sensors. The facial nerve plus the three nerves of the trigeminal ganglion, the ophthalmic, maxillary, and mandibular carry sensory information from and motor commands to the face and mouth and control the tear and salivary glands. The largest nerve bundle projecting forward is the optic nerve that carries visual information from the eye to the lateral geniculate body of the thalamus. The anterior commissure is the smaller of two nerve bundles that connect the two sides of the cortex. The larger is the corpus callosum, which crosses just above the thalamus. Shown next to the anterior commissure is the cerebral peduncle, the bundle of neurons from the motor cortex down through the pyramids to the motor neurons in the spinal cord. At the back of the brain stem are the cerebellar peduncles, nerve bundles carrying information into and out of the cerebellum. Just above the cerebellar peduncles are the two bumps of the inferior and superior colliculi.

THE MEDULLA

The lowest major segment of the brain stem is called the medulla oblongata. Among the most important structures in the medulla are the vestibular nuclei. Figure 4.13 illustrates the pathways of the vestibular system. The information from the hair cells in the vestibular sensors is transmitted via the vestibulocochlear nerve to the vestibular nuclei where the computations necessary to maintain equilibrium are performed. Some fibers also go directly to the cerebellum. As can be seen in figure 4.13, output from the vestibular nuclei goes to the motor computational centers for the eyes, the neck muscles, and the body and limb muscles. Outputs from the vestibular nuclei also go to the cerebellum, the computational center for rapid, precise motor activity.

An example of one of the many functions of the vestibular system related to balance and equilibrium is the automatic stabilization of the gaze of the eyes. As the head turns, the vestibular reflex causes the eyes to turn the opposite direction by an equal amount so that the gaze remains fixed. If the head continues to turn, the eyes jump rapidly ahead and then rotate back at the rate of head turning, thus fixing the gaze on another spot. This action is known as "nystagmus."

The vestibular nuclei also receive input from the joint receptors in the neck. This allows the vestibular nuclei to subtract a tilt of the head in the computation of tilt of the body. The commands sent to the body muscles thus can maintain the balance of the body in spite of motions of the head.

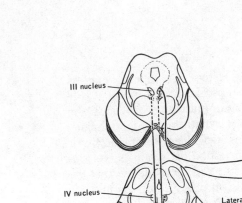
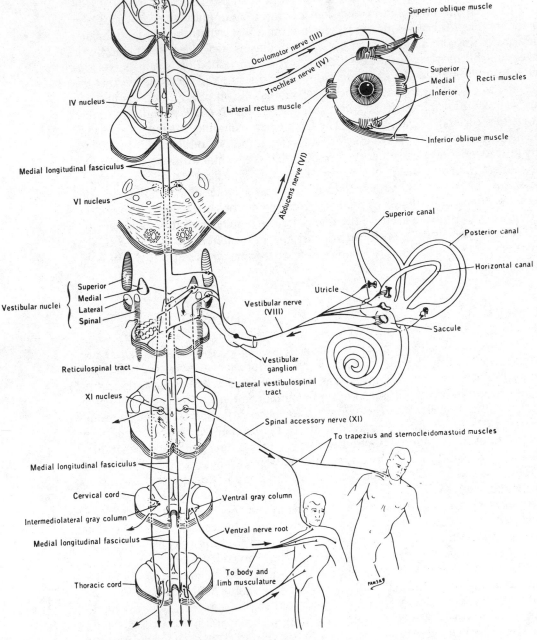

Figure 4.13: *Pathways of the vestibular reflex.*

THE RETICULAR FORMATION

The center core of the brain stem from the medulla up to the thalamus consists of a diffuse mass of cells and fibers called the reticular formation, one of the most primitive brain structures. In the course of phylogenetic development, distinct cell masses and fiber bundles have arisen to overlay and surround the reticular formation. To a large extent these have taken over the command and control duties of the more primitive reticular formation. Nevertheless, many specific functions remain, including some basic motor responses. Stimulation of the reticular formation may elicit movements and even affect complete postural adjustments. More typically, the reticular formation acts to facilitate or inhibit spinal motor mechanisms and thus control the intensity rather than initiate or direct movements. The reticular formation is also involved in the processing of sensory information from a variety of sources. It controls habituation and arousal and has the ability to filter, modify, and direct attention to sensory input. It has a profound influence on sleep and waking and even performs some higher level integrative processes related to motivation, emotion, and learning. Specific groups of cells in the reticular formation are known to control such activities as gastrointestinal secretions, vasoconstrictor tone, and respiration.

Surrounded on all sides by the fiber tracts and nuclei of the specific sensory pathways as well as by the pyramidal and extrapyramidal motor systems, the reticular formation receives input from the basal ganglia and from the cerebellum. It also receives a profusion of collaterals from many ascending sensory pathways. In addition, some axons from the spinal sensory neurons travel directly to the reticular formation and synapse on cells scattered throughout its longitudinal extent. It is not uncommon to find a single cell of the reticular formation that will fire or stop firing in response to sensory input from a variety of modalities.

The pons is a large bulge on the front of the brain stem, containing a number of computing centers that service the facial muscles, including the jaws and lips. It is perhaps significant that the pons is well-developed in primitive creatures, whose jaws and lips are principal manipulatory organs.

The cerebellum is attached to the brain stem just behind the pons by three large fiber tracts called the cerebellar peduncles. The cerebellum is involved in the control of rapid, precise muscular activities such as running, jumping, typing, or playing the piano. It is not surprising that birds have a large cerebellum because of the requirement for rapid, precise movements involved in flying.

The cerebellum receives motor-command inputs from the motor cortex by way of the pons as well as feedback inputs from muscle spindles, Golgi tendon organs, and tactile receptors in the skin and joints. These convey information as to the status of muscle contraction, degree of tension in muscles, positions of the limbs, and forces acting on the surface of the body.

The cerebellum transmits its outputs to the motor cortex through the thalamus, as well as to the basal ganglia, the red nucleus, the reticular formation of the brain stem, and the vestibular nuclei. A more complete description of the neural structure and computational properties of the cerebellum is presented in Chapter 6.

THE MIDBRAIN

Just above the pons and cerebellum is a region called the midbrain. The midbrain is the smallest portion of the brain stem. Located on the back of the midbrain are two pairs of small bumps called the inferior and superior colliculi. The inferior colliculi are among the principal computing centers in the auditory pathway. The inferior colliculi receive input from the cochlear nuclei and transmit output to the medial geniculate nuclei of the thalamus. Neurons in the inferior colliculi are arranged in an orderly manner with respect to frequencies. It is thought that the inferior colliculi play a significant role in the localization of sound.

The superior colliculi are related to vision. In submammalian vertebrates the primary visual processing center is the optic tectum, a precursor to the mammalian superior colliculi. The superior colliculi have a complex, laminated structure resembling the cerebral cortex. Beginning with reptiles, the importance of the optic tectum (superior colliculi) diminishes progressively as an increasing number of optic fibers establish more extensive connections with the thalamus and cortex. In man the superior colliculi have become greatly reduced in size, receiving only about 20 percent of the fibers from the optic nerve. They serve primarily as reflex centers concerned with eye movements. The superior colliculi receive input from the lateral geniculate, the retina, and the visual cortex. Output goes to the oculomotor nucleus and the other midbrain structures that control the muscles moving the eyes. The superior colliculi are thought to compute the functions necessary to fixate the eyes on an object of attention. The part of the visual scene of special interest is computed in the visual areas of the occipital cortex, primarily in the visual association areas. From there it passes to the visual pointing centers of the superior colliculi. Decisions made in the superior colliculi then travel to the reticular areas around the oculomotor nuclei and thence into the motor nuclei themselves.

Red Nucleus

Forward of the superior colliculi, in the center of the midbrain, is the red nucleus. The red nucleus is an important part of the extrapyramidal motor system. It receives input from the caudate nucleus and the putamen as well as from the prestitial nucleus and the nucleus commissuralis. It also receives input from the cerebellum. Output from the red nucleus goes to the spinal motor neurons and to the reticular nuclei of the brain stem, which then project to the spinal motor neurons.

Next to the red nucleus is the substantia nigra, a large pigmented region that is only partially understood. The substantia nigra is thought to have an important role in the extrapyramidal motor system. It receives input from the basal ganglia and the cerebral cortex. Output goes primarily to the thalamus.

THE THALAMUS

The thalamus, the gateway to the cerebral cortex, is technically not part of the brain stem but of the forebrain. It is the computational and switching center through which all sensory information, with the exception of smell, is routed. From the thalamus, sensory information is passed to the specific cortical regions dedicated to the early and intermediate stages of sensory processing.

Every thalamic nucleus that sends fibers to a particular cortical region also receives in turn some fibers from that same region. Thus, there is a great deal of looping circuitry between the thalamus and cortical regions to which it sends input. The consequence of this is that the cortex can send the thalamus instructions for filtering the incoming data, separating the important from the inconsequential. Signals, or portions of images that contain priority information, can be amplified, and other regions can be filtered to suppress that which is not relevant to current behavioral activity. In some cases, the cortex may even supply the thalamus with expectations or predictions of what sensory data to expect, so that differences between the expected and the observed can be passed to the motor-generating modules in the forebrain.

The thalamus consists of a cluster of 29 separate nuclei. Figure 4.14 illustrates the origin of input and destination of output of some of the major thalamic nuclei. Among the most important thalamic nuclei is the lateral geniculate nucleus, the relay station of the optic tract. The lateral geniculate, like all the other thalamic relay stations, also receives inputs from the cortical area to which it projects, in this case, the visual cortex. This allows visual perceptions made in the cortex to influence and modify the incoming visual data.

A second important thalamic nucleus is the medial geniculate. This is the relay station for audio data. The medial geniculate receives audio information from the inferior colliculus as well as directly from the cochlear nucleus. It sends its output to the auditory cortex located mainly in the upper part of the temporal lobe.

A third principal thalamic region is the ventral posterolateral nucleus. This is the relay station for most of the sensory information from the spinal cord. Touch, position, pain, heat, and cold are all relayed to the sensory cortex through the ventral posterolateral nucleus.

The ventral lateral nucleus is the relay station for information from the cerebellum on its way to the premotor cortex. The anterior nucleus passes communications between the hypothalamus and the limbic cortex. The ventral anterior nucleus transmits signals from the globus pallidus and the substantia nigra to various regions in the frontal and temporal cortex.

In addition to these specific relay nuclei of the thalamus, there are a number of so-called association nuclei that receive no direct fibers from the sensory systems, but have abundant connections with other structures in the forebrain. These send fibers to the association areas of the cerebral cortex in the frontal and parietal lobes and, to a lesser extent, in the occipital and temporal lobes.

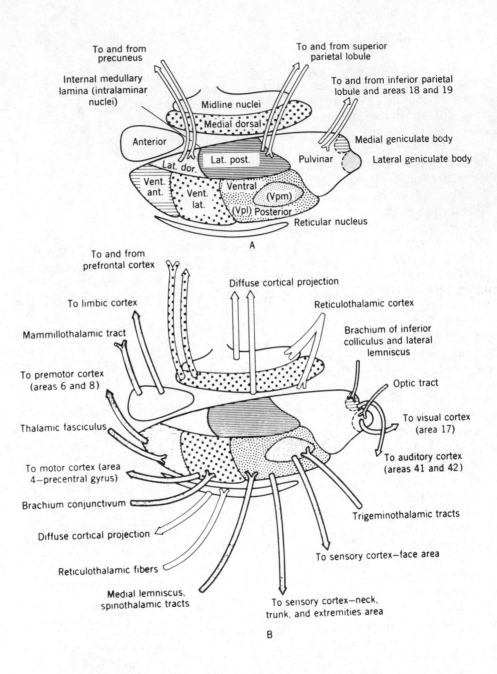

Figure 4.14: *Major nuclei of the thalamus showing the origin and destination of fibers entering and leaving. The thalamus is the final processing station for all sensory information (except smell) before it reaches the cerebral cortex.*

THE FOREBRAIN

The forebrain contains the highest levels of the computational hierarchy we call the brain. The forebrain contains the thalamus, the basal ganglia, the cerebral cortex, and the limbic system, including the hypothalamus.

The Basal Ganglia

Located to either side and slightly above the thalamus are the large subcortical nuclei of the basal ganglia. The basal ganglia consist of two large clusters of cells: the caudate nucleus and the lenticular nucleus, which is sometimes further divided into the globus pallidus and the putamen. These are shown in relationship to the rest of the brain in figure 4.15.

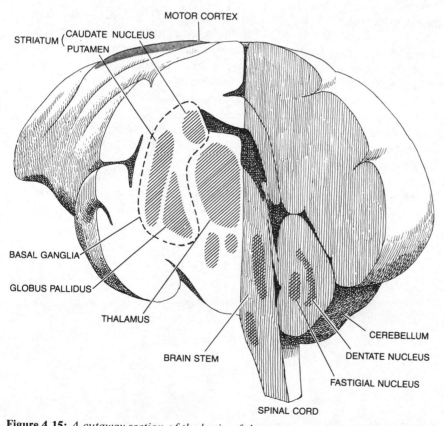

Figure 4.15: *A cutaway section of the brain of the macaque monkey showing the relative position of the thalamus to the three components of the basal ganglia, the putamen, the globus pallidus, and the caudate nucelus. [From "Brain Mechanisms of Movement," by E. V. Evarts. Copyright © 1979 by Scientific American, Inc. All rights reserved.]*

The basal ganglia are the highest levels in the motor systems of the lower vertebrates. For example, in birds, where the cerebral cortex is poorly developed, the basal ganglia perform all the higher motor functions. Even in cats, and to a lesser extent in dogs, removal of the cerebral cortex does not interfere with the ability to perform many complex behavioral patterns such as walking, eating, fighting, showing anger, and performing sexual activities. Only if large portions of the basal ganglia are also destroyed is the animal reduced to the simple stereotyped movements generated in the brain stem. Even in very young humans, destruction of the cortex does not destroy the ability to walk crudely, to control equilibrium, or to perform simple "unconscious" movements.

In humans, the basal ganglia, together with the premotor cortex, the thalamus, the substantia nigra, and the red nucleus, make up the principal part of the extrapyramidal motor system. Figure 4.16 illustrates functional pathways of the extrapyramidal system.

The basal ganglia appear to be able to control the initiation and cessation of action primarily through the inhibition and modulation of muscle tone produced by the lower motor centers of the brain stem. Destruction of the basal ganglia releases these lower centers from inhibition and produces muscle rigidity.

The effects of lesions and electrical stimulation of the basal ganglia are complex. In some cases stimulation elicits complete motor sequences of coordinated movement. In other cases, stimulation causes an animal to cease its ongoing behavior and hold its position for many seconds while the stimulation continues. Destruction of the globus pallidus results in a severe decrease of motor activity; the subject remains passive and immobile. Lesions in the caudate nucleus can lead to hyperactivity such as the "obstinate progression" phenomenon where an animal will continue the effort to make walking movements even after encountering a wall, if the floor is slippery enough to permit its feet to slide backward.

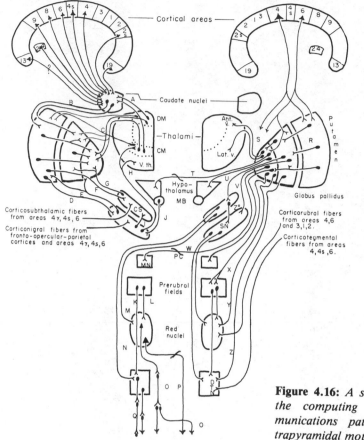

Corticosubthalamic fibers
from areas 4γ, 4s, 6

Corticonigral fibers from
fronto-opercular-parietal
cortices and areas 4γ, 4s, 6

Corticorubral fibers
from areas 4,6
and 3,1,2.

Corticotegmental
fibers from areas
4,4s,6.

Figure 4.16: *A schematic diagram of the computing centers and communications pathways of the extrapyramidal motor system.*

THE CEREBRAL CORTEX

At the very top of the brain, covering all the lower level structures, is the cerebral cortex, or cerebrum. Cortex means "bark," and the cerebral cortex covers the cerebral hemispheres like the bark of a tree. In humans the cortex is convoluted, or wrinkled like the surface of a prune, which greatly enlarges the surface area of the cortex: a human brain contains approximately 20 square feet of cortical area. The cerebrum is the most recent phylogenetic area in the brain. As can be seen in figure 4.17, it is largest in humans, smaller in chimpanzees and monkeys, smaller still and less convoluted in cats and opossums, and decreasingly apparent in birds, reptiles, amphibians, and fish.

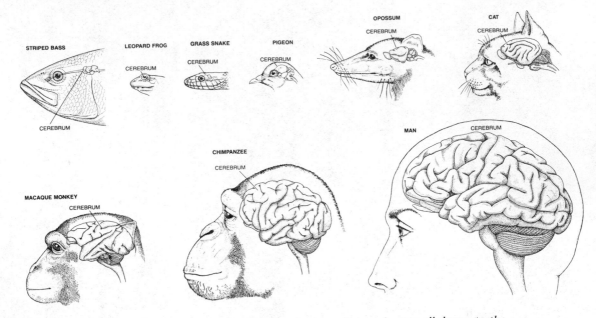

Figure 4.17: *Progressive increase in the size of the cerebrum in vertebrates, all drawn to the same scale. In carnivores, and particularly in primates, the cerebrum increases dramatically in size and complexity. [From "The Brain," by D. H. Hubel. Copyright © 1979 by Scientific American, Inc. All rights reserved.]*

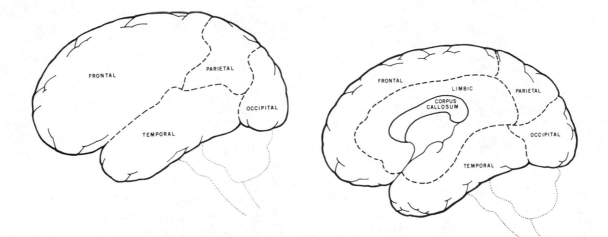

Figure 4.18: *The five major regions of the cerebral cortex. At the left is the left side of the brain seen from the left side. At the right is the right side seen from the left.*

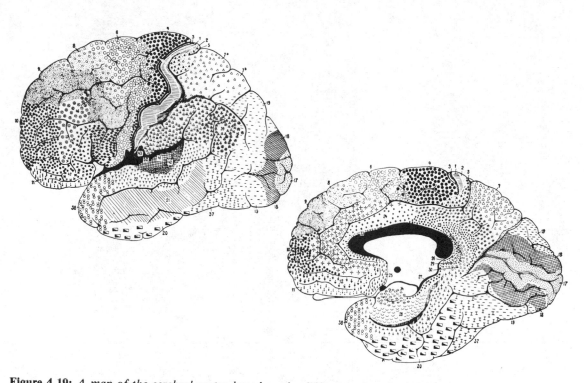

Figure 4.19: *A map of the cerebral cortex based on the differences in cell architecture compiled by Brodmann in 1914. This map is in remarkably good agreement with functional regions discovered in subsequent years.*

In humans the cortex is divided into five major regions, or lobes: frontal, parietal, temporal, occipital, and limbic as shown in figure 4.18. These divisions are based partly on function and partly on anatomical features. A much more detailed map of the cerebral cortex that delineates over fifty different regions is shown in figure 4.19.

The Frontal Lobe

The best understood region of the frontal cortex is the primary motor cortex (Brodmann area 4). This area contains the giant pyramidal cells, discovered by Betz, that give rise to many of the long, myelinated fibers of the pyramidal tract. These fibers carry motor commands directly from the cortex to the motor neurons in the spinal cord. There is a point-to-point mapping from area 4 to the muscles in various regions of the body. Figure 4.20 illustrates the destination of motor commands from the various parts of area 4.

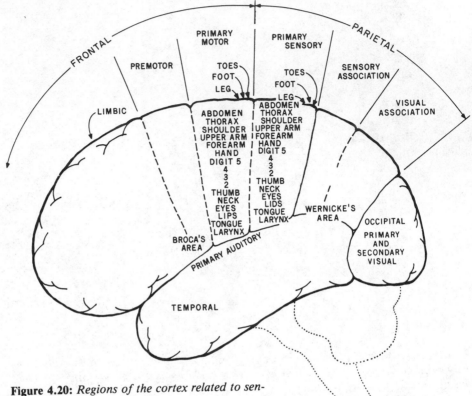

Figure 4.20: *Regions of the cortex related to sensory input and motor output for various parts of the body.*

The cells in the motor cortex are arranged in columns normal to the surface of the cortex. These columns are about 1 millimeter in diameter and have several thousand neurons in each column. The cells in each column are themselves arranged in six distinct layers, distinguished by the origin of the axonal input to them. Each column of cells seems to perform a specific motor function, such as stimulating a particular muscle or several synergistic muscles. Specific cells within a column are responsive to different types of input signals. Some cells respond to sensory signals reporting joint movement, others to touch stimuli, and still others to signals from the cerebellum, basal ganglia, and premotor cortex.

Direct electrical stimulation of a single output neuron in the motor cortex will almost never excite a muscle contraction. At least several output neurons need to be stimulated simultaneously. When barely threshold stimuli are used, only small segments of the peripheral musculature contract at one time. In the "finger" and "thumb" regions, threshold stimuli can sometimes cause single muscles to contract.

Conversely, in the "leg" region a threshold stimulus may cause some gross movement of the leg.

The area just forward of the primary motor cortex is called the premotor cortex (area 6). Stimulation of this area will often elicit complex contractions of groups of muscles. Vocalization or rhythmic movements, such as alternate thrusting of a leg forward and backward, coordinated moving of the eyes, chewing, swallowing, or contortion of parts of the body into different postural positions, may occasionally occur.

The premotor area next to the mouth, lips, and tongue area on the left side of the brain is known as Broca's speech area. Damage to this region results in speech defects related to the ordering of sequences of sounds and with the transition from one sound to another. Damage does not prevent a person from vocalizing or responding to questions with answers that are semantically meaningful. However, the victim usually cannot encode thoughts into well-formed grammatical sentences. Words may be uttered out of order, or the victim may be unable to move from one word to another, resulting in the repetition of sounds. There is particular difficulty with the inflection of verbs, with pronouns and connective words, and with complex grammatical constructions.

Just above Broca's area is the premotor area for the eyes. Damage here will prevent a person from voluntarily moving the eyes to a new target once they fixate on an object. The premotor cortex has direct input connections from the sensory association areas of the parietal lobe and sends output to the primary motor cortex and the basal ganglia.

The area forward of the premotor cortex is known to have functions related to the brain's ability to sequentially organize complex motor tasks and to deal with complex spatial relationships. It is also deeply involved in the formulation of long-range plans and conceptual abstractions. Damage to this area can cause disruption in the ability to plan and execute extended sequences of action. Fragmented motor sequences can appear but may be out of order, or they might show repetition or inability to proceed to the next part of a sequence of conceptual abstractions. This part of the brain is the youngest phylogenetically. The high forehead of humans is the result of the skull expanding to accommodate this latest addition to the brain. As a general rule, damage to the more forward areas of the frontal cortex produces more global defects in planning and symbolic reasoning, while damage to regions nearer the primary motor cortex tends to interfere with more primitive elements of motor behavior.

The premotor area just forward of Broca's area appears to be involved with the initiation of sentences rather than with the sequential organization of words. Damage here may interfere with the patient's ability to initiate speech.

The Parietal Lobe

The parietal lobe of the cerebral cortex lies just behind the frontal lobe and contains the primary tactile sensory areas (Brodmann areas 1, 2, and 3). These areas receive sensory input from the same parts of the body controlled by the immediately adjacent portions of the motor cortex. The front part of the sensory areas primarily receives touch information. The rear part of the sensory area receives information about the position, force, and velocity of movement in the body.

Just to the rear of the primary sensory area is the sensory association area. Electrical stimulation in this area can occasionally cause a person to experience a complex sensation, sometimes even the "feeling" of a specific object such as a knife or a ball.

To a large extent the sensory-processing activities of the parietal cortex seem to mirror the motor-generating activities of the frontal cortex. The more rearward regions correspond to higher level, more abstract processing activities. The parts of areas 39 and 40 that lie next to the sensory association area for the lips, tongue, and pharynx are related to the interpretation of speech. Lesions in this region produce marked speech disturbances and an impairment in the ability to understand spoken words.

Electrical stimulation in areas 39 and 37 occasionally produces a highly complex thought—a detailed scene from one's childhood might be seen, or a passage from a specific musical composition or a discourse by a specific person might be heard. Destruction of this area causes a great diminution in intellect because of the inability to interpret the meaning of experiences.

The Occipital Lobe

The occipital lobe lies behind and below the parietal lobe at the very rear of the brain and contains the first three cortical visual processing areas, 17, 18, and 19. The operation of these areas can best be understood by viewing them in the context of the overall visual-processing system outlined in figure 4.21. Area 17 receives the primary visual input directly from the first relay station in the visual pathway, the lateral geniculate nucleus of the thalamus. Area 17 contains a point-to-point map of the visual field as seen by the retinae of the eyes. Area 17 computes information about visual features such as the lines, edges, and motion of lines and edges which is transmitted to area 18 and to some extent to area 19. Damage to area 17 causes blindness, but of a very peculiar nature: a person or animal retains the ability to avoid obstacles and to fixate and reach for an object accurately, even though it is reported that the object can neither be seen nor identified. Apparently, the visual pathway through the superior colliculi provides spatial information about objects to the higher levels of the visual-processing system, even though the primary visual cortex does not report such visible features as outlines, shapes, or patterns.

Damage to areas 18 or 19 does not cause blindness, but impairs a person's ability to interpret what he sees. Damage in area 18 may prevent a person from organizing various visual features into objects. Such a person often loses the ability to recognize the meaning of written words. Damage in the outer layers of area 18 eliminates the ability to perceive visual spatial relationships. Damage to the inner layers produces defects in object recognition. In area 19 there is no point-to-point mapping of the retina. At this level in the visual-processing system, only the nature of the stimulus is important, not the position. Damage in area 19 may impair the ability to perceive the relationship between objects or to recognize more than one object at a time.

The output of areas 18 and 19 projects to 20 and 21 of the temporal cortex.

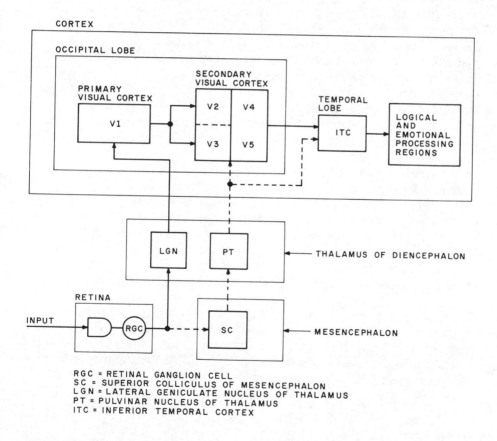

RGC = RETINAL GANGLION CELL
SC = SUPERIOR COLLICULUS OF MESENCEPHALON
LGN = LATERAL GENICULATE NUCLEUS OF THALAMUS
PT = PULVINAR NUCLEUS OF THALAMUS
ITC = INFERIOR TEMPORAL CORTEX

Figure 4.21: *A schematic diagram of the major computational centers and data-flow pathways in the visual perceptual system. Two major pathways, which diverge at subcortical levels, are apparent.*

The Temporal Lobe

The temporal lobe is on the side of the brain and is best known for the auditory input, areas 41 and 42, but it also contains regions 20, 21, and 22, the highest levels in the visual-processing system. Damage in the posterior part of regions 20, 21, and 22 interferes with the ability to discriminate between visual patterns or objects, while damage in the forward portions impairs the ability to make perceptual classifications.

Output from the inferior temporal cortex goes to the limbic lobe where emotional evaluations and value judgments are made based on the results of the visual perception process.

Auditory stimuli arrive in the superior temporal lobe regions 41 and 42 from the auditory processing modules in the inferior colliculus and the cochlear nuclei. As was shown in figure 3.28, information is represented in the temporal lobe in a pattern that matches the pitch of the audio input. Damage to area 42 produces an inability to recognize spoken words or interpret sounds.

Output from the primary auditory areas travels to a region called Wernicke's area, located at the junction of areas 39, 37, and 22. It is here that strings of words are organized into and recognized as thoughts. Input related to written words may also come to Wernicke's area from a region between the visual cortex area 19 and the parietal association area 39.

Following damage to Wernicke's area, a person might be able to hear or see and recognize individual words but be unable to organize these words into a coherent thought. Spoken or written output can be grammatically correct but semantically deviant. Words are often strung together with considerable facility with the proper inflection so that the result has the grammatical form of a sentence. However, the words chosen are often inappropriate and include nonsense syllables and words.

Output from Wernicke's area is carried to Broca's area by a bundle of axons called the arcuate fasciculus. Thus, language perceptions generated in Wernicke's area are transmitted to Broca's area where they are encoded into grammatically correct phrases. These are then transmitted to the premotor cortex regions for the lips, tongue, and larynx where the words are broken down into strings of phonemes and the motor commands are generated that produce speech behavior. This hierarchical interaction of speech generating and understanding modules corresponds very closely to the hierarchical model shown in figure 7.7.

The Limbic Lobe

The limbic lobe of the cortex is located on the inner surface of the deep cleft between the two hemispheres. It lies just above the corpus callosum, which is the massive bundle of axons that connects the two sides of the brain and loops around the thalamus front and back. The limbic cortex, together with the subcortical limbic nuclei such as the septal nuclei, the amygdala, the hypothalamus, the hippocampus, the anterior thalamus, the preoptic region and parts of the basal ganglia, make up what is called the limbic system.

The limbic system is the geographical seat of the emotions. In humans it is comprised of a complicated network of about 53 regions linked together by 35 major nerve bundles. The anatomy of the limbic system is shown in figure 4.22. The hypothalamus, an important but small part of the limbic system, is further subdivided in figure 4.23.

In recent years much has been learned about the function of the various nuclei in the limbic system. It has been discovered that specific regions in the limbic lobe evaluate sensory input in terms of good-bad, pleasant-painful, rewarding-punishing, satisfactory-aversive. Electrical stimulation of certain regions of the limbic system pleases, rewards, or satisfies the subject. Stimulation of other areas causes pain, fear, defense or escape reactions, and all the other elements of punishment.

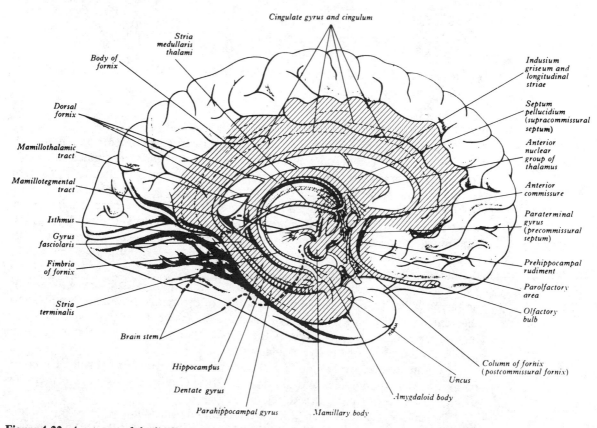

Figure 4.22: *Anatomy of the limbic system. The regions in the shaded area make up the limbic system.*

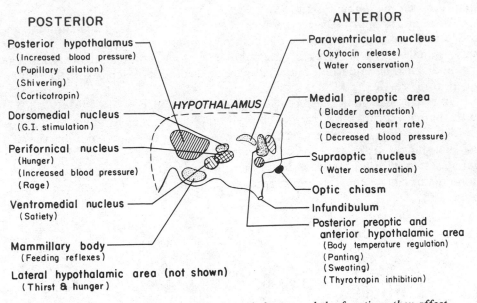

POSTERIOR

Posterior hypothalamus —
(Increased blood pressure)
(Pupillary dilation)
(Shivering)
(Corticotropin)

Dorsomedial nucleus —
(G.I. stimulation)

Perifornical nucleus —
(Hunger)
(Increased blood pressure)
(Rage)

Ventromedial nucleus —
(Satiety)

Mammillary body —
(Feeding reflexes)

Lateral hypothalamic area (not shown)
(Thirst & hunger)

HYPOTHALAMUS

ANTERIOR

Paraventricular nucleus
(Oxytocin release)
(Water conservation)

Medial preoptic area
(Bladder contraction)
(Decreased heart rate)
(Decreased blood pressure)

Supraoptic nucleus
(Water conservation)

Optic chiasm

Infundibulum

Posterior preoptic and
anterior hypothalamic area
(Body temperature regulation)
(Panting)
(Sweating)
(Thyrotropin inhibition)

Figure 4.23: *The principal nuclei of the hypothalamus and the functions they affect.*

The technique of self-stimulation has been used in experiments on animals. An electrode is positioned in some part of the limbic system and the animal is allowed to control the stimulus by pressing a lever. If the stimulus produces a pleasurable result, the animal will press the lever repeatedly to obtain the stimulus again and again. The degree of pleasure can be measured by testing how hard the animal will work to press the lever, or how much pain it will endure to get to the lever. If the stimulus produces an unpleasant result, the animal can be given a lever to turn the stimulus off. The intensity of the aversion can be measured by testing how quickly the animal will move to turn the stimulus off.

The major reward centers, found with this technique, are located in the septum and hypothalamus, primarily along the course of the medial forebrain bundle and in the ventromedial nuclei of the hypothalamus. Punishment centers have been found in the periventricular structures of the hypothalamus and the thalamus and the perifornical nucleus of the hypothalamus.

In humans, electrical stimulation of the pleasure centers have produced reports of joy, elation, happiness, and satisfaction. Stimulus of the aversive centers has produced feelings of pain, dread, terror, and rage.

The ability to discriminate good from bad and to evaluate whether a particular activity is rewarding or punishing is critical to the selection and control of behavior. The emotional centers of the limbic system provide this capacity for evaluation.

These regions of the brain provide the value judgments as to whether the results reported by the sensory-processing regions of the brain are good or bad. These are the centers that tell us whether what we are doing (or are thinking of doing) is rewarding or punishing. If the evaluation is positive, we will tend to continue our ongoing action (or begin our contemplated action). If the evaluation is negative, we will stop what we are doing or refrain from what we had planned to do.

Such evaluations are also useful in the control of memory storage. Some events are very important to remember; others are not. The emotions tell us what is worth remembering. Animal experiments have shown that sensory experiences causing neither reward nor punishment will hardly be remembered at all, even if repeated a number of times. However, a single event that arouses extreme pain, pleasure, or fear will be remembered very clearly.

The part of the limbic system called the hippocampus is involved with memory storage. Destruction of the hippocampus on both sides of the brain leads to loss of the ability to remember anything new. Old memories stored before the hippocampal damage are not affected, but there is a total loss of the ability to remember anything afterwards, even events only a few minutes old. The hippocampus has numerous connections with almost all parts of the limbic system. Stimulation of the hippocampus at times causes rage or other emotional reactions. At other times it causes a total loss of attention. For example, stimulation of the hippocampus in people while they are talking can result in their completely losing contact with the conversation.

The hippocampus is believed to make the emotional judgments as to what is worth remembering. This allows the brain to be selective in what it stores, carefully recording those experiences that are memorable and discarding those that are insignificant. Destruction of this selection center would therefore result in everything being forgotten as if unimportant.

There are other areas of the limbic system, particularly in the hypothalamus, that perform a somewhat different type of evaluation. For example, the ventromedial nucleus of the hypothalamus tells the brain when the body has had enough to eat. When this center is stimulated, an animal eating food suddenly stops eating and shows complete indifference to food. On the other hand if this area is destroyed, the animal cannot be satiated and will eat voraciously, becoming quickly obese. The lateral hypothalamus produces feelings of hunger and thirst.

Other areas in the hypothalamus produce visceral responses such as increased blood pressure, pupillary dilation, shivering, changes in heart rate and body temperature, panting, and sweating. Figure 4.23 illustrates the various bodily functions controlled or influenced by stimulation of various regions in the hypothalamus.

PROSPECTS FOR MODELING THE BRAIN

This concludes our review of the structure and function of the brain. Perhaps the most obvious feature of this amazing organ is that many different computations are going on simultaneously in many different places: each sensory-motor system is a separate computational structure; each neuron is a separate computing device; each nucleus or patch of cortex is a computing module capable of calculating a mathematical function on the multiple variables that are its inputs. The brain is not a computer; it is a network of millions, even billions of computers, each operating on its own set of inputs and transmitting its outputs to a specific set of other computers in the net. The computers of the brain are slow compared to modern digital computers, but there are so many of them operating in parallel that the number of computations per second far exceeds the capacity of the fastest electronic computer ever built.

Attempting to model the entire brain in any single computer is hopeless. There are limits to the speed of computation and the complexity of software that certainly would doom any such effort. However, the emerging technology of large-scale integrated circuitry that makes it possible to build entire computers, or even arrays of computers, on a single chip of silicon raises the possibility of constructing networks of hundreds, or even hundreds of thousands, of computers operating in parallel. These would operate independent of each other except for the input and output information shared by a number of computing centers. Such modularity would permit the programs in the various computers to be debugged and optimized separately. This would limit the complexity of the software in any single computer to a manageable level. No computer would have to manage more than one task or sub-task at a time. Eventually, as more and more computers were added, the rate of computation in such a structure might well approach that of the human brain.

A structure with the computational power of the brain will probably need to be almost as complex as the brain. We often heard that we use only X percent of our brains (where X may be any number from 10 to 80). This is an old wives' tale, often retold in the context of self-fulfillment lectures encouraging people to more fully utilize their mental powers. It may have originated with frustrated parents or schoolmasters in response to the perennial reluctance of children to do their studies. Whatever its origin and regardless of its popular acceptance, this notion is clearly absurd. The brain consumes approximately 20 percent of the heart's blood flow on a top-priority basis. The demands of survival in a hostile world would not permit individuals of any species to prosper or survive very long while wasting so much of their most precious resources. The brain is complex because the computational tasks it performs are complex and multitudinous. If we would duplicate or model the performance of even a small brain, we must devise a complex structure.

The entire brain is made up of neurons. Each cluster of neurons computes a relatively simple function on a well-defined set of variables. Thus, no part of the model need be very complex, certainly no more complex than a single board microcomputer, perhaps backed up by a disc or bubble memory. The problem is how to partition the functions of the brain so that they can be modeled, and how to interconnect a network of computers so that it corresponds to that partition.

In order to even begin thinking about these questions, we must first devise some concise and precise way of describing the behavior we want our model to produce and the computations required to produce it. We need a mathematical notation that can deal with many variables, indeed, many thousands of variables, and that can explicitly represent the flow of time. We also need a graphical notation that can help us visualize the stream of consciousness and the behavior that arises from its swirling currents. The creation of such mathematical tools is a task we'll examine in the next chapter.

CHAPTER **5**

Hierarchical Goal-Directed Behavior

In order to discuss an engineering design for a robot-control system modeled after the brain, we must first devise a mathematical convention and notation to enable us to describe behavior precisely and concisely. Otherwise, we will be overwhelmed by the sheer number of words needed to describe what we are modeling, and our designs will not be precise enough to translate into electronic circuits and software programs. Our notation must be capable of dealing with many different variables and processes simultaneously and of describing all the various aspects of behavior and perception.

VECTORS

One way to describe many variables and deal with many simultaneous multivariant computations is to use *vector* notation. A vector is simply an ordered set, or list of variables. The vector **V** in figure 5.1b has two components, v_x along the X axis and v_y along the Y axis. The ordered set, or list of components, defines the vector so that we can write $\mathbf{V} = (v_x, v_y)$.

The components of a vector can also be considered as the coordinates of a point (v_x, v_y) that correspond to the tip of the vector. The locus of all pairs of components that can exist defines a vector space (for two dimensions the vector space is a surface). A vector can have more than two components. A vector with three components defines a volume (figure 5.1c), and a vector with four or more components defines a hyperspace (figure 5.1d). A hyperspace is impossible to visualize, but is an essential concept for our discussion.

A vector in a higher dimensional space can usually be visualized as a projection onto a lower dimensional space. For example, typical mechanical drawings portray front, side, and top views of a three-dimensional form projected onto a two-dimensional sheet of paper. Each projection can either illustrate a cut through the object at a particular plane along the projection axis, or a superposition of all the salient features of the object collapsed into the plane of the illustration. In the collapsed version, the fact that two points or lines intersect in the projected image does not necessarily mean that they coincide or intersect in the higher dimensional space—they may simply lie behind each other along the projection axis. The projection operator ignores variable differences that correspond to distance along the projection axis.

It is not necessary to make the projection axis coincident with any of the coordinate axes. For example, in the oblique projection (perspective drawing) of figure 5.1c, the projection axis (the normal line to the paper through the origin of the coordinate system) is not aligned with any of the coordinate axes. The lines in the drawing represent the projections of lines in a three-dimensional space onto the two-dimensional surface of the paper. In a similar way we can project higher dimensional vectors and hyperspaces of any dimension onto a two-dimensional drawing. Figure 5.1d illustrates a four-dimensional vector projected onto a two-dimensional drawing.

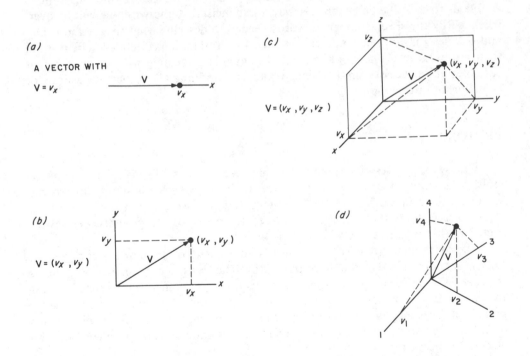

Figure 5.1: *Defining space with vectors. A vector is an ordered list of variables which defines a point in space; (a), (b), (c), and (d) depict vectors representing 1, 2, 3, and 4 dimensions, respectively. The number of dimensions in the space is equal to the number of variables in the list. (The illustration in (d) is meant only to be symbolic of a four-dimensional vector, which cannot be visualized in three dimensions.)*

STATES AND TRAJECTORIES

A vector can specify a state. This is the primary use we will make of vectors in this discussion. A state is defined by an ordered set of variables. For example, the state of the weather might be characterized by a state vector $\mathbf{W} = (w_1, w_2, w_3, w_4)$ where:

w_1 = temperature
w_2 = humidity
w_3 = wind speed
w_4 = rate of precipitation

The state vector $\mathbf{W}$ exists in a space that consists of all possible combinations of values of variables in the ordered set (w_1, w_2, w_3, w_4). We can thus say that the vector $\mathbf{W}$ defines a space S_W. Every point in the space corresponds to a particular, unique weather condition. The entire space corresponds to all possible weather conditions.

The weather, like many things, is not constant; it varies with time. Each of the state variables (temperature, humidity, wind speed, and rate of precipitation) is time-dependent. Thus, as time passes, the point defined by $\mathbf{W}$ will move through the four-dimensional space. Figure 5.2 illustrates the locus of the point traced out by $\mathbf{W}$ as it moves to define a trajectory $\mathbf{T}_W$.

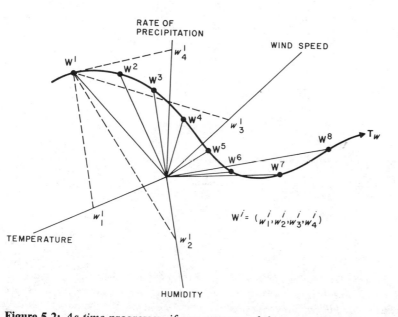

Figure 5.2: *As time progresses, if one or more of the components of a vector $\mathbf{W}$ change, the vector will move through space, tracing out a trajectory $\mathbf{T}_W$.*

It will often be convenient to represent time explicitly in our notation. We can easily do this by simply adding one more variable, time (t), to our state vector, thus increasing by one the number of dimensions in the space defined by the state vector. For example $\mathbf{W}^t = (w_1, w_2, w_3, w_4, t)$.

As time progresses, any point defined by the state vector moves along the time axis. A state vector whose w_i components do not vary with time will now trace out a straight line trajectory parallel to the time axis as shown in figure 5.3a. If, however, any of the w_i components is time-dependent, the state trajectory will contain velocity components that are orthogonal as well as parallel to the time axis, as shown in figure 5.3b.

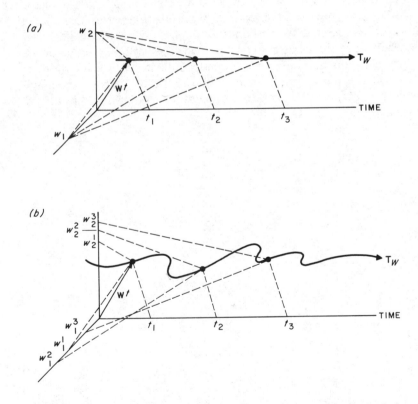

Figure 5.3: *If the ordered list of variables which define a vector includes time, the space defined by the vector will have time as one of its axes. As time progresses, the vector will move along the time axis. If none of the other variables is time dependent, the trajectory will be a straight line parallel to the time axis, as in (a). If any of the other variables change with time, the trajectory will be some curve with a component along the time axis as in (b).*

If we project the state space of all the variables except time onto a two-dimensional surface, we can represent the passage of time by the motion of this two-dimensional plane along the time axis normal to it, as in figure 5.4. The state trajectory $\mathbf{T}_s$ is the locus of points traced out by the state vector as time passes.

A large variety of things can be represented as vectors. For example, we can represent a picture as a vector. Any picture can be represented as a two-dimensional array of points, each with a particular brightness and color hue. Thus each point can be represented as three numbers corresponding to three primary color brightnesses: the first for red, the second for blue, and the third for green. If all three brightnesses are zero, the color is black. If all three are large and equal, the color is white. As long as the number of points is large and the spacing is closer than the eye can readily make out, the eye cannot distinguish such an array from a scene made up of the real object. This is, of course, the principle by which pictures are printed in books and transmitted over television. If the numbers corresponding to the color and brightness of each resolution element are simply arranged in a list, then that list is a vector. Any picture can be represented by a vector, and any series of pictures, like those on a motion picture film, can be represented by a trajectory. The space is defined by the set of all possible pictures capable of being printed or projected by a two-dimensional array of brightness elements with a particular resolution.

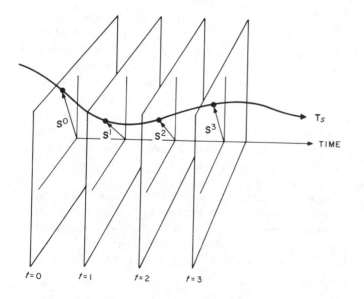

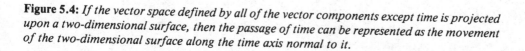

Figure 5.4: *If the vector space defined by all of the vector components except time is projected upon a two-dimensional surface, then the passage of time can be represented as the movement of the two-dimensional surface along the time axis normal to it.*

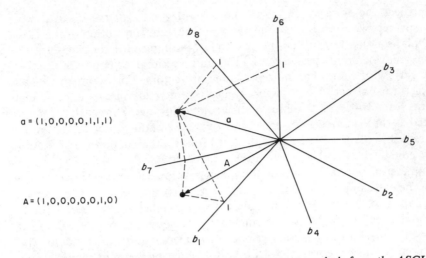

Figure 5.5: *A vector can represent a symbol. Here two symbols from the ASCII character set, an uppercase A and a lowercase a, are represented as vectors (or points) in an eight-dimensional space. The values of the eight bits in the ASCII code are plotted along the eight axes (*b_8 *is the even parity bit).*

A particular sound, note, or musical chord can also be represented as a vector by specifying the amplitude and phase of the output of a set of frequency filters. A tone, a melody, or a string of phonemic sounds representing a word or phrase can be represented as a trajectory. The space is defined by the set of all possible sounds that can be produced by different combinations of frequencies and phase relationships.

Symbols can also be represented as vectors. We can, for example, represent an American Standard Code for Information Interchange (ASCII) character as a vector as shown in figure 5.5. The ordered set of binary digits in the ASCII representation corresponds to the components of a binary vector. Each symbol in the ASCII alphabet is uniquely paired with a vector in an eight-dimensional hyperspace. Each symbol thus corresponds to a point in the hyperspace.

This is an important concept, because it allows us to define any set of symbols as vectors or points in hyperspace. Any string of symbols then becomes a trajectory through the hyperspace. For example, the string of symbols, "the cat chased the rat," can be described as a trajectory through a hyperspace defined by a set of variables defining the English alphabet (plus a blank character). This also applies to the string *WXYZ* when

W is the command: reach to Position *A*
X is the command: grasp
Y is the command: move to Position *C*
Z is the command: release

We need not restrict ourselves to binary vectors. Symbols may be represented by vectors with continuously variable components as well. This allows us to introduce the concept of fuzzy symbols. If the hyperspace is continuous, then each point which corresponds to a symbol has some neighborhood of points around it which are much closer to it than any other symbol's points. This is illustrated in figure 5.6. We may view the points in such a neighborhood in one of two ways:

1. The difference between the neighborhood points and the exact symbol point derives from noise on the channel transmitting variables denoting the vector components. This is useful in signal detection theory, where the detection of a vector within some neighborhood of a symbol vector corresponds to the recognition of that symbol against a noisy background.
2. The difference from the exact symbol derives from distortions or variations in the symbol itself. This makes the best sense if the components of the symbol's vector are values of attributes or features of the symbol, rather than arbitrary digits as in the ASCII convention. In this case, a neighborhood of points corresponds to a cluster of feature vectors from a symbol set which is not identical, but very nearly so.

For example, a vector of features from the printed character e will be slightly different for each instance of that symbol on a page due to variations in the paper on which it is printed. However, if these e feature vectors fall in compact clusters far

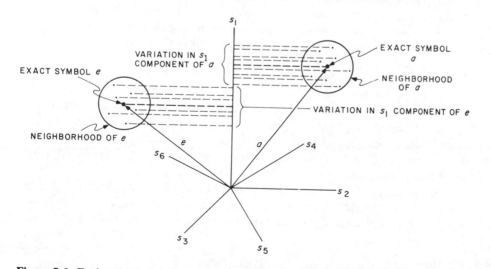

Figure 5.6: *Each point in hyperspace, corresponding to a particular symbol such as* a *or* e, *has some neighborhood of points around it which are closer to it than to any other symbol. Variations from the exact or ideal position of a symbol vector may derive from noise in a transmission channel or from differences between the observed symbol and the ideal.*

from the feature vectors of other symbols, the letter *e* will be easily recognized, despite the fact that no two specimens are exactly alike.

This is a fundamental concept in pattern-recognition theory. Hyperspace is partitioned into regions, and the existence of a feature vector in a particular region corresponds to the recognition of a pattern or symbol. By definition, the best set of features is the one that maximizes the separability of pattern vectors. In the design of pattern recognizers it is important to select a set of features that is easily measured and that produces widely separated and compact clusters in feature space.

A vector can also be used to describe the state of a set of neurons. At any instant, each neuron has some voltage value that produces some firing rate. If we select a set of neurons and make a list of their firing rates, that list defines a vector. Thus, we can describe the state of any set of neurons by a vector whose components are the voltage values or firing rates of the individual neurons in the set.

This can be done for any set of neurons. If, for example, we pick the set of neurons that make up the retina of the eye, then the pattern of neural activity generated by a particular visual image can be described as a vector. Any particular visual image will generate a particular pattern of neural activity on the retina and hence a particular vector corresponding to the state of the retinal neurons. As time progresses and the image changes, the vector traces out a trajectory. This trajectory corresponds to a visual experience. Of course, the incoming image itself can be described by a set of values, such as an array of brightness values, or even of color, texture, or depth values.

Similarly, we can describe the state of any other set of neurons in the brain as a vector and the sequence of states of these neurons over a period of time as a trajectory of that vector through the vector space of all possible states of those neurons. We can, for example, describe the state of the neurons in the motor system by a vector and a sequence of neuronal activity producing a behavioral action as a trajectory. We can describe the state of the neurons in the pain system as a vector and the experience of pain from an injury as a trajectory. We can describe the state of the neurons in the hypothalamus that produce the feeling of hunger as a vector, or the neurons in the septum that produce the feeling of joy by a vector. Thus we can define the mental feelings corresponding to pain and pleasure, the sensory experiences, and behavioral activities as trajectories of state vectors through multidimensional space.

We can, in fact, define a vector containing the value of every neuron in the entire central nervous system. Such a vector then describes the state of the mind, and the trajectory of that vector corresponds to the stream of consciousness.

FUNCTIONS AND OPERATORS

In the physical world, functions are usually defined as relationships between physical variables. For example, we could say that the climate over a particular geographical region is a function of the heat input, the prevailing wind conditions, and other factors. The seasons are a function of the position and orientation of the earth relative to the sun. Similarly, we can say that the level of our hunger is a function of the signals on nerve fibers reporting on the state of the stomach, chemistry of the blood, the time of day as indicated by internal biological rhythms, and so on.

In mathematics, a function defines, and is defined by, a relationship between symbols. Sometimes the relationship can be set in one-to-one correspondence to physical variables. A function often implies a directional relationship. For example, in the physical world there is a one-way direction in the relationship between cause and effect. In traditional terms a function can be expressed as an equation, such as

$$y = f(x)$$

which reads: y equals a function f of x. The function

$$y = 2x^2 + 3x + 6$$

is a relationship between y and x.

Functions can also be expressed as graphs. Figure 5.7 is a plot of the equation $y = 2x^2 + 3x + 6$. Functions may sometimes be defined by tables. The table in figure 5.8a defines the Boolean AND function $Z = X \cdot Y$. This function can also be drawn as a circuit element (see figure 5.8b) which performs the AND function on two inputs.

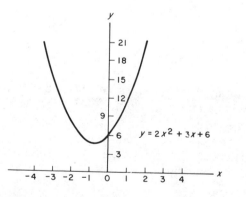

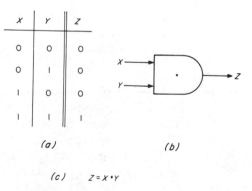

Figure 5.7: *Functions can be expressed in a number of different ways. Here the functional relationship between y and x is expressed as an equation and a graph.*

Figure 5.8: *Functions can also be expressed as tables and circuits. Here the Boolean function* z = x • y *is expressed as a table, a circuit, and an equation.*

Tables can also be used to define non-Boolean functions. Tables of logarithms or trigonometric functions are good examples of this. Of course, a table defines a continuous function exactly and only at the discrete points represented in the table. Thus, the accuracy of a continuous function represented by a table depends on the number of table entries (i.e., the resolution on the input variables). Accuracy can, of course, be increased by interpolation techniques. In general, the number of entries required to compute a function by a table lookup is proportional to R^N, where R is the resolution of each input variable and N is the number of input variables. This exponential increase in size of the table required is the principal reason that multidimensional functions are seldom computed by table lookup.

Modern mathematics often expresses functional relationships in terms of *mappings* from a set of states defined by independent variables onto a set of states defined by dependent variables. In one notation, this is expressed by the string f

$$f: C \rightarrow E$$

which reads, "f is a relationship which maps the set of causes C into the set of effects E." It means that for any particular state in the set C, the relationship f will compute a state in the set E. This is shown in figure 5.9.

We have already shown that states can be denoted by vectors and sets of states by sets of points in vector hyperspaces. Thus, the notion of a function being a mapping from one set of states to another naturally extends to a mapping of points in one vector hyperspace onto points in another.

Suppose, for example, we define an operator h as a function which maps the input $\mathbf{S} = (s_1, s_2, s_3, \ldots s_N)$ onto the output scalar variable p. We can write this as

$$p = h(\mathbf{S})$$

or

$$p = h(s_1, s_2, \ldots s_N)$$

We can also draw the functional operator as a circuit element or "black box" as in figure 5.10. (A black box is an engineering concept sometimes used to depict a process with inputs and outputs. The viewer sees the effects on the output of changes to the input, but the internal workings of the process remain hidden in a black box.)

If we assume that we have L such operators, $h_1, h_2, \ldots h_L$, each operating on the input vector $\mathbf{S}$ as in figure 5.11, we have a mapping

$$H: \mathbf{S} \rightarrow \mathbf{P} \qquad \text{or} \qquad \mathbf{P} = H(\mathbf{S})$$

where the operator $H = (h_1, h_2, \ldots h_L)$ maps every input vector $\mathbf{S}$ into an output vector $\mathbf{P}$. Now since $\mathbf{S}$ is a vector (or point) in input space, we can represent the function H as a mapping from input space onto output space.

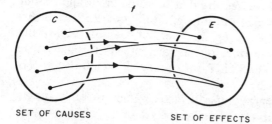

SET OF CAUSES   SET OF EFFECTS

Figure 5.9: *A function can also be expressed as a mapping from one set onto another. Here the function f maps the set of causes C onto the set of effects E such that for every cause in C there is an effect in E. In our discussion we will be concerned only with single-valued functions such that there is only one effect for each cause. We will, however, allow more than one cause to have the same effect (i.e., more than one point in C can map onto the same point in E).*

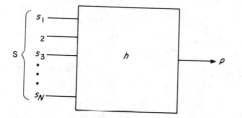

Figure 5.10: *We will define the operator* h *as a function which maps the input vector* S *into the output scalar variable* p.

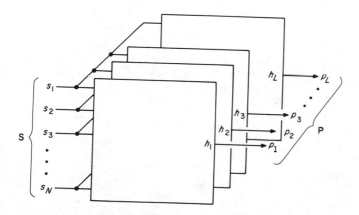

Figure 5.11: *We will define the set of operators* $H = (h_1, h_2, \ldots, h_L)$ *as a function which maps the input vector* **S** *into the output vector* **P**.

For the purposes of our discussion we require that both the input and output space be bounded and that each **S** will map into one and only one **P**. Several different **S** vectors may map into the same **P** vector, however. Of course, if any of the variables in **S** are time-dependent, **S** will trace out a trajectory $\mathbf{T}_s$ through input space. The operator H will map each point **S** on $\mathbf{T}_s$ into a point **P** on a trajectory $\mathbf{T}_P$ in output space, as shown in figure 5.12.

A function can also describe the operation performed by a neuron on its inputs or by a cluster of neurons on their inputs. If we define the vector **S** such that $(s_1, s_2, \ldots, s_n)$ are the firing rates on the synaptic inputs of a particular neuron, then we can say the output $p = h(\mathbf{S})$ is the firing rate on the axon of that neuron. The function h is defined by the strengths and types of the various synaptic connections and their position on the dendrites and cell body of the neuron. If we define the vector **S** such that $(s_1, s_2, \ldots, s_n)$ are the firing rates on all the input fibers to a cluster of neurons, then we can say the output $\mathbf{P} = H(\mathbf{S})$ is the firing rate of all the axons leaving that cluster; that is, p_1 is the firing rate of the first neuron in the cluster, p_2 is the firing rate of the second neuron, and so on to p_L, the firing rate of the last neuron in the cluster.

Thus we can define a function H as the mathematical transformation performed by a cluster of neurons on a set of input fibers. As the input vector **S** traces out a trajectory $\mathbf{T}_s$ through input space, the function H performs a transformation on each input **S** so that the output vector **P** traces out a trajectory $\mathbf{T}_P$ through output space. For example, if we label all the inputs to a motor control module in the spinal cord so that they define a vector **S**, then the output firing rates to the muscles can be labeled to define the vector **P**. The transformation performed by the spinal motor control module on the input vector **S** is the function H, which computes the output $\mathbf{P} = H(\mathbf{S})$.

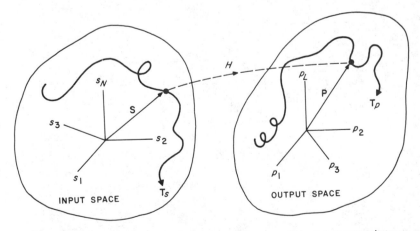

Figure 5.12: *The operator* H *maps every input vector* **S** *in input space into an output vector* **P** *in output space.* H *thus maps the trajectory* $\mathbf{T}_S$ *into the trajectory* $\mathbf{T}_P$.

This notation gives us a means of talking about the states, computations, and sequences of states (or trajectories) which make up the activity of the brain. We can define the instantaneous state of any neuron, or cluster of neurons, or even of the entire brain as a vector. We can describe any experience, behavior pattern, or any thought or idea as a trajectory. This is an extremely powerful concept, for it enables us to visualize graphically the internal activity of the brain, as well as the external activity of behavior. It gives us a mathematically precise and concise notation for describing the activity of individual neurons, clusters of neurons, and the entire brain. Furthermore, it gives us a way to partition the activities of different areas of the brain into different vector spaces and represent them simultaneously along the time axis. Thus, we can decompose the enormous complexity of many simultaneous computations into intellectually comprehensible modules and then systematically recombine them into an integrated whole.

GOAL-SEEKING CONTROL SYSTEMS

We are now ready to consider the structure of control systems for sensory-interactive goal-directed behavior. The simplest form of goal-seeking device is the *servomechanism*. The setpoint, or reference input to the servomechanism, is a simple form of command. Feedback from a sensing device, which monitors the state of the output or the results of action produced by the input, is compared with the command. If there is any discrepancy between commanded action and the results, an error signal is generated that acts on the output in the proper direction and by the proper amount to reduce the error. The system thus follows the setpoint, or, put another way, it seeks the goal set by the input command.

Almost all servomechanism theory deals with a one-dimensional command, a one-dimensional feedback, and a one-dimensional output. Our vector notation will allow us to generalize from this one-dimensional case to the multidimensional case with little difficulty.

Assume we have the multivariable servomechanism shown in figure 5.13. The function H operates on the input variables in S and computes an output $P = H(S)$. Note that we have partitioned the input vector S into two vectors: $C = (s_1, s_2 \ldots, s_i)$ and $F = (s_{i+1}, \ldots s_N)$, such that $S = C + F$. If $i = 1$, $N = 2$, $L = 1$, and H computes some function of the difference between C and F, we have a classical servomechanism.

In our more general case, C may be any vector, and in some cases it may be a symbolic command. The feedback vector may contain information of many different types. It may simply report position or velocity of the controlled outputs, but for a complicated system such as a robot manipulator or the limb of an animal, it may also report the resistance to movement by the environment, the inertial configuration of the manipulator structure, and other parameters relevant to the problem of making rapid and precise movements.

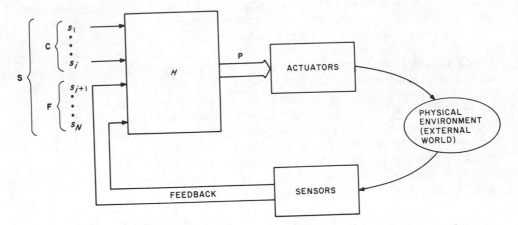

Figure 5.13: *A multivariable servomechanism. The reference or command input is the vector* **C** *consisting of the variables* s_1 *through* s_i. *The feedback is the vector* **F** *consisting of sensory variables* s_{i+1} *through* s_N. *The function* H *computes an output vector* **P** *consisting of* P_1 *through* P_L *that drives actuators, thus affecting the physical environment.*

Figure 5.14 illustrates the situation when a stationary command vector **C** establishes a setpoint, and as time progresses the feedback vector **F** varies, creating an input trajectory T_s. The *H* operator computes an output vector for each input and so produces an output trajectory T_P. The variation in **F** may be caused by external forces imposed by the environment, by actions produced by the output, or by both. One or more of the variables in the feedback vector **F** may even be taken directly from the output vector **P**. In the latter case the *H* operator becomes the transition function for a finite state automaton. In any of these cases the result is that a single command vector **C** produces a sequence of output vectors T_P. The process is driven by the sequence of feedback vectors F^1, F^2, F^3. The superscript F^k denotes the vector **F** at time t_k.

The sequence of operations illustrated in figure 5.14 can also be viewed as a decomposition of a command **C** into a sequence of subcommands P^1, P^2, P^3. The vector **C** may be a symbol standing for any number of things such as a task, a goal, or a plan. In such cases the output string P^1, P^2, P^3 represents a sequence of subtasks, subgoals, or subplans, respectively.

Whether figure 5.14 is a servomechanism or a task-decomposition operator, there are many practical problems concerned with stability, speed, gain, delay, and phase shift. In our notation these are all embedded in the *H* functions. If the *H* functions are correctly formulated and defined over the entire space traversed by the **S** input, then the output T_P will drive the physical actuators in such a way that the goal is achieved (i.e., the error between the command **C** and the result **P** is nulled) and stability is maintained under all conditions.

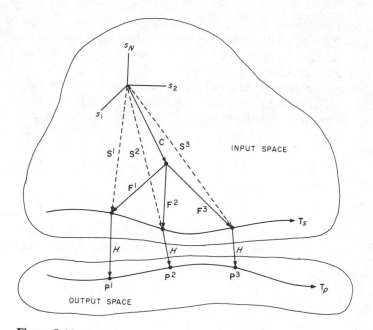

Figure 5.14: *A stationary **C** vector establishes a setpoint, and as time progresses the feedback vector varies from **F**¹ to **F**² to **F**³. The **S** vector thus traces out a trajectory **T**_S. The **H** operator computes an output **P** for each input **S** and so produces an output trajectory **T**_P. The result is that the input command **C** is decomposed into a sequence of output subcommands **P**¹, **P**², **P**³.*

Servomechanisms are, of course, only the simplest form of sensory-interactive goal-seeking devices. By themselves they are certainly not capable of explaining the much more complex forms of goal-seeking commonly associated with purposive behavior in biological systems. However, when connected together in a nested (or hierarchical) structure, the complexity of behavior in feedback control systems increases dramatically.

HIERARCHICAL CONTROL

Assume that the command vector C in figure 5.14 changes such that it steps along the trajectory T_C as shown in figure 5.15. The result is that the sequence of input commands C^1, C^2, C^3, followed by the sequence C^4, C^5, produces the sequence of output vectors P^1, P^2, P^3, P^4, P^5. In this case the subsequence P^1, P^2, P^3 is called by the commands C^{1-3} and driven by the feedback F^1, F^2, F^3. The subsequence P^4, P^5 is called by C^{4-5} and driven by F^4, F^5, etc.

If we now represent time explicitly, the C, F, and P vectors and trajectories of

116

figure 5.15 appear as shown in figure 5.16. The fact that **C** remains constant while the feedback changes from $\mathbf{F}^1$ to $\mathbf{F}^2$ to $\mathbf{F}^3$ means that the trajectory $\mathbf{T}_c$ is parallel to the time axis over that interval. The jump from $\mathbf{C}^{1\text{-}3}$ to $\mathbf{C}^{4\text{-}5}$ causes an abrupt shift in the $\mathbf{T}_c$ trajectory in the time interval between $\mathbf{F}^3$ and $\mathbf{F}^4$.

Note that each instant can be represented by a plane (or set of coplanar regions) perpendicular to the time axis. Each plane contains a point from each trajectory and represents a snapshot of all the vectors simultaneously at a specific instant in time.

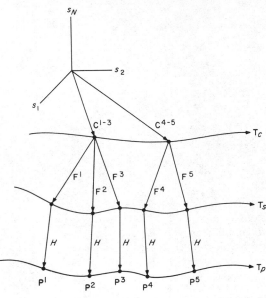

Figure 5.15: *If the command vector* **C** *also changes from time to time, it will trace out a trajectory* $\mathbf{T}_C$.

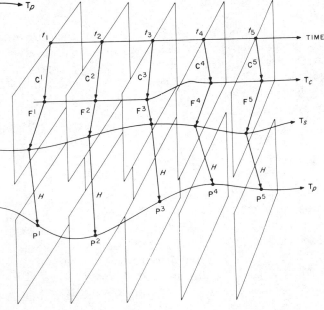

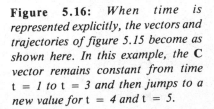

Figure 5.16: *When time is represented explicitly, the vectors and trajectories of figure 5.15 become as shown here. In this example, the* **C** *vector remains constant from time* t = 1 *to* t = 3 *and then jumps to a new value for* t = 4 *and* t = 5.

We are now ready to consider a hierarchy of servomechanisms, or task-decomposition operators, as shown in figure 5.17a. Here the highest level input command C_4 is a symbolic vector denoting the complex task <ASSEMBLE AB>. Some of the components in C_4 may denote modifiers and arguments for the assemble task. The subscript C_k denotes the C vector at the kth level in the hierarchy.

The feedback F_4 may contain highly processed visual scene analysis data which identifies the general layout of the work space and thereby determines which output vectors P_4 (and hence which simple task commands C_3) are generated and in which order. F_4 may also contain data from P_4 and P_3 which indicates the state of completion of the decomposition of C_4. F_4 combines with C_4 to define the complete input vector S_4. The H_4 operator produces an output vector $P_4 = H_4(S_4)$.

At least part of the output P_4 becomes part of the input command vector C_3 to the next lower level. C_3 is also a symbolic vector which identifies one of a library of simple task commands together with the necessary modifiers and arguments. As the feedback F_4 varies with time, the input vector S_4, and hence the output vector P_4, move along a trajectory generating a sequence of simple task commands at C_3, such as <FETCH A>, <FETCH B>, <MATE B TO A>, <FASTEN B TO A>. The trajectory represented by this sequence is shown in figure 5.17b.

Note that in figure 5.17b vectors are not repeatedly drawn for each instant of time during the trajectory segments when they are reasonably constant. Thus, C_4 is shown only at the beginning and end of the trajectory segment labeled <ASSEMBLE AB>. C_2 is shown only at the transition points between <REACH TO A>, <GRASP>, <MOVE TO C>, etc. It should be kept in mind, however, that H_4 computes P_4 continuously and produces an output at every instant of time, just as H_1 computes P_1.

Feedback at F_3 may identify the position and orientation of the parts A and B and may also carry state sequencing information from outputs P_3 and P_2. As F_3 varies with time, it drives the input S_3 (and hence P_3) along a trajectory generating a sequence of elemental movement commands at C_2, such as <REACH TO A>, <GRASP>, <MOVE TO X>, <RELEASE>.

Feedback at F_2 may contain information from proximity sensors indicating the fine positioning error between the fingers and the objects to be manipulated, together with state sequencing information derived from P_2 and P_1. The operator H_2 produces P_2, which denotes the proper velocity vectors C_1 for the manipulator hand in work-space coordinates. Feedback F_2 also provides work-space position data necessary for the sequencing of action primitives in H_2. P_2 provides velocity or force commands C_1 to the coordinate transformations in H_1. F_1 provides position, velocity, and force information for the traditional servocomputations. The output P_1 is a set of drive signals to the actuators.

Feedback enters this hierarchy at every level. At the lowest levels, the feedback is unprocessed (or nearly so) and hence is fast-acting with very short delays. At higher levels, feedback data passes through more and more stages of an ascending sensory-processing hierarchy. Feedback thus closes a real-time control loop at each

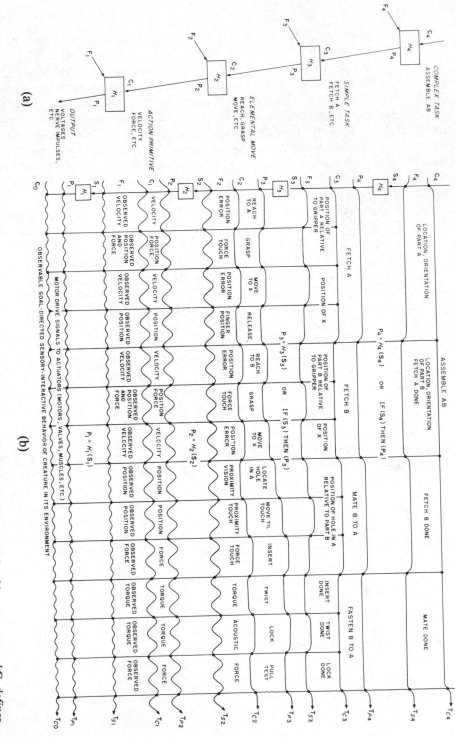

Figure 5.17: *A hierarchy of H operators produces sensory interactive goal-directed behavior. The highest level input command* C_4 *defines a goal, which in this example is* $<ASSEMBLE\ AB>$. *The feedback* F_4 *carries highly processed sensory data describing the state of enivronment in which the assemble command must operate, including the state of the lower level* P *vectors. The* H_4 *operator maps each input* S_4 *into an output* P_4. *As* F_4, *changes the goal* $<ASSEMBLE\ AB>$ *is decomposed into a sequence of subgoals* $<FETCH\ A>$, $<FETCH\ B>$, $<MATE\ B\ TO\ A>$, $<FASTEN\ B\ TO\ A>$. *At each level in the hierarchy a different type of feedback data with a different rate-of-change drives the decomposition of a higher level command into a sequence of lower level subcommands. Finally, at the lowest level the* P_0 *vector consists of motor drive signals which actuate observable behavior* C_0.

level in the hierarchy. The lower level loops are simple and fast-acting. The higher level loops are more sophisticated and slower.

At each level the feedback vector $\mathbf{F}$ drives the output vector $\mathbf{P}$ along its trajectory. Thus, at each level of the hierarchy, the time rate of change of the output vector $\mathbf{P}_i$ will be of the same order of magnitude as the feedback vector $\mathbf{F}_i$ and considerably more rapid than the command vector $\mathbf{C}_i$. The result is that each stage of the behavior-generating hierarchy effectively decomposes an input task represented by a slowly changing $\mathbf{C}_i$ into a string of subtasks represented by a more rapidly changing $\mathbf{P}_i$.

At this point we should emphasize that the difference in time rate of change of the vectors at various levels in the hierarchy does *not* imply that the H operators are computing more slowly at the higher levels than at the lower. We will, in fact, assume that every H operator transforms $\mathbf{S}$ into $\mathbf{P}$ with the same computational delay $\triangle t$ at all levels of the hierarchy. That is,

$$\mathbf{P}_i(t) = H_i[\mathbf{S}_i(t - \triangle t)] \quad \text{or} \quad \mathbf{P}_i^k = H_i(\mathbf{S}_i^{k-1})$$

at every level. The slower time rate of change of $\mathbf{P}$ vectors at the higher levels stems from the fact that the $\mathbf{F}$ vectors driving the higher levels convey information about events that occur less frequently. In some cases certain components of higher level $\mathbf{F}$ vectors may require the integration of information over long time intervals or the recognition of symbolic messages with long word lengths.

When we represent time explicitly as in figure 5.17b, we can label the relatively straight segments of the $\mathbf{T}_C$ trajectories as tasks and subtasks. Transitions between the subtasks in a sequence correspond to abrupt changes in $\mathbf{T}_C$.

If we do not represent time explicitly, the relatively constant $\mathbf{C}$ vectors correspond to nodes, as in figure 5.15. The resulting tree structure represents a classical AND/OR decomposition of a task into sequences of subtasks, where the discrete $\mathbf{C}_i$ vectors correspond to OR nodes and the rapidly changing sequences of $\mathbf{P}_i$ vectors become sets of AND nodes *under* those OR nodes.

INTENTIONAL OR PURPOSIVE BEHAVIOR

Figure 5.17 illustrates the power of a hierarchy of multivariant servomechanisms to generate a lengthy sequence of behavior that is both goal-directed and appropriate to the environment. Such behavior appears to an external observer to be intentional or purposive. The top-level input command is a goal, or task, successively decomposed into subgoals, or subtasks, at each stage of the control hierarchy until at the lowest level, output signals drive the muscles (or other actuators) producing observable behavior.

To the extent that the $\mathbf{F}$ vectors at the various levels contain sensory information from the environment, the task decompositions at those levels will be capable of responding to the environment. The type of response to each **F** vector depends on the *H* function at that level. If the **F** vector at any level is made up solely of internal variables, then the decomposition at that level will be stereotyped and insensitive to conditions in the environment.

Whether or not the hierarchy is driven by external or internal variables, or both, the highest level input command commits the entire structure to an organized and coordinated sequence of actions that will achieve the goal or accomplish the task under normal conditions. The selection of a high-level input command in a biological organism thus corresponds to an intent or purpose, which, depending on circumstances, may or may not be successfully achieved through the resulting hierarchical decomposition into action.

GOAL-DIRECTED BEHAVIOR

The concept of purpose or intent is not scientifically respectable among many psychologists. In particular, the behaviorist school of B.F. Skinner has attempted to banish the very concept of goal-directedness from all scientific descriptions of animal and even human behavior. This might puzzle the layman, since goal-seeking activity of one kind or another seems to lie at the very core of almost all animal behavior. The reason for this viewpoint can only be understood in the context of the historical beliefs and misunderstandings concerning the essence of intent and purpose. In Greek philosophy the notion of purposive behavior implied a mystical concept of "soul." To the Greeks, the soul was an abstract "principle of life," sometimes bestowed on the behavior of inanimate objects. For example, Aristotle argued that a falling object accelerated because it grew more "jubilant" as it found itself nearer home, and later authorities taught that a projectile was carried forward by its "impetuosity." Early Christian theologians defined both soul and mind to be something outside of the body—indeed outside of the natural world. The appearance of purpose in nature became evidence of something outside of nature, a supernatural power, a divine creator, an intelligent sustainer of the natural order.

Consider, for example, the following passage from St. Thomas Aquinas' *Summa Theologica:*

> The fifth [argument for the existence of God] begins from the guidedness of things. For we observe that some things which lack knowledge, such as natural bodies, work towards an end. This is apparent from the fact that they always or most usually work in the same way and move towards what is best. From which it is clear that they reach their end not by chance but by intention. For those things which do not have knowledge do not tend to an end, except under the direction of someone who knows and understands: the arrow, for example, is shot by the archer. There is therefore an intelligent personal being by whom everything in nature is ordered to this end, and this we call God.

In more recent times, Descartes fused mind, soul, and rationality into a single entity, which like God, is of a substance that is nowhere and unextended. This kind of thinking does indeed place the notion of intent and purpose outside the realm of scientific investigation. Against such a historical backdrop, it is not surprising that the behaviorist school fought to purge the concept of purpose and intent from the science of behavioral psychology. The point was to divorce the study of behavior from the supernatural and establish it as a natural science.

Yet such nonphysical things as purposes, intents, goals, plans, and values have objective reality. They are a part of our everyday experience and the fact that the Greeks or medieval philosophers attributed them to supernatural causes is no reason for modern science to pretend that they do not exist. Ideas, goals, and dreams play a great part in the generation of behavior, and any theory of behavior that does not take these nonphysical realities into account is very limited in scope.

Every since the development of modern servo-control theory during World War II, it has been clear that there is no need to appeal to the supernatural or to any life principle in order to explain goal-directed behavior. Goal-seeking is the natural behavior of any system that uses feedback information to steer behavior along a course leading to a goal. The simplest case of this is the servomechanism. No one today would cite the operation of a thermostat, or even a guided missile, as proof for the existence of God. We do not need to appeal to any life principle in order to explain servo-control theory. Neither should we feel any need to invoke the supernatural to explain the behavior of hierarchical goal-seeking systems with several levels in biological systems. To be sure, the addition of complex sensors, sophisticated sensory processing, internal world models, and multiple levels of feedback into the hierarchy produces an exponential increase in the complexity of possible behavior patterns; but this is not magic. It is predictable and deterministic.

In the following pages we will try to show how the study of robotics can provide an experimental tool for the study of hierarchical control systems and their relationship to goal-seeking and purposive behavior. With the advent of inexpensive and powerful microprocessors, robot-control systems can be made sufficiently complex so their behavior casts considerable light on many difficult issues of intention, perception, and cognition. Yet the robot is a machine; the variables that control it can be isolated and measured. Thus, robotics offers a way to make the study of purposive behavior into a hard science. Mathematically precise theories can be formulated and quantitatively tested with a rigor not achievable with biological subjects. By synthesizing purposive behavior, robotics may aid our understanding of it.

OBTAINING SUCCESSFUL PERFORMANCE

We can describe the success or failure of goal-seeking behavior in any particular task performance in terms of whether the H functions at each level are capable of providing the correct mappings so as to maintain the output trajectory within a region of successful performance despite perturbations and uncertainties in the environment.

At all levels, variations in the F vectors due to irregularities in the environment cause T_s trajectories to vary from one task performance to the next. This implies that while there may exist a set of ideal trajectories through S and P space at each level of the hierarchy corresponding to an ideal task performance, there also must be an envelope of nearly ideal trajectories that correspond to successful, but not perfect, task performance. This is illustrated in figure 5.18.

The H functions must not only be defined along the T_s trajectories corresponding to ideal performance, but also in the regions around the ideal performance. Consequently, any deviation from the ideal is treated as an error signal that generates an action designed to restore the actual trajectory to the ideal, or at least to maintain it within the region of successful performance.

Small perturbations can usually be corrected by low-level feedback loops, as shown in figure 5.19. These involve relatively little sensory data processing and hence are fast-acting. Larger perturbations in the environment may overwhelm the lower level feedback loops and require strategy changes at higher levels in order to maintain the system within the region of successful performance. This is illustrated in figure 5.20. Major changes in the environment are detected at higher levels after being processed through several levels of pattern recognizers. This produces differences in the F vector at the higher level which in turn produces different C vectors to lower levels. The result is an alternative higher level strategy to cope with the perturbation.

Of course, if the H functions do not provide stability, or if the environment is so perverse that the system is overwhelmed, then the trajectories diverge from the region of successful performance and failure occurs.

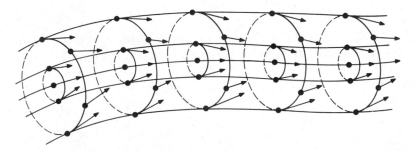

Figure 5.18: *Around each trajectory representing an ideal task performance there exists an envelope of nearly ideal trajectories which correspond to successful, but not perfect, task performance. If the H functions are defined throughout these envelopes such that the system can drive back toward the ideal whenever it deviates, then the trajectory will be stable and task performance can be successful despite perturbations and unexpected events.*

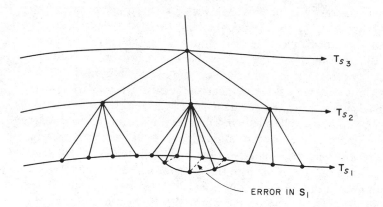

Figure 5.19: *If the* H *functions at the lower levels are sufficiently well defined, small perturbations from the ideal performance can be corrected by low-level feedback without requiring any change in the command from higher levels.*

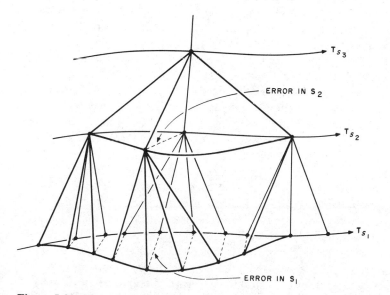

Figure 5.20: *If the lower level* H *functions are not adequately defined, or if the perturbations are too large for the lower level to cope, then feedback to the higher levels produces changes in the task decomposition at a higher level. The result is an alternative strategy.*

Note that it is not necessary for the feedback vector **F** to explicity represent an error signal. It is merely necessary for it to convey information that indicates the state of the current task performance. The H function at each hierarchical level is defined on the multidimensional space of all possible commands and all possible task states. In order to generate successful behavior, the H function must compute the correct control signals for every **S** vector near the ideal trajectory to steer the behavior trajectory back toward the center of the success envelope.

The **F** vector can, of course, explicitly represent an error signal. In this case, the H function must be defined over the space of all possible commands and all possible error signals. In either case, the dimensionality of the **S** vector is the same. However, in the second case the range of the variables in the **F** vector is reduced and centered at zero. This is sometimes computationally convenient, but not logically significant.

Overlearned tasks correspond to those for which the H functions at the lower levels are sufficiently well defined so as to maintain the terminal trajectory successfully without requiring intervention by the higher levels for strategy modification. Thus, a highly skilled and well-practiced performer, such as a water skier, can execute extremely difficult maneuvers with apparent ease despite large perturbations, such as waves. His lower level H functions are well defined over large regions of space corresponding to large perturbations in the environment. He is thus capable of compensating for these perturbations quickly and precisely to maintain successful performance without intervention by higher levels. Such a performance is characterized by a minimum amount of physical and mental effort.

We say, "He skis effortlessly without even thinking." What we mean is that his lower level corrections are so quick and precise that his performance never deviates significantly from the ideal. There is never any need for higher level loops to make emergency changes in strategy. On the other hand, a novice skier (whose H functions are poorly defined, even near the ideal trajectory, and completely undefined elsewhere) may have great difficulty maintaining a successful performance at all. He is continually forced to bring higher levels into play to prevent failure, and even the slightest perturbation from the ideal is likely to result in a watery catastrophe. He works very hard and fails often, because his responses are late and often misdirected. His performance is erratic and hardly ever near the ideal.

However, practice makes perfect, at least in creatures with the capacity to learn. Each time a trajectory is traversed, if there is some way of knowing what mistakes were made, corrections can be made to the H functions in those regions of input spaces that are traversed. The degree and precision of these corrections and the algorithm by which they are computed determine the rate of convergence (if any) of the learning process to a stable and efficient success trajectory.

There are many interesting questions about learning, generalization, and the mechanisms by which H functions are created and modified at the various hierarchical levels in biological brains. However, we will defer these issues until later.

ALTERNATIVE TRAJECTORIES

Note that figure 5.17 illustrates only a single specific performance of a particular task. None of the alternative trajectories that might have occurred under different circumstances with a different set of **F** vectors is indicated. Alternatives that might have occurred can be illustrated in a plane orthogonal to the time axis.

Figure 5.21 illustrates the set of alternative **C** vectors available at various levels in the behavior-generating hierarchy of the male three-spined stickleback fish. This figure represents a snapshot, or single cut through space orthogonal to the time axis. C_6, the highest level goal, is survival. The feedback F_6 consists of variables indicating water temperature and depth, blood chemistry, and hormone levels generated by length-of-day detectors. When the hormone levels indicate the proper time of year and the blood chemistry does not call for feeding behavior, then migratory behavior will be selected until warm, shallow water is detected. The F_6 vector will then trigger the reproduction subgoal.

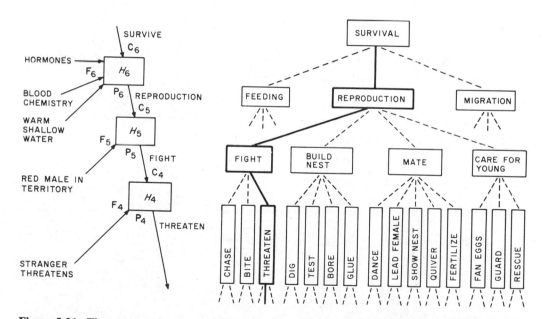

Figure 5.21: *The command and control hierarchy proposed by Tinbergen to account for the behavior of the male three-spined stickleback fish. The heavy line indicates the particular type of behavior vector actually selected by the feedback shown at the various levels of the hierarchy on the left. This figure represents a snapshot in time corresponding to one of the two-dimensional surfaces shown in figure 5.16.*

126

When C_5 indicates <REPRODUCTION>, an F_5 vector indicating a red male in the territory will cause the <FIGHT> command to be sent to C_4. When C_4 indicates <FIGHT> and the intruder threatens, a C_3 will be selected, and so on. At each level, a different feedback vector would select a different lower level subgoal. For example, if F_5 indicates a female in the territory, C_4 will become <MATE>, and the type of mating behavior selected will depend on F_4.

In simple creatures like the stickleback fish, the sensory stimuli that produce F_4 and F_3 vectors that trigger specific behavioral trajectories are called *innate releasing mechanisms*. Innate releasing mechanisms and their associated behavioral patterns have been studied extensively in a number of insects (i.e., the digger wasp and various bee and ant species), several fish, and many birds (i.e., the herring gull, turkey, and golden-eye drake). A behavior-generating hierarchy for a bird is shown in figure 5.22.

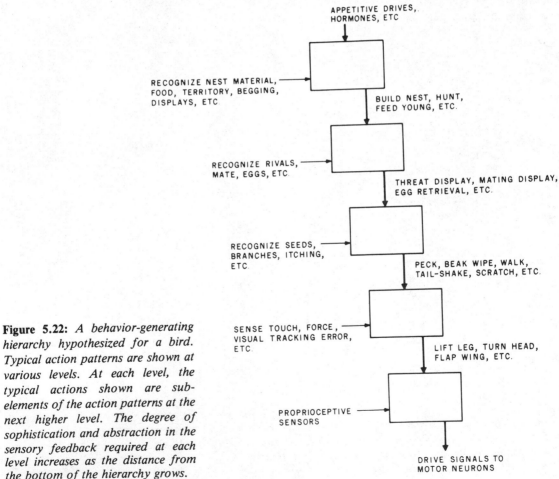

Figure 5.22: *A behavior-generating hierarchy hypothesized for a bird. Typical action patterns are shown at various levels. At each level, the typical actions shown are sub-elements of the action patterns at the next higher level. The degree of sophistication and abstraction in the sensory feedback required at each level increases as the distance from the bottom of the hierarchy grows.*

In these relatively simple creatures, behavior is sufficiently stereotyped that it can be described in terms of a small set of behavioral patterns triggered by an equally small set of sensory stimuli. This suggests that insects, fish, and birds have only a few levels in their control hierarchies and a small set of behavioral patterns stored as H functions at each level. It further implies that there are few externally driven components in the F vectors at each level. Behavior trajectories are internally driven, with only a few branch points controlled by sensory data processed through simple pattern recognizers. The trajectory segments driven entirely by internal variables are called fixed action patterns, or *tropisms*. The external variables that control the relatively few branch points are the innate releasing mechanisms.

In higher animals, behavior is more complex and much less stereotyped. This implies more levels in the hierarchy, more external sensory variables in the F vectors at each level, and hence many more possibilities for branching of the resulting trajectories.

Figure 5.23 illustrates a set of trajectories in which there is opportunity for branching at *several* different levels at *every* step along each trajectory. At each instant in time the C vector to any particular level depends upon what the C and F vectors were to the next higher level at the previous instant. Thus, a change in the F vector at any level causes an alternative C vector to be sent to the level below. Behavior is continuously modified at all levels by external variables and hence does not appear stereotyped at all.

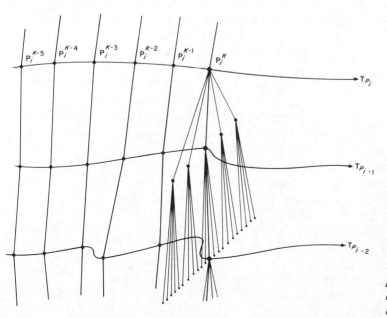

Figure 5.23: *A set of T_P trajectories in which there is opportunity for branching at many points in time. If behavior can be modified by feedback at many different levels and in many different ways, it appears to be adaptive and flexible. If there are only a few branch points with only a few alternative actions available at each branch, behavior will appear stereotyped.*

Many degrees of freedom place great demands on the H functions for maintaining stability and precision of control in such a large space of possibilities. Since successful behavior is only a tiny subset of all possible behaviors, it is clear that most of the potential branches will lead to disaster unless the H functions produce actions which steer the $\mathbf{S}$ and $\mathbf{P}$ vectors back into the narrow regions surrounding success trajectories. For a multilevel hierarchy with sensory interaction at many different levels, this is extremely complex. However, if the H functions are trainable, then performance can improve through practice. Complex tasks can be learned, imitated, and communicated from one individual to another.

It is clear from the illustrations in figures 5.17, 5.21, and 5.23 that the complexity of behavior resulting from a hierarchical control system depends on

1. the number of levels in the control hierarchy
2. the number of feedback variables that enter each level
3. the sophistication of the H functions that reside at each level
4. the sophistication of the sensory-processing systems that extract feedback information for use by the various H functions

THE SENSORY-PROCESSING HIERARCHY

The sensory feedback that enters each level of the behavior-generating hierarchy comes from a parallel sensory-processing hierarchy, as shown in figure 5.24. Sensory data enters this hierarchy at the bottom and is filtered through a series of sensory-processing and pattern-recognition modules arranged in a hierarchical structure that runs parallel to the behavior-generating hierarchy. Each level of this sensory-processing hierarchy processes the incoming sensory data stream, extracting features, recognizing patterns, and applying various types of filters to the sensory data. Information relevant to the control decisions being made at each level is extracted and sent to the appropriate behavior-generating modules. The partially processed sensory data that remains is then passed to the next higher level for further processing.

As was discussed in the section on vectors, any spatial pattern such as a picture, a sound, or a symbol can be represented as a vector; any visual or auditory sequence or any string of symbols can be represented by a trajectory.

The fundamental problem in pattern recognition is to name the patterns. All patterns called by the same name are in the same class. When a pattern has been given a name, we say it has been recognized. For example, when the image of a familiar face falls on my retina and I say "That's George," I have recognized the visual pattern by naming it.

Many patterns have the same name or fall in the same class, as shown in figure 5.25. For example, the same face casts many identifiable images. George's profile casts quite a different image on our retina than George's face seen straight on. Two identical positions of George's face will cast different images if the lighting is different, or if George is closer or further away. Yet these are all recognized as George.

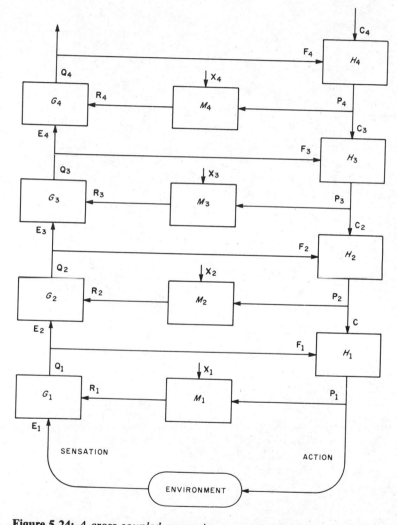

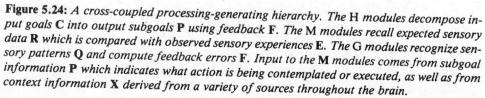

Figure 5.24: *A cross-coupled processing-generating hierarchy. The* **H** *modules decompose input goals* **C** *into output subgoals* **P** *using feedback* **F**. *The* **M** *modules recall expected sensory data* **R** *which is compared with observed sensory experiences* **E**. *The* **G** *modules recognize sensory patterns* **Q** *and compute feedback errors* **F**. *Input to the* **M** *modules comes from subgoal information* **P** *which indicates what action is being contemplated or executed, as well as from context information* **X** *derived from a variety of sources throughout the brain.*

The name of a pattern is itself a vector. "George" is a vector. So is the name "tree" or "cow" or "typewriter." Thus, the recognition process is a function, or a vector mapping from pattern space into name space. Each pattern vector is transformed by the recognition operator into a name vector. Many different pattern vectors can be mapped into the same name vector as illustrated in figure 5.26.

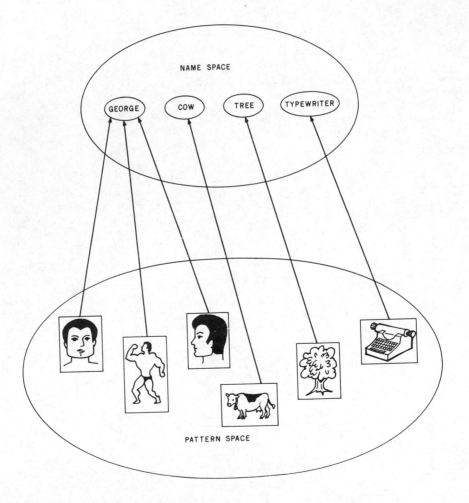

Figure 5.25: *The process of pattern recognition is one of naming the patterns. Typically many different patterns will be classified by the same name.*

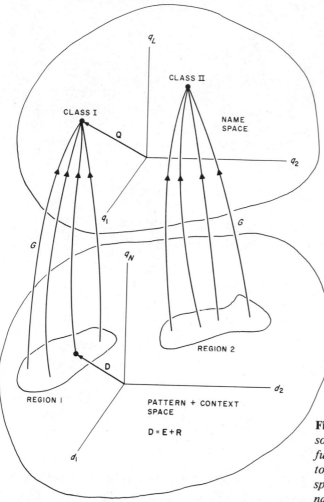

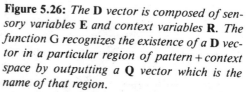

Figure 5.26: *The* **D** *vector is composed of sensory variables* **E** *and context variables* **R**. *The function G recognizes the existence of a* **D** *vector in a particular region of pattern + context space by outputting a* **Q** *vector which is the name of that region.*

At this point we need to introduce some new symbols to clearly distinguish between vectors in the sensory-processing hierarchy and those in the behavior-generating hierarchy. We will define the input vector to a pattern-recognizer module as

$$\mathbf{D} = \mathbf{E} + \mathbf{R}$$

where $\mathbf{E} = (d_1, d_2, \ldots, d_i)$ is a vector, or list, of data variables derived from sensory input from the external environment

and $\mathbf{R} = (d_{i+1}, \ldots, d_N)$ is a vector of data variables derived from recalled experiences, or internal context.

The functional operator in the sensory-processing hierarchy will be denoted G and the output $\mathbf{Q}$ such that

$$\mathbf{Q} = G(\mathbf{D})$$

The $\mathbf{D}$ vector represents a sensory pattern plus context, such that each component d_i represents a feature of the pattern or the context. The existence of the $\mathbf{D}$ vector within a particular region of space therefore corresponds to the occurrence of a particular set of features or a particular pattern in a particular context. The recognition problem then is to find a G function that computes an output vector:

$\mathbf{Q} = G(\mathbf{D})$ such that
$\mathbf{Q}$ is the name of the pattern and context $\mathbf{D}$ as shown in figure 5.26

In other words, G can recognize the existence of a particular pattern and context (i.e., the existence of $\mathbf{D}$ in a particular region of input space) by outputting the name $\mathbf{Q}$. For example, in figure 5.26

$\mathbf{Q} = $ Class I whenever $\mathbf{D}$ is in region 1
$\mathbf{Q} = $ Class II whenever $\mathbf{D}$ is in region 2

.
.
.

etc.

The G function in the sensory-processing module can be chosen to define the size and shape of the regions in the input space. As long as the regions of input space corresponding to pattern classes are reasonably well separated, a G function can usually be found that can reliably distinguish one region of input space from another and hence correctly classify the corresponding sensory patterns.

In the case where the $\mathbf{D}$ vector is time-dependent, an extended portion of a trajectory $\mathbf{T}_D$ may map into a single name $\mathbf{Q}$ as shown in figure 5.27. It is then possible by integrating $\mathbf{Q}$ over time and thresholding the integral to detect, or recognize, a temporal pattern $\mathbf{T}_D$ such as a spoken phrase or a visual movement.

Note that the recognition, or naming, of a temporal pattern as illustrated in figure 5.27 is the inverse of the decomposition of a task as illustrated in figures 5.14-5.17. In task decomposition a slowly varying command $\mathbf{C}$ is decomposed into a rapidly changing output $\mathbf{P}$. In pattern recognition a rapidly changing sensory experience $\mathbf{E}$ is recognized by a slowly varying name $\mathbf{Q}$.

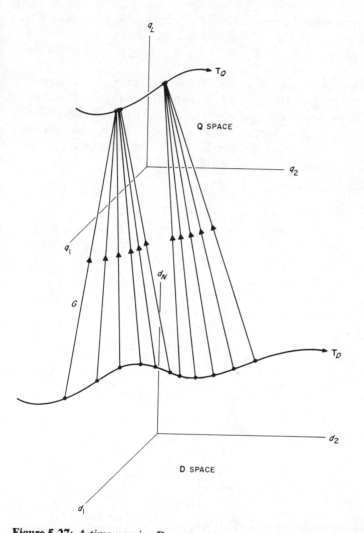

Figure 5.27: *A time-varying* **D** *vector traces out a trajectory* $\mathbf{T}_D$ *which represents a sensory experience* $\mathbf{T}_E$ *taking place in the context* $\mathbf{T}_R$. *A section of a* $\mathbf{T}_D$ *trajectory which maps into a small region of* **Q** *space corresponds to the recognition of an extended temporal pattern as a single event.*

THE USE OF CONTEXT

In pattern recognition, or signal detection, the instantaneous value of the sensory input vector **E** is frequently ambiguous or misleading. This is particularly true in noisy environments or in situations where data dropouts are likely to occur. In such cases the ambiguity can often be resolved or the missing data filled in if the context can be taken into account or if the classification decision can make use of some additional knowledge or well-founded prediction regarding what patterns are expected.

The addition of context or prediction variables $\mathbf{R}$ to the sensory input $\mathbf{E}$ such that $\mathbf{D} = \mathbf{E} + \mathbf{R}$ increases the dimensionality of the pattern input space. The context variables thus can shift the total input (pattern) vector $\mathbf{D}$ to different parts of input space depending on the context. Thus, as shown in figure 5.28, the ambiguous patterns $\mathbf{E}_1$ and $\mathbf{E}_2$, too similar to be reliably recognized as in separate classes, can be easily distinguished when accompanied by context $\mathbf{R}_1$ and $\mathbf{R}_2$.

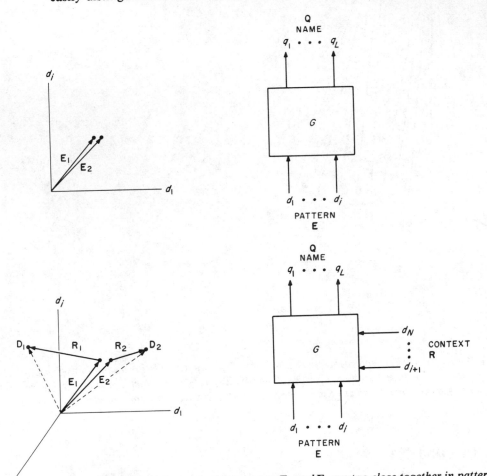

Figure 5.28: *In (a) the two pattern vectors $\mathbf{E}_1$ and $\mathbf{E}_2$ are too close together in pattern space to be reliably recognized (i.e., named) as in different classes. In (b) the addition of context $\mathbf{R}_1$ to $\mathbf{E}_1$ and $\mathbf{R}_2$ to $\mathbf{E}_2$ makes the vectors $\mathbf{D}_1$ and $\mathbf{D}_2$ far enough apart in pattern + context space to be easily recognized as in separate classes.*

In the brain many variables can serve as context variables. In fact, any fiber carrying information about anything occurring simultaneously with the input pattern can be regarded as context. Thus context can be data from other sensory modalities as well as information regarding what is happening in the behavior-generating hierarchy. In many cases, data from this latter source is particularly relevant to the pattern-recognition task, because the sensory input at any instant of time depends heavily upon what action is currently being executed.

For example, information from the behavior-generating hierarchy provides contextual information necessary for the visual-processing hierarchy to distinguish between motion of the eyes and motion of the room about the eyes. In a classic experiment, von Holst and Mittelstaedt demonstrated that this kind of contextual data pathway actually exists in insects. They observed that a fly placed in a chamber with rotating walls will tend to turn in the direction of rotation so as to null the visual motion. They then rotated the fly's head 180° around its body axis (a procedure which for some reason is not fatal to the fly) and observed that the fly now circled endlessly because by attempting to null the visual motion it was now actually increasing it. Later experiments with motion perception in humans showed that the perception of a stationary environment despite motion of the retinal image caused by moving the eyes is dependent on contextual information derived from the behavior-generating hierarchy. The fact that the context is actually derived from the behavior-generating hierarchy rather than from sensory feedback can be demonstrated by anesthetizing the eye muscles and observing that the effect depends on the *intent* to move the eyes and not on the physical act of movement. The perceptual correction occurs even when the eye muscles are paralyzed so that no motion actually results from the conscious intent to move.

EXPECTATIONS AND PREDICTION

Contextual information can also provide predictions of what sensory data can be expected. This allows the sensory-processing modules to do predictive filtering, to compare incoming data with predicted data, and to detect patterns obscured by noise or data dropouts.

The mechanism by which such predictions or expectations can be generated is illustrated in figure 5.24. Here contextual input for the sensory-processing hierarchy is shown as being processed through an M module before being presented to the sensory pattern-recognition G modules at each level. Input to the M modules derives from the $\mathbf{P}$ vector of the corresponding behavior-generating hierarchy at the same level as well as an $\mathbf{X}$ vector, which includes context derived from other areas of the brain such as other sensory modalities or other behavior-generating hierarchies. These M modules compute $\mathbf{R} = M(\mathbf{P} + \mathbf{X})$. Their position in the links from the behavior-generating to the sensory-processing hierarchies allows them to function as a predictive memory. They are in a position to store and recall (or remember) sensory experiences (**E** vector trajectories) which occur simultaneously with **P** and **X** vector trajectories in the behavior-generating hierarchy and other locations within the brain. For example, data may be stored in each M_i module by setting the desired output $\hat{\mathbf{R}}_i$ equal to the sensory experience vector $\mathbf{E}_i$. At each instant of time $t = k$ sensory data represented by $\mathbf{E}_i^k$ will then be stored in an address selected by the $\mathbf{P}_i^k + \mathbf{X}_i^k$ vector. The result will be that the sensory experience represented by the sensory data trajectory $\mathbf{T}_{E_i}$ will be stored in association with the context trajectory $\mathbf{T}_{P_i + X_i}$.

Any time afterwards, $t = k + j$, a reoccurrence of the same address vector $\mathbf{P}_i^{k+j} + \mathbf{X}_i^{k+j} = \mathbf{P}_i^k + \mathbf{X}_i^k$ will produce an output $\mathbf{R}_i^{k+j}$ equal to the $\mathbf{E}_j^k$ stored at time $t = k$. Thus a reoccurrence of the same address trajectory $\mathbf{T}_{P_i + x_i}$ will produce a recall trajectory $\mathbf{T}_{R_i}$ equal to the earlier sensory experience $\mathbf{T}_{E_i}$. These predictive memory modules thus provide the sensory-processing hierarchy with a memory trace of what sensory data occurred on previous occasions when the motor-generating hierarchy (and other parts of the brain) were in similar states along similar trajectories. This provides the sensory-processing system with a prediction of what sensory data to expect. What is expected is whatever was experienced during similar activities in the past.

In the ideal case, the predictive memory modules M_i will generate an expected sensory data stream $\mathbf{T}_{R_i}$ which exactly duplicates the observed sensory data stream $\mathbf{T}_{E_i}$. Even if the match is only approximate, it enables the G_i modules to apply very powerful mathematical techniques to the sensory data. For example, the G_i modules can use the expected data $\mathbf{T}_{R_i}$ to

1. Perform cross-correlation or convolution algorithms to detect sync patterns and information-bearing sequences buried in noise.
2. Flywheel through data dropouts and noise bursts.
3. Detect deviations or even omissions from an expected pattern as well as the occurrence of the pattern in its expected form.

If we assume, as shown in figure 5.24, that predictive recall modules exist at all levels of the processing-generating hierarchy, then it is clear that the memory trace itself is multileveled. In order to recall an experience precisely at all levels, it is necessary to generate the same $\mathbf{P}_i + \mathbf{X}_i$ address at all levels as existed when the experience was recorded.

If the M_i modules have the property of generalization, they will produce a recall vector $\mathbf{R}_i$ which is similar to the stored experience as long as the context vector $\mathbf{P}_i + \mathbf{X}_i$ is within the neighborhood of the context vector during storage. The more the context vector during recall resembles the context vector during storage, the more the recall vector $\mathbf{R}_i$ will resemble the experience vector $\mathbf{E}_i$ which was stored. We will examine this property of generalization in greater detail in the next chapter and show how a neurological model of an M module can produce it.

INTERNAL WORLD MODELS

We can say that the predictive memory modules M_i define the brain's internal model of the external world. They provide answers to the question, "What will happen if I do such and such?" The answer is that whatever happened before when such and such was done will probably happen again. What happened before is what is stored in the M_i modules. In short, IF I do Y, THEN Z will happen; Z is whatever was stored in predictive memory the last time (or some statistical average over the last N times) that I did Y, and Y is some action such as performing a task or pursuing a goal in a particular environment or situation. This is represented internally by the **P** vectors at the various different levels of the behavior-generating hierarchy and the **X** vectors describing the states of various other sensory-processing, behavior-generating hierarchies.

Any creature with such a memory structure can hypothesize an action and receive a mental image of the results of that action before it is performed. Furthermore, while the activity of behavior is proceeding, the M modules provide expectations to be compared with the observed sensory data. This allows the sensory processing modules to detect deviations between the expected and the observed and to modify behavior on the basis of the difference between the current experience and previously stored memories.

The M_i modules (as well as the H_i or G_i modules) can be thought of as storing knowledge in the form of IF/THEN rules. The $\mathbf{P}_i + \mathbf{X}_i$ input is the IF premise, and the recalled $\mathbf{R}_i$ vector is the THEN consequent. Much of the best and most exciting work now going on in the field of artificial intelligence revolves around IF/THEN production rules and how to represent knowledge in large computer programs based on production rules. Practically any kind of knowledge, or set of beliefs, or rules of behavior can be represented as a set of production rules. We will explore this topic in greater depth in later chapters.

CONCLUSIONS

By defining a vector and trajectory notation for describing states and events, we have completed the first major step in our development. We have suggested a hierarchical computing structure that can execute goals, or intended tasks, in an unpredictable environment. We have applied our vector notation to this hierarchy to mathematically and graphically describe the resulting goal-directed behavior. We have shown how a sensory-processing hierarchy that runs parallel to the behavior-generating hierarchy can recognize patterns and detect errors, thus steering behavior along trajectories that lead to success. Finally, we have shown how memory modules, addressed by the state of the behavior hierarchy, can recall previous experiences and generate expectations and predictions of future results.

In the next chapter we will examine a neurological model that has the properties of the H, G, and M modules we have discussed here. In later chapters we will suggest how the brain might use such modules to create plans, solve problems, imagine the future, understand knowledge, and produce language.

CHAPTER **6**

A Neurological Model

In the last chapter, we described how sensory-interactive goal-directed behavior can be generated and controlled by a multilevel hierarchy of computing modules. At each level of the hierarchy, input commands are decomposed into strings of output subcommands that form the input commands to the next lower level. Feedback from the external environment or from internal sources drives the decomposition process and steers the selection of subcommands so that the task of reaching the goal can be successfully achieved. In this chapter we are going to attempt to model some of the neurological structures that are believed to exist in the brain and to simulate the kind of computations, memory storage methods, and associative recall effects these structures seem to be performing.

Unfortunately, any such model must necessarily be speculation: definitive experimental evidence about the structure and function of neurological circuitry in the brain is extremely difficult to obtain. Because neurons are very tiny and delicate, it is hard to measure what is happening in them without damaging them or otherwise interfering with the flow of information related to their operation. There are techniques for measuring the activity of individual neurons and sometimes even observing the behavior of several neurons simultaneously. There are also techniques for monitoring synchronized changes in the activity of large numbers of neurons. But the brain is such a complicated anatomical structure, with such a jumbled interconnection of different kinds of neurons being excited and inhibited by such a broad variety of chemical and electrical stimuli, that it is impossible to infer from these measurements anything very sophisticated about the mathematical functions that are being computed or the procedures being executed.

Neurons are as intricately interconnected as a bramble patch overgown with vines, and many of their most important information-processing properties are statistical in nature. These statistics may apply over ensembles of thousands of neurons.

The flow of information is further complicated by multiple feedback loops, some of which are confined to small, local clusters of neurons, and others which may thread through several entirely different regions of the brain. As a result, no one has yet been able to construct a clear picture of the overall information-processing architecture in the brain. At present, there is no widely accepted theory that can bridge the gap between hard neurophysiological measurements and psychological concepts, such as perception and cognition.

Nevertheless, much is known about the structure and function of at least some parts of the brain, particularly in the periphery of the sensory and motor systems, and a great deal can be inferred from this knowledge. In one area, the cerebellar cortex, the geometry is sufficiently regular to enable researchers to identify positively a number of important neurophysiological relationships.

The cerebellum, which is attached to the midbrain and nestles up under the visual cortex as shown in figure 6.1, is intimately involved with control of rapid, precise, coordinated movements of limbs, hands, and eyes. Injury to the cerebellum results in motor deficiencies such as overshoot in reaching for objects, lack of coordination, and the inability to execute delicate tasks or track precisely with the eyes.

During the 1960s, advances in the technology of single-cell recordings and electron microscopy made possible an elegant series of experiments by Sir John Eccles and a number of others that identified the functional interconnections between the principal components in the cerebellar cortex. A brief outline of the structure and function of the cerebellar cortex appears in figure 6.2.

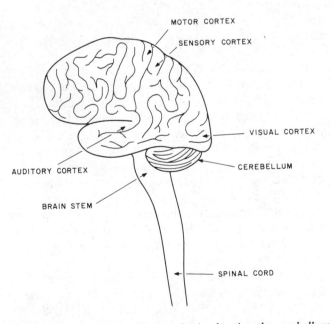

Figure 6.1: *Side view of human brain showing the cerebellum attached to the brain stem and partially hidden by the visual cortex.*

The principal input to the cerebellar cortex arrives via mossy fibers (so named because they looked like moss to the early workers who first observed them through a microscope). Mossy fibers carry information from a number of different sources such as the vestibular system (balance), the reticular formation (alerting), the cerebral cortex (sensory-motor activity), and sensor organs that measure such quantities as position of joints, tension in tendons, velocity of contraction of muscles, and pressure on skin. Mossy fibers can be categorized into at least two classes based on their point of origin: those carrying information that may include commands from higher levels in the motor system, and those carrying feedback information about the results of motor outputs. Once these two sets of fibers enter the cerebellum, however, they intermingle and become virtually indistinguishable.

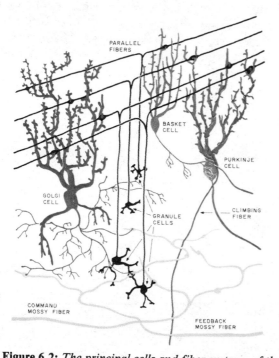

Figure 6.2: *The principal cells and fiber systems of the cerebellar cortex. Command and feedback information arrives via mossy fibers, each of which makes excitatory (+) contact with several hundred granule cells. Golgi cells sample the response of the granule cells via the parallel fibers and suppress by inhibitory (−) contacts all but the most highly excited granule cells. Purkinje cells are the output of the cerebellar cortex. They sum the excitatory (+) effect of parallel fibers through weighted connections. They also receive inhibitory (−) input from parallel fibers via basket cell inverters. The strengths of these weights determine the transfer function of the cerebellar cortex. Climbing fibers are believed to adjust the strength of these weights so as to train the cerebellum.*

The feedback mossy fibers tend to exhibit a systematic regularity in the mapping from point of origin of their information to their termination in the cerebellum. It is thus possible to sketch a map of the body on the surface of the cerebellum corresponding to the origins of feedback mossy fiber information as shown in figure 6.3. This map is not sharply defined, however, and has considerable overlap between regions, due in part to extensive intermingling and multiple overlapping of terminations of the mossy fibers in the cerebellar granule cell layer. Each mossy fiber branches many times and makes excitatory (+) contact with several hundred granule cells spaced over a region several millimeters in diameter.

Granule cells, the most numerous cells in the brain, are estimated to number more than 10^{10} in the human cerebellum alone. There are 100 to 1000 times as many granule cells as mossy fibers. Each granule cell is contacted by one to twelve mossy fibers and gives off a single output axon which rises toward the surface of the cerebellum. When it nears the surface this axon splits into two parts which run about 1.5 millimeters in opposite directions along the folded ridges of the cerebellum, making contact with a number of different kinds of cells in passage. These axons from the granule cells run parallel to each other in a densely packed sheet—hence the name "parallel fibers."

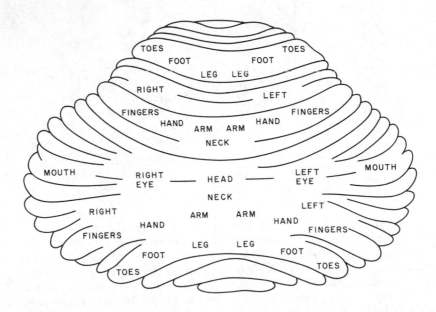

Figure 6.3: *A map of the surface of the cerebellar cortex showing the point of origin of mossy fiber feedback and ultimate destination of Purkinje cell ouput.*

One of the cell types contacted by parallel fibers is Golgi cells, named for their discoverer. These cells have a widely spread dendritic tree and are excited by parallel fibers over a region about 0.6 millimeters in diameter. Each Golgi cell puts out an axon that branches extensively, making inhibitory ($-$) contact with up to 100,000 granule cells in its immediate vicinity, including many of the same granule cells that excited it. The dendritic trees and axons of neighboring Golgi cells intermingle, blanketing the entire granular layer with negative feedback. The general effect is that of an automatic gain control on the level of activity in the parallel fiber sheet. The Golgi cells are thought to operate such that only a small and controlled percentage (perhaps one percent or less) of the granule cells are allowed above threshold at any one time regardless of the level of activity of the mossy fiber input. Any particular pattern of activity on the mossy fiber input will produce a few granule cells that are maximally excited and many others that are less than maximally stimulated. The Golgi cells suppress the outputs of all but the few maximally stimulated granule cells. The result is that every input pattern, or vector, is transformed by the granule layer into a small and relatively fixed percentage, or subset, of active parallel fibers.

These fibers not only contact Golgi cells, but also make excitatory contact with Purkinje cells and basket and stellate cells (named for their shapes) through weighted connections (synapses). Each Purkinje cell performs a summation over its inputs and produces an output that is the output of the cerebellar cortex. The basket and stellate cells are essentially inverters that provide the Purkinje with negative weights that are summed along with the positive weights from parallel fibers.

A second set of fibers entering the cerebellar cortex are the climbing fibers, so named because they climb the Purkinje cells like ivy on a tree. Typically, there is one climbing fiber for each Purkinje cell, and these climbing fibers are believed to have some role in adjusting the strength of the weighted synaptic connections with the parallel fibers so as to alter the Purkinje output. Climbing fibers are thus hypothesized to provide the information required for learning.

THE CEREBELLAR MODEL ARITHMETIC COMPUTER (CMAC)

The availability of detailed knowledge regarding the structure and function of the various cell and fiber types in the cerebellum has led a number of theoreticians to propose mathematical models to explain the information-processing characteristics of the cerebellum. One model was developed independently in Great Britain by David Marr and in the United States by this author. The general outlines of this model are shown in figure 6.4. Further work by the author has produced the more abstract version illustrated in figure 6.5 as well as a mathematical formalism called the Cerebellar Model Arithmetic Computer (CMAC).

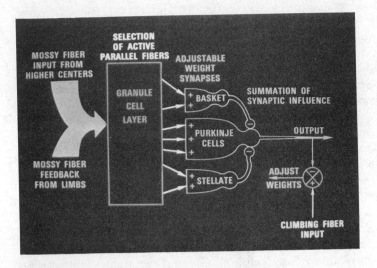

Figure 6.4: *A theoretical model of the cerebellum.*

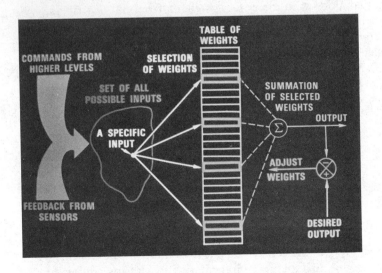

Figure 6.5: *A schematic representation of CMAC (Cerebellar Model Arithmetic Computer).*

CMAC is defined by a series of mappings,

$$S \rightarrow M \rightarrow A \rightarrow p$$

where S is an input vector
$\quad$ M is the set of mossy fiber used to encode S
$\quad$ A is the set of granule cells contacted by M
and p is an output value

The overall mapping

$$S \rightarrow p$$

has all of the properties of a function

$$p = h(S)$$

as described in Chapter 5. A set of L CMACs operating on the same input produces a mapping

$$S \rightarrow P$$

which has the properties of the function

$$P = H(S)$$

We may describe the information encoded by mossy fibers as a vector $S = C + F$

where $C = (s_1, s_2, \ldots, s_i)$ is a vector, or list, of command variables
$\quad$ and $F = (s_{i+1}, \ldots, s_N)$ is a vector, or list, of feedback variables
$\quad$ "$+$" is an operator denoting the combination of two vectors defined by two lists of variables into a single vector or list of variables;

that is,

$$S = C + F$$

means that $S = (s_1, s_2, \ldots, s_i, s_{i+1}, \ldots, s_N)$

Some of the elements of the command vector C may define symbolic motor commands such as <REACH>, <PULL BACK>, or <PUSH>. The remainder of the elements in C define arguments, or modifiers, such as the velocity of motion desired, the force required, or the position of the terminal point of a motion. Elements of the feedback vector **F** may represent physical parameters such as the position of a particular joint, the tension in a tendon, the velocity of contraction of a muscle, or the pressure on a patch of skin.

The S → M Mapping

The vector components of **S** must be transmitted from their various points of origin to their destination in the cerebellar granular layer. Distances may range from a few inches to more than a foot. This presents a serious engineering problem because, like all nerve axons, mossy fibers are noisy, unreliable, and imprecise information channels with limited dynamic range. Pulse frequency and pulse phase modulation (which the brain uses for data transmission over long distances) are subject to quantization noise and are bandwidth limited. Nerve axons typically cannot transmit pulse rates above five hundred pulses per second. Nevertheless, high-resolution high-bandwidth data is required for precise control of skilled actions.

The brain solves this problem by encoding each of the high-precision variables to be transmitted so that it can be carried on a large number of low-precision channels. Many mossy fibers are assigned to each input variable such that any one fiber conveys only a small portion of the information content of a single variable.

The nature of this encoding is that any particular mossy fiber will be maximially active over some limited range of the variable that it encodes and less than maximally active over the rest of its variable's range. For example, the mossy fiber labeled *a* in figure 6.6 is maximally active whenever the elbow joint is between 90° and 120°

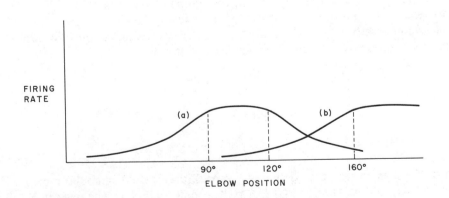

Figure 6.6: *Typical responses of mossy fibers to the sensory variable they encode.*

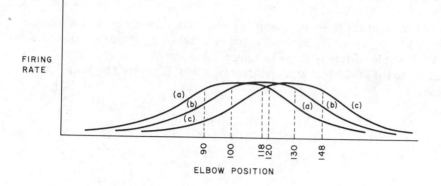

FIRING RATE

(a)
(b)
(c)

(a) (b) (c)

90 100 118 120 130 148

ELBOW POSITION

Figure 6.7: *Three different mossy fibers encoding a single sensory variable (elbow position). All three fibers maximally active simultaneously indicate that the elbow lies between 118° and 120°.*

and is less than maximally active for all other elbow positions. The mossy fiber labeled *b* in figure 6.6 is maximally active whenever the elbow angle is greater than 160°. If there are a large number of mossy fibers whose responses have a single maximum but which are maximally active over different intervals, then it is possible to tell the position of the elbow quite precisely by knowing which mossy fibers are maximally active. For example, in figure 6.7, the fact that mossy fibers *a*, *b*, and *c* are maximally active indicates that the elbow joint is between 118° and 120°.

CMAC models this encoding scheme in the following way. Define m_i to be the set of mossy fibers assigned to convey the value of the variable s_i. Define $m_i{}^*$ to be the mossy fibers in m_i which are maximally stimulated by a particular value of s_i. If for every value of s_i over its range there exists a unique set $m_i{}^*$ of maximally active mossy fibers, then there is a mapping $s_i \rightarrow m_i{}^*$ such that knowing $m_i{}^*$ (i.e., which fibers in m_i are maximally active) tells us what is the value of s_i. If such a mapping is defined for every component s_i in the vector **S**, then we have a mapping:

$$\mathbf{S} \rightarrow M = \begin{cases} s_1 \rightarrow m_1{}^* \\ s_2 \rightarrow m_2{}^* \\ \cdot \\ \cdot \\ \cdot \\ s_N \rightarrow m_N{}^* \end{cases}$$

where M is the set of all mossy fibers in all of the sets m_i where $i = 1, \ldots, N$. In other words, M is the set of all mossy fibers which encode the variables in the vector S.

In CMAC each of the $s_i \rightarrow m_i{}^*$ mappings may be defined by a set of K quantizing functions ${}^iC_1, {}^iC_2, \ldots, {}^iC_k$, each of which is offset by $1/K$th of the quantizing interval. An example of this is given in figure 6.8 where $K = 4$ and $N = 2$. s_1 is represented along the horizontal axis and the range of s_1 is covered by four quantizing functions

$$
\begin{aligned}
{}^1C_1 &= \{A, B, C, D, E\} \\
{}^1C_2 &= \{F, G, H, J, K\} \\
{}^1C_3 &= \{M, N, P, Q, R\} \\
{}^1C_4 &= \{S, T, V, W, X\}
\end{aligned}
$$

Each quantizing function is offset from the previous one by one resolution element. For every possible value of s_i there exists a unique set $m_1{}^*$ consisting of the set of values produced by the K quantizing functions. For example, in figure 6.8 the value $s_1 = 7$ maps into the set $m_1{}^* = \{B, H, P, V\}$.

A similar mapping is also performed on s_2 by the set of quantizing functions

$$
\begin{aligned}
{}^2C_1 &= \{a, b, c, d, e\} \\
{}^2C_2 &= \{f, g, h, j, k\} \\
{}^2C_3 &= \{m, n, p, q, r\} \\
{}^2C_4 &= \{s, t, v, w, x\}
\end{aligned}
$$

For example, the value $s_2 = 10$ maps into the set $m_2{}^* = \{c, j, q, v\}$. If the s_1 in figure 6.8 corresponds to the position of the elbow joint, the mossy fiber labeled B will be maximally active whenever the elbow is between 4 and 7, and less than maximally active whenever the elbow position is outside that region. Similarly, the mossy fiber labeled H is maximally active when the elbow is between 5 and 8; the fiber P is maximally active between 6 and 9, and V between 7 and 10, etc. The combination of mossy fibers in the set $m_1{}^* = \{B, H, P, V\}$ thus indicates that the variable $s_1 = 7$. If s_1 changes one resolution element, from 7 to 8 for example, the mossy fiber labeled B will drop out of the maximally active set $m_1{}^*$ to be replaced by another labeled C.

This encoding scheme has a number of advantages. The most obvious is that a single precise variable can be transmitted reliably over a multiplicity of imprecise information channels. The resolution, or information content, of the transmitted variable depends on the number of channels. The more mossy fibers dedicated to a particular variable, the greater the precision with which it is represented.

A second equally important result is that small changes in the value of the input variable s_i have no effect on most of the elements in $m_i{}^*$. This leads to a property known as generalization, crucial for learning and recall in a world where no two situations are ever exactly the same. In CMAC the extent of the neighborhood of

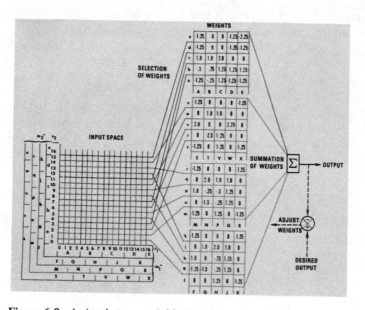

Figure 6.8: *A simple two-variable CMAC with four quantizing functions on each variable. A detailed explanation is in the text.*

generalization along each variable axis depends on the resolution of the CMAC quantizing functions. In the brain this corresponds to the width of the maximally active region of the mossy fibers.

The $M \to A$ Mapping

Just as we can identify mossy fibers by the input variables they encode, so can we identify granule cells by the mossy fibers that provide them input. Each granule cell receives input from several different mossy fibers, and no two granule cells receive input from the same combination of mossy fibers. This means that we can compute a unique name, or address, for each granule cell by simply listing the mossy fibers that contact it. For example, a granule cell contacted by two mossy fibers B and c can be named, or addressed, Bc.

In the CMAC example in figure 6.8, 25 granule cells are identified by their contacts with mossy fibers from the quantizing functions $^1C_1$ and $^2C_1$. Another 25 granule cells are identified by $^1C_2$ and $^2C_2$, 25 by $^1C_3$ and $^2C_3$, and 25 more by $^1C_4$ and $^2C_4$. There are, of course, many other possible combinations of mossy fiber names that might be used to identify a much larger number of granule cells. For this simple example, however, we will limit our selection to the permutation of corresponding quantizing functions along each of the coordinate axes. This provides a large and representative sample that uniformly spans the input space. Furthermore, this particular naming algorithm is simple to implement in either software or hardware.

We can define A to be the set of all granule cells identified by their mossy fiber inputs. All of the granule cells in A are not active at the same time. As was previously noted, most granule cells are inhibited from firing by Golgi-cell gain control feedback. Only the small percentage of granule cells whose input mossy fibers are *all* maximally active can rise above threshold. We will define the set of active granule cells as A^*.

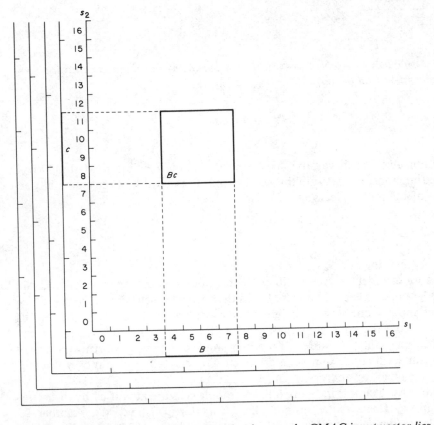

Figure 6.9: *The weight* Bc *will be selected as long as the CMAC input vector lies in the region bounded by* $4 \leq s_1 \leq 7,\ 8 \leq s_2 \leq 11.$

Since we already know which mossy fibers are maximally active (i.e., those mossy fibers in the sets m_i^*), we can compute names of granule cells in A^*. For example, in figures 6.8 and 6.10, if $s_1 = 7$ and $s_2 = 10$, then $m_1^* = \{B, H, P, V\}$ and $m_2^* = \{c, j, q, v\}$. The active granule cells in A^* can now be computed directly as $A^* = \{Bc, Hj, Pq, Vv\}$. All other granule cell names in the larger set A involve at least one mossy fiber which is not maximally active—i.e., not in m_1^* or m_2^*.

Note that, as illustrated in figure 6.9, the granule cell Bc will be active as long as the input vector remains in the region of input space $4 \leq s_1 \leq 7$ and $8 \leq s_2 \leq 11$. Thus, the generalizing property introduced by the $S \rightarrow M$ mapping carries through to the naming of active granule cells. A particular granule cell is active whenever the input vector S lies within some extended region, or neighborhood, of input space.

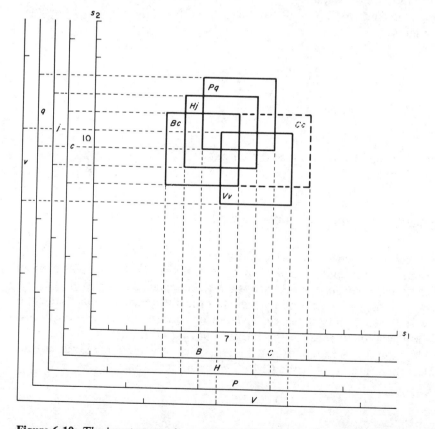

Figure 6.10: *The input vector* $(s_1, s_2) = (7, 10)$ *selects weights* Bc, Hj, Pq, *and* Vv. *These all overlap only at the point (7, 10). If the input vector* (s_1, s_2) *moves to (8, 10) the weight* Bc *will drop out to be replaced by* Cc.

Other granule cells are active over other neighborhoods. These neighborhoods overlap, but each is offset from the others so that for any particular input **S**, the neighborhoods in $A*$ all overlap at only one point, namely the point defined by the input vector. This is illustrated in figure 6.10. If the input vector moves one resolution element in any direction, for example, from (7,10) to (8,10), one active granule cell (*Bc*) drops out of $A*$ to be replaced by another (*Cc*).

The $A \rightarrow p$ Mapping

Granule cells give rise to parallel fibers which act through weighted connections on the Purkinje output cell, varying its firing rate. To each cell in A, then, is associated a weight which may be positive or negative in value. Only the cells in $A*$ have any effect on the Purkinje output cell. Thus, the Purkinje output sums only the weights selected, or addressed, by $A*$. This sum is the CMAC output scalar variable p. For example, in figure 6.8, **S** = (7,10) maps into $A* = \{Bc, Hj, Pq, Vv\}$ which selects the weights

$$W_{Bc} = 1.0$$
$$W_{Hj} = 2.0$$
$$W_{Pq} = 1.0$$
$$W_{Vv} = 0.$$

These weights are summed to produce the output

$$p = 4.0$$

Thus the input **S** = (7,10) produces the output $H(\mathbf{S}) = 4.0$.

In figure 6.8 four weights are selected for every **S** vector in input space. Their sum is the value of the output p. As the input vector moves from any point in input space to an adjacent point, one weight drops out to be replaced by another. The difference in value of the new weight minus the old is the difference in value of the output at the two adjacent points. Thus, the difference in adjacent weights is the partial derivative, or partial difference, of the function at that point.

As the input vector **S** moves over the input space, a value p is output at each point. We can therefore say that the CMAC computes the function

$$p = h(\mathbf{S})$$

The particular function h computed depends on the particular set of values stored in the table of weights. For example, the set of weights shown in figure 6.8 computes the function shown in figure 6.11.

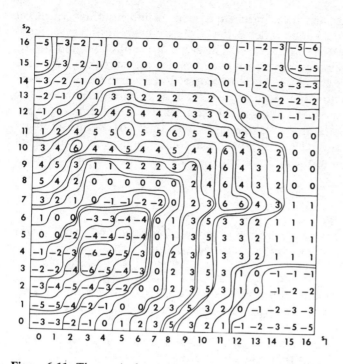

Figure 6.11: *The particular set of weights shown in figure 6.8 will compute the function shown here.*

In the cerebellum there are many Purkinje cells that receive input from essentially the same mossy fibers. Thus, there are many CMACs all computing on the same input vector **S**. We can therefore say that a set of L CMACs computing on the same input vector produces a vector mapping

$$\mathbf{P} = H(\mathbf{S})$$

DATA STORAGE IN CMAC

One of the most fascinating, intensively studied, and least understood features of the brain is memory, and how data is stored in memory. In the cerebellum each Purkinje cell has a unique fiber, a climbing fiber, which is believed to be related to learning. Recently discovered fibers from an area called the locus coeruleus also appear to be related to learning. In addition, a number of hormones have profound effects on learning and retention of learned experiences.

Although the exact mechanism, or mechanisms, for memory storage are as yet unknown, the cerebellar model upon which CMAC is based hypothesizes that climbing fibers carry error-correction information. The coincidence of climbing fiber error signals with Purkinje cell output punishes synapses that participate in erroneous firing of the Purkinje cell. The amount of error correction occurring at any one experience may depend on factors such as the state of arousal or emotional importance attached by the brain's evaluation centers to the data being stored during the learning process. Other plausible assumptions that input from the locus coeruleous might mediate learning by reward/punishment signals, that some chemical or hormonal input might occur, or that all of the above are involved await the future attention of serious investigation.

In the work to date, cerebellar learning has been modeled in CMAC by the following procedure:

1. Assume that $\hat{H}$ is the function we want CMAC to compute. Then $\hat{\mathbf{P}} = \hat{H}(\mathbf{S})$ is the desired value of the output vector for each point in the input space.
2. Select a point $\mathbf{S}$ in input space where $\hat{\mathbf{P}}$ is to be stored. Compute the current value of the function at that point $\mathbf{P} = H(\mathbf{S})$.
3. For every element in
    $\mathbf{P} = (p_1, p_2, \ldots, p_L)$ and in
    $\hat{\mathbf{P}} = (\hat{p}_1, \hat{p}_2, \ldots, \hat{p}_L)$
    if $\quad |\hat{p}_i - p_i| \leq \xi_i$

where $|\hat{p}_i - p_i|$ is the absolute value of $\hat{p}_i - p_i$ and ξ_i is an acceptable error, then do nothing; the desired value is already stored.

However, if $|\hat{p}_i - p_i| > \xi_i$ then add $\triangle_i$ to every weight which was summed to produce p_i

where $\triangle_i = g\dfrac{\hat{p}_i - p_i}{|A^*|}$

$|A^*|$ is the number of weights in the set A^* which contributed to p_i.

and g is a gain factor which controls the amount of error correction produced by one learning experience.

If $g = 1$, then CMAC produces "one-shot" learning which fully corrects the observed error in one data storage operation. If $0 < g < 1$, then each learning experience only moves the output p_i in the direction of the desired value $\hat{p}_i$. More than one memory storage operation is then required to achieve correct performance.

An example of how an arbitrary function such as

$$\hat{p} = \sin x \sin y$$
$$\text{where } x = 2\pi s_1/360$$
$$\text{and } y = 2\pi s_1/360$$

can be stored in CMAC is shown in figure 6.12. In this example the input is defined with unity resolution over the space $0 < s_1 \leq 360$ and $0 < s_2 \leq 180$ and the number of weights selected by each input is $|A^*| = 32$.

All the weights were initially equal to zero. The point $S_1 = (90,90)$ was chosen for the first data entry. The value of the desired function $\hat{p} = h(90,90)$ is 1. By formula (1), where $g = 1$, each of the weights selected by $S = (90,90)$ is set to $1/32$ causing the proper value to be stored at $S = (90,90)$ as shown in figure 6.12a. After two data storage operations, one at (90,90), the other at (270,90), the contents of the CMAC memory are as shown in figure 6.12b. The results of 16 storage operations along the $s_2 = 90$ axis are shown in figure 6.12c. Figure 6.12d shows the contents of the CMAC memory after 175 storage operations scattered over the entire input space.

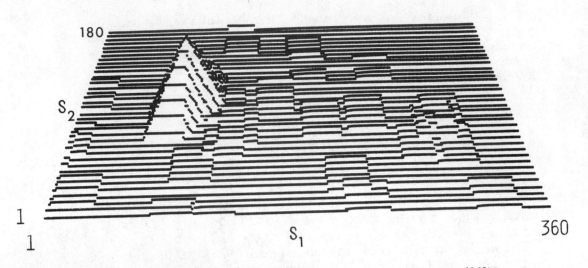

Figure 6.12: *The effect of training CMAC on the function* $\hat{p} = sin\,(2\pi\,s_1/360)\,sin\,(2\pi\,s_2/360).$
a: *One training at* $(s_1,\ s_2) = (90,\ 90).$

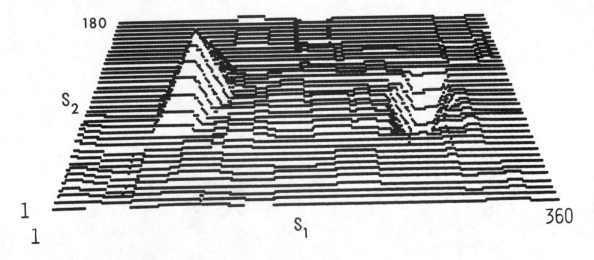

Figure 6.12b: *A second training at* $(s_1,\ s_2) = (270,\ 90).$

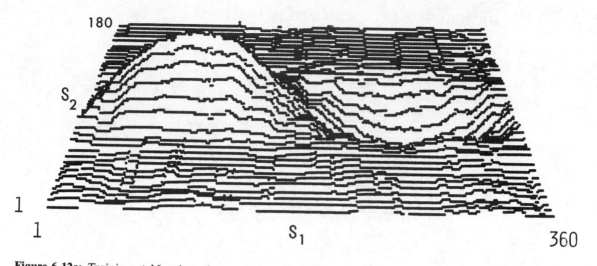

Figure 6.12c: *Training at 16 points along a trajectory defined by* $s_2 = 90$.

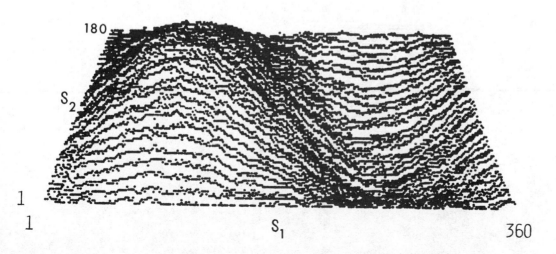

Figure 6.12d: *Training at 175 selected points scattered over the input space.*

MEMORY SIZE REQUIREMENTS IN CMAC

The CMAC $S \rightarrow A^*$ mapping corresponds to an address decoder wherein S is the input address and the active granule cells in A^* are select lines. These access weights whose sum can be interpreted as the contents of the address S. In a conventional memory each possible input address selects a unique single location wherein is stored the contents of that address, as illustrated in figure 6.13a. In CMAC each possible input address selects a unique *set* of memory locations, the sum of whose contents is the contents of the input address, as shown in figure 6.13b.

This suggests that CMAC might require considerably less memory than a conventional look-up table in storing certain functions. The reason is that the number of ways that x elements can be selected from a table of y entries always exceeds y and, in some cases, it does so by orders of magnitude.

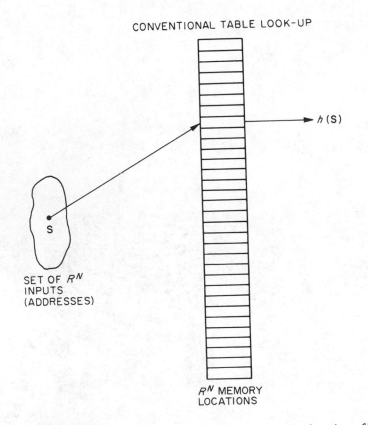

CONVENTIONAL TABLE LOOK-UP

$h(S)$

SET OF R^N
INPUTS
(ADDRESSES)

R^N MEMORY
LOCATIONS

Figure 6.13a: *In a conventional memory, storage of a function of* N *variables with resolution* R *on each input variable requires* R^N *memory locations.*

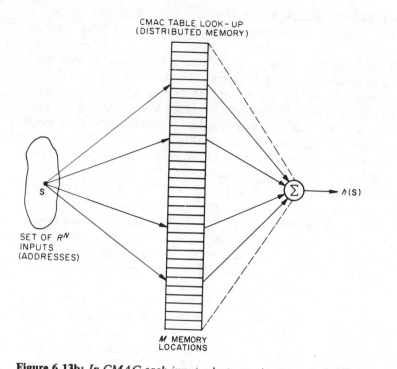

CMAC TABLE LOOK-UP
(DISTRIBUTED MEMORY)

S

SET OF R^N
INPUTS
(ADDRESSES)

$h(S)$

M MEMORY
LOCATIONS

Figure 6.13b: *In CMAC each input selects a unique set of memory locations. The number of unique sets which can be selected from* M *locations is much larger than* M.

A conventional memory requires R^N memory locations to store a function of N variables, where R is the number of resolution elements on each variable. CMAC requires at most KQ^N memory locations, where K is the number of quantizing functions and Q the number of resolution elements on each quantizing function.

A modest example of CMAC's reduced memory requirements can be seen in figure 6.8 where $N = 2$ and $R = 17$. Here, then, are 17^2, or 289, possible input vectors. The CMAC shown has only 100 weights since $K = 4$ and $Q = 5$. Thus $KQ^N = 100$.

This savings in memory size becomes increasingly significant for large N. It allows CMAC to store a large class of low resolution functions of up to twelve variables over the entire input space with computer memory of practical size (less than 100 K bytes), whereas conventional table look-up becomes impractical for similar functions of more than four variables.

For some cases an even greater savings in memory requirements can be achieved by the use of hash coding techniques in the selection of addresses for the elements in A^*. Hash coding allows CMAC to store functions of many variables as long as the information content of the portion of the function stored does not exceed the number of bits in the CMAC memory. For example, in figure 6.12, the 360×180 (over 64,000) element input space is represented in a 1024 location CMAC memory by hash coding.

Hash coding is a commonly used memory-addressing technique for compressing a large but sparsely populated address space into a smaller, more densely populated one. Many addresses in the larger space are mapped onto each of the addresses in the smaller one. One method is simply to overlay pages. Hashing works as long as the probability of a collision (i.e., more than one filled location in the large memory mapping into the same address in the small) is low.

In most cases of computations performed in the brain, the address space is very sparsely populated. Skilled movements are not learned over the entire space of possible positions, orientations, velocities, and magnitudes. They are learned over only a small percentage of the space that is narrowly clustered around the success envelope of the trajectories involved in the skilled movement. CMAC thus does not violate any law of information theory. It is not a method for reducing the amount of storage required to store a particular amount of information, but a method for using the available memory to store the function required to produce successful behavior over just the regions of S space where those actions occur.

In short, CMAC computes by table look-up. It stores a response to those states and inputs which occur during learning of various skills. It recalls from memory a response to every state and input that occurs during practice. The results of any computation can be modified, and sometimes improved, by learning, i.e., by changing the contents of the memory.

CMAC can tolerate a fairly high incidence of collisions because of its distributed memory, i.e., its output is the sum of many locations. Thus a collision, which in a conventional memory would make the output completely incorrect, in CMAC only introduces a small amount of noise into the output. Hash coding noise can be seen in the base plane in figure 6.12a through c.

In CMAC hashing noise occurs randomly over the input space each time new data is stored. Thus each new data storage operation somewhat degrades previously stored data. The effect is that the contents of a CMAC memory are most accurately defined in the regions where they are most recently stored. Old data gets hashed over and tends to gradually fade or be "forgotten."

GENERALIZATION IN THE CMAC MEMORY

The fact that each possible CMAC input vector selects a unique *set* of memory locations rather than a single location implies that any particular location may be selected by more than one input vector. In fact, the $S \rightarrow A^*$ mapping insures that any two input vectors which are similar (i.e., close together in input space) will activate many of the same granule cells and hence select many of the same weights. This is what causes CMAC to generalize.

In figure 6.14a the input vector S_2 selects three out of four of the same memory locations as S_1. Thus, the output $h(S_2)$ will be similar to $h(S_1)$, differing only by the contents of the single location which is not in common. The $S \rightarrow A^*$ mapping controls the amount of overlap between sets of selected memory locations such that as the input space distance between two input vectors increases, the amount of overlap decreases. Finally, at some distance the overlap becomes zero (except for random hashing collision) as in figure 6.14b, and the sets of selected memory locations are disjoint. At that point, input S_2 can be said to be outside the neighborhood of generalization of S_1. The value of the output $h(S_2)$ is thus independent of $h(S_1)$.

The extent of the neighborhood of generalization depends upon both the number of elements in the set $|A^*|$ and the resolution of the $s_i \rightarrow m_i^*$ mappings. It is possible in CMAC to make the neighborhood of generalization broad along some

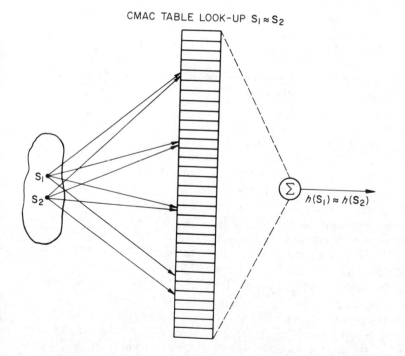

Figure 6.14a: *The CMAC memory generalizes.* S_2 *selects three out of four of the same weights as* S_1. *Thus output* h(S_2) *will be similar to* h(S_1), *differing only by the contents of the location not in common.*

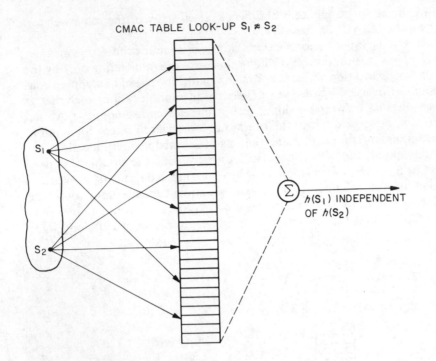

CMAC TABLE LOOK-UP $S_1 \neq S_2$

$h(S_1)$ INDEPENDENT
OF $h(S_2)$

Figure 6.14b: *When* S_2 *is outside of the neighborhood of generalization of* S_1, *the overlap goes to zero (except for random hashing collisions).*

variable axes and limited along others by using different resolution quantizing functions for different input variables. This corresponds to the effect in the cerebellum where some input variables are finely resolved by many mossy fibers and others resolved more coarsely by fewer mossy fibers.

A good example of generalization can be seen in figure 6.12a. Following a single data storage operation at $S_1 = (90,90)$ we find that an input vector $S_2 = (91,90)$ will produce the output $p = 31/32$ even though nothing had ever been explicitly stored at (91,90). This occurs because S_2 selects 31 of the same weights as S_1. A third vector $S_3 = (92,90)$ or a fourth $S_4 = (90,92)$ will produce $p = 30/32$ because of sharing 30 weights with S_1. Not until two input vectors are more than 32 resolution elements apart do they map into disjoint sets of weights.

As a result of generalization, CMAC memory addresses in the same neighborhood are not independent. Data storage at any point alters the values stored at neighboring points. Pulling one point to a particular value as in figure 6.12a produces the effect of stretching a rubber sheet.

Generalization has the advantage that data storage, or training, is not required at every point in the input space in order for an approximately correct response to be obtained. This means that a good first approximation to the correct H function can be stored for a sizable envelope around a T_s trajectory by training at only a few points along that trajectory. For example, figure 6.12c demonstrates that training at only 16 points along the trajectory defined by $s_2 = 90$ generalizes to approximately the correct function for all 360 points along that trajectory plus a great many more points in an envelope around that trajectory. Further training at 175 points scattered over the entire space generalizes to approximately the correct response for all 360×180 (over 64,000) points in the input space as shown in figure 6.12d.

Generalization enables CMAC to predict on the basis of a few representative learning experiences what the appropriate behavioral response should be for similar situations. This is esential in order to cope with the complexities of real world environments where identical T_s trajectories seldom, if ever, reoccur.

THE LEARNING OF BEHAVIOR

An example of how CMAC uses generalization to learn trajectories in a high-dimensional space is shown in figure 6.15. A seven-degrees-of-freedom manipulator arm was controlled by seven CMACs, one for each joint actuator, such that the output vector $P = H(S)$ had seven components. The input vector S to each CMAC contained 18 variables corresponding to position and velocity feedback from each of the seven joints of the arm plus four binary bits defining the Elemental Move Command. The resolution on the feedback variables was different for each of the seven CMACs, being highest from the joint driven by the output p_i and lower for other joints in inverse proportion to their distance along the arm from the controlled joint.

The desired output trajectory $T_{\hat{P}_a}$ is shown as the set of solid curves marked a in figure 6.16. This trajectory corresponds to the Elemental Movement $<\text{SLAP}>$, which is a motion an arm might make in swatting a mosquito.

The (i) curve in figure 6.17 shows the learning performance with no previous learning over 20 complete $T_{\hat{P}_a}$ "slap" motions. At the beginning of each motion the arm was positioned at the correct starting point and driven from there by the P output computed by the CMAC H function. Differences between $\hat{P}$ and P at 20 points along the slap trajectory were corrected (with g set to 1/20). Each point on the curves in figure 6.17 represents the sum of all the errors for all the joints during an entire slap motion. Note that learning is rapid despite the high-dimensional input space in which no two T_s trajectories were ever exactly the same. This is due to CMAC's ability to generalize from a relatively small number of specific teaching experiences to a large number of similar but not identical trajectories.

The (ii) curve in figure 6.17 shows the learning performance on the same 20 $T_{\hat{P}_a}$ trajectories when preceded by 20 training sessions on the $T_{\hat{P}_b}$ trajectory indicated by the dotted set of curves marked b in figure 6.16. Note that performance on $T_{\hat{P}_a}$ is consistently better following prior learning on a similar trajectory $T_{\hat{P}_b}$. This shows that the learning on $T_{\hat{P}_b}$ generalizes to the similar trajectory $T_{\hat{P}_a}$.

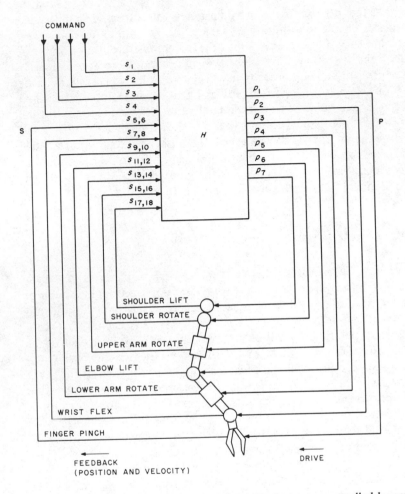

Figure 6.15: *Information flow diagram for a robot arm controlled by seven CMACs.*

Needless to say, predictions based on generalization are not always correct and sometimes need to be refined by further learning. The ability of CMAC to discriminate (i.e., to produce different outputs for different inputs, S_1 and S_2,) depends upon how many weights selected by S_1 are *not* also selected by S_2, and how different in value those weights are. If two inputs which are close together in input space are desired to produce significantly different outputs, then repeated training may be required to overcome the (in this case erroneous) tendency of CMAC to generalize by building up large differences in the few weights not in common.

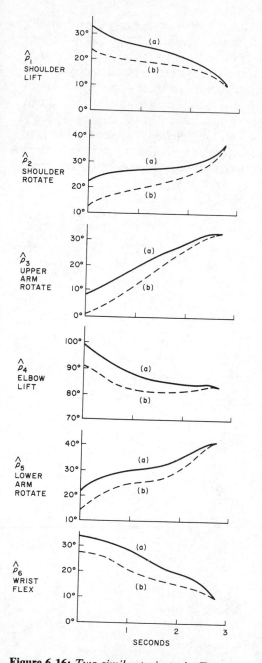

Figure 6.16: *Two similar trajectories* $\mathbf{T}_{\hat{P}_a}$ *and* $\mathbf{T}_{\hat{P}_b}$ *which have different starting points but the same endpoint. Both trajectories define a version of an Elemental Movement* <SLAP> *which was taught to the CMACs of figure 6.15.*

In most behavioral control situations, sharp discontinuities requiring radically different outputs for highly similar inputs do not occur. Indeed, most servo-control functions have simple S-shaped characteristics along each variable axis. The complexity in control computation in multivariant servo systems typically derives from cross-products which affect the slope of the function or produce skewness, and non-symmetrical hills and valleys in various corners of the N-dimensional space. As can be seen from figure 6.11, these are the type of functions CMAC can readily store and hence compute. Nevertheless, even on smooth functions, generalization may sometimes introduce errors by altering values stored at neighboring locations which were already correct. This type of error corresponds to what psychologists call learning interference, or retroactive inhibition.

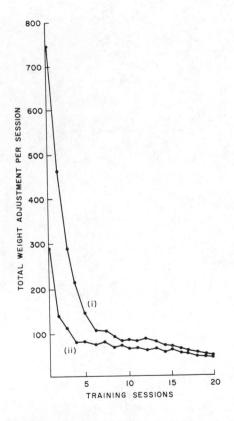

Figure 6.17: *CMAC learning and generalization performance on the $<SLAP>$ motion $T_{\hat{p}_a}$. Curve* i *is with no previous training. Curve* ii *is after 20 training sessions on the similar trajectory* $T_{\hat{p}_b}$. *The improvement of* ii *over* i *is due to generalization.*

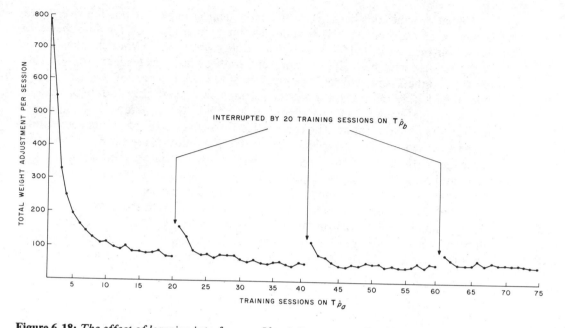

Figure 6.18: *The effect of learning interference. If training on* $T_{\hat{P}_a}$ *is interrupted by training on the similar trajectory* $T_{\hat{P}_b}$, *a degradation in performance on* $T_{\hat{P}_a}$ *is observed. Repeated iterations gradually overcome this learning interference.*

For example, in the learning of the two similar trajectories in figure 6.16, training on $T_{\hat{P}_b}$ causes degradation or interference with what was previously learned on $T_{\hat{P}_a}$. This can be seen in figure 6.18 where after 20 training sessions on $T_{\hat{P}_a}$, the CMAC is trained 20 sessions on $T_{\hat{P}_b}$. Following this, the performance on $T_{\hat{P}_a}$ is degraded. However, the error rate on $T_{\hat{P}_a}$ quickly improves over another 20 training sessions. Following this, another 20 training sessions are conducted on $T_{\hat{P}_b}$. Again, degradation in $T_{\hat{P}_a}$ due to learning interference occurs, but not as severely as before. Another set of 20 training sessions on $T_{\hat{P}_a}$ followed by another 20 on $T_{\hat{P}_b}$ shows that the amount of learning interference is declining due to the buildup of values in the few weights which are not common to both $T_{\hat{P}_a}$ and $T_{\hat{P}_b}$. Thus, learning interference, or retroactive inhibition, is overcome by iterative repetition of the learning process.

The type of learning thus described might be called learning by error correction. In this case, the H function is learned by comparing its output with a desired result. When the behavior produced is correct, no change is made. When the behavior produced deviates from the ideal, changes are made in synaptic strengths to move the output toward the ideal. Learning by error correction requires the existence of an ideal vector $\hat{P}$ which traces out an ideal trajectory $T_{\hat{P}}$.

What provides this ideal vector in a biological system? One possibility is the existence of an external teacher. In many learning situations we have a teacher who, like a golf instructor, tells us what we are doing wrong: hold your shoulder down, keep your arm straight, lean over more, etc. In these cases the teacher provides the $\hat{\mathbf{P}}$ vectors and the $\mathbf{T}_{\hat{P}}$ trajectories. The promise of reward or threat of punishment provides the alerting motivation to set the learning gain coefficient to a high value.

A simple example of this type of learning is the programming of a first-generation industrial robot. The robot is led through a series of points corresponding to a desired trajectory $\mathbf{T}_{\hat{P}}$, and a set of selected points is recorded. This training procedure defines an H function on a two-dimension space where $s_1 =$ the task name and $s_2 =$ the program step counter. H is defined such that $P = \hat{P}$ at every point in the table defining the space as shown in figure 6.19.

Even if we assume an external teacher, however, there is still a problem of how the individual components of the $\hat{\mathbf{P}}$ vectors could be generated in the brain. The simplest case to understand is the storage of $\mathbf{R}$ vectors in the M modules. The M modules record memories of events that occur in the sensory data stream. This is

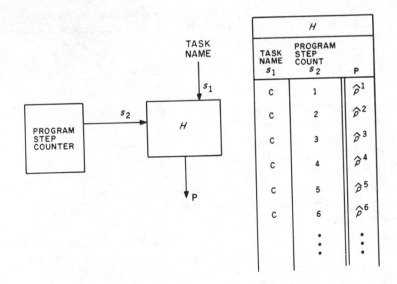

Figure 6.19: *A simple controller for an industrial robot. Input s_1 defines the name of a task, and input s_2 defines the step in the task. The H function is defined by the table. For every set of inputs (s_1, s_2) there is some point to which the robot should go. The entire set of points in the order defined constitutes the robot's programmed trajectory. The robot is taught by leading it through a desired trajectory $\mathbf{T}_{\hat{P}}$ defined by the set of desired points $\hat{p}_i$ and recording them.*

represented by the **E** vectors and the T_E trajectories. Thus, the **E** vector can provide the $\hat{\mathbf{R}}$ teacher for the learning that takes place in the M modules as shown in figure 6.20. Memories of past experiences **E** are recorded in the M modules as $\hat{\mathbf{R}}$ vectors. Errors in recalled **R** vectors are corrected by repeated learning experiences.

Learning in the M modules can be rapid and precise. Often a single learning experience is sufficient to remember a lengthy and detailed record of a complex experience. Repeated learning experiences refine what is stored in the manner suggested by figures 6.17 and 6.18. Memories of sensory experiences are addressed by the state of the brain and particularly by the state of the behavior-generating hierarchy that existed when the memory was stored. Learning interference is dependent upon the degree of similarity between the states of the brain during two learning experiences.

For the H function in the behavior-generating hierarchy, on the other hand, there is no readily discernible internal mechanism that can provide the $\hat{\mathbf{P}}$ vectors and the $T_{\hat{P}}$ trajectories for error-correction learning. How is it, then, that the learning takes place in the H modules so that input command can produce strings of outputs strung together in such a way that skilled movements result?

One possible mechanism for training the H modules is instrumental conditioning, the type of learning which is most closely associated with B.F. Skinner. In this kind of learning there is no example: the teacher gives no information as to what should be done, what the error is, or what should be done to correct it. The teacher (or the contingencies of the environment) simply rewards whatever behavior is desirable or successful when it occurs and punishes whatever behavior is undesirable

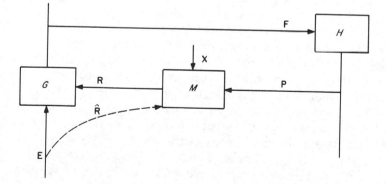

Figure 6.20: *Learning in the* M *modules is accomplished by using the observed experience vector* **E** *as the desired output* $\hat{\mathbf{R}}$ *of the* M *module. Thus, memories of experiences are stored on addresses provided by the action decomposition vector* **P** *plus the whole brain context vector* **X**. *Recall of the stored experience is most precise when the* **P** + **X** *vector is the same as when the experience was stored.*

or unsuccessful when it occurs. There may be additional information conveyed by the intensity of the reward or punishment indicating how good or how bad the results are, but nothing more.

In terms of the CMAC model, instrumental conditioning can be explained in the following way: if a **P** vector occurs just prior to a reward, all the weights contributing to it will be strengthened; if a **P** vector occurs just prior to a punishment, all the weights contributing to it will be reduced. One of the principal characteristics of instrumental conditioning is that learning never stops. Even after a behavior pattern is fully learned, it is reinforced every time it is performed. This must eventually drive the weights into saturation. Thus, the **P** vectors produced by instrumental conditioning eventually become binary all-or-none vectors.

There is, of course, evidence that saturation does occur in the learning of behavior patterns. Habit, addiction, and compulsive behavior are all symptoms of saturation. Virtually all self-rewarding behavior patterns from sex to eating chocolate bon-bons are habit-forming, and except for the mechanism of satiety, would rapidly progress to the saturation state of addiction.

Saturated binary **P** vectors are adequate at the levels of the brain where yes–no decisions are being made: <GO LEFT>, <TURN RIGHT>, <PRESS THE LEVER>, <SIT>, <JUMP>, <FIGHT>, <FLEE>. However, binary **P** vectors are not in themselves adequate for telling how far right or left to turn, how hard to press the lever, or how high to jump. A multiplicity of binary **P** vectors, each with a different threshold, might produce the effect of a smoothly graded response, but the mechanisms of how this would work do not spring immediately to mind.

In order to produce skilled dexterous behavior, the higher levels must not only select the proper behavioral patterns, but the lower levels must learn the proper amount of force to apply to the legs in a jump, the proper angle to set the wings while landing on a branch, etc. It is difficult to see how these features of the *H* functions could be learned by the instrumental conditioning method alone. These are the type of graded responses that must be learned by error correction.

In lower level learning, we may assume that the selection of a goal vector has already taken place. The learning problem, then, is to produce the proper output in response to the goal vector input to produce the correctly modulated action. This might be accomplished by a series of successive approximations. Assume, for example, that the process starts with massive and effortful motions, involving much if not all of the relevant musculature. In many cases, such as in the learning of a manipulatory task, the initial stage of acquiring a complex skilled movement relies heavily on feedback from the eyes. Corrections are made as a result of visually perceived deviations of the limb from the target. As a skill is learned, the amount of effort involved gradually decreases. The unneccessary muscle contractions are reduced, and the amount of concentration of all the body's sensory feedback systems is also reduced. Eventually, the visual system is used only to select the target and intialize motion. The rest of the action can be carried out under proprioceptive feedback guidance.

This suggests that the learning of lower level skills in the H modules may occur by making all the outputs fire when an unlearned input command first occurs, and then finding out by trial and error which outputs improve performance by being reduced in value. This also suggests that the M modules in the vision system may have first stored an example of how an action of the arm or leg should look, and that the sensory-processing system has available some mechanism for evaluating how well the visual observation compares with the ideal. Thus, the M modules of one modality, such as vision, may store ideal sensory trajectories and teach the H modules of another modality, such as a limb, to produce actions that result in sensory observations that match the stored ideals.

This is a form of error-correction learning. However, it does not necessarily require that the sensory system produce $\hat{P}$ vectors for training the H modules. In this type of learning, we can assume the sensory modules can only detect whether the results are good or bad and by how much. They don't need to have a way of computing which neurons in the H modules are firing too fast and which are firing too slow. Thus, the sensory system of vision can only provide instrumental conditoning reinforcement signals to the H modules of the limb, and if these signals are primarily negative reinforcers upon the detection of errors, the learning process will terminate when the errors are reduced to zero. This prevents the saturation effects which are otherwise associated with instrumental conditioning.

Even at the higher levels, however, instrumental conditioning would not work without the assumption of a hierarchy. This is because the reinforcing signal usually comes only at the end of a lengthy and complex sequence. For example, in figure 6.21, we see diagrammed the set of trajectories generated by the actions of a cat, which upon seeing a wind-up toy mouse, pursues it, captures it, and only then learns that it is not a real mouse. The disappointment is a negative reinforcement. If there were no hierarchy, the negative reinforcement would be applied only to the set of synapses involved in the capture phase of the activity. In this case, the cat would never learn to ignore the fake mouse. This is because the set of synapses that are active during the capture phase are different from the set which are active in the goal-selection process. Even if the negative reinforcement were applied to every action over the entire <HUNT> task, then all the activities such as <TRACK> and <PURSUE> which occurred during the <HUNT> activity would be inhibited indiscriminately.

However, if the activity is generated in a hierarchy, there can be different time constants for reinforcement at the different levels. A long time constant at the higher level will cause the discovery of the fake to affect the set of weights which are active when the goal <HUNT> is selected. At this level the weights generating the <HUNT> action are activated during the entire <HUNT> sequence. Therefore, the corresponding synapses are well marked by actually being active when the reinforcing signal is received. These same synapses will again be active the next time the mouse runs. A short time constant at the lower level will leave the <TRACK> and <PURSUE> subgoals unaffected. The learning of the proper behaviorial response

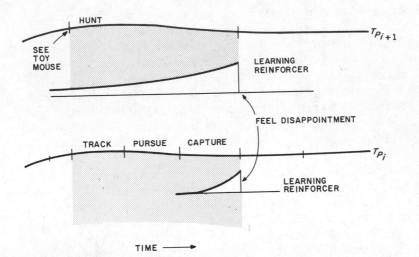

Figure 6.21: *A pair of trajectories generated in the behavior of a cat upon being fooled by a wind-up toy mouse. The cat tracks, pursues, and captures it, only then to learn that it is not a real mouse. This diagram illustrates how the cat can learn not to pursue a toy mouse even though the reinforcer occurred during the capture phase, and not immediately following the pursuit phase. Explanation is in text. Learning occurs at many different levels in the hierarchy. At all levels, learning works by storing what just occurred in the recent past. Memory storage is accomplished by altering synaptic sites that were active shortly before the storage signal, or learning reinforcer, occurred. Different levels have different time constants. At higher levels, the time rate of change of behavior and sensory vectors is slower. Thus, the learning reinforcer at higher levels can operate over longer time intervals. Learning of high-level behavioral patterns can therefore be effective even when reinforcement occurs after a lengthy delay.*

for the real and fake mouse is made at the higher level on the set of synapses that are different in the real and fake situations. Those evoked only by the real mouse are increased by the reward of capturing the prey. Those evoked only by the fake mouse are decreased by the disappointment of capturing a fake. Thus, the cat quickly learns to select the <HUNT> goal only in the case of the real mouse.

This, of course, assumes that the cat can distinguish between the real and the fake. In learning situations where there is no distinguishable difference between stimuli leading to reward and punishment, the subject becomes uncertain and incapable of decisive action.

A third kind of learning is stimulus-response, or classical conditioning. This type of learning is most often associated with Pavlov. It consists of the procedure of presenting a conditioned stimulus (CS) such as the ringing of a bell just before an unconditioned stimulus (US) such as the taste of food. The unconditioned stimulus produces an unconditioned response (UR) such as salivation. However, after a sufficient number of trials, the animal learns to associate the bell with the presentation of food and hence to salivate upon hearing the bell before the food is presented. The learned response to the bell is called the conditioned response (CR).

Classical conditioning can occur in the cross-coupled hierarchy by the following sequence: a conditioned stimulus (such as a bell) is recognized, thereby putting the behavior-generating hierarchy into a particular state. This state addresses the M module into which the sensory experience of an unconditoned stimulus (such as the taste of food) is stored. Thus, when the bell is again recognized, the same state is induced in the behavior-generating hierarchy. This again addresses the M module which now contains the memory of food. The recognition of the conditioned stimulus thus creates a state of mind which recalls the image and expectation of food. This, in turn, is injected into the sensory-processing hierarchy where it produces the conditioned response of salivation.

It is assumed here that learning of all types and at all levels works by altering synaptic weights. The reinforcing or error-correction signal arrives after the act takes place and either strengthens or weakens the synapses that took part in generating the action or in experiencing the sensation. This implies that some physical quantity at the synaptic level remembers which synapses were active so that these can be altered by reinforcement. This "short-term memory" may be caused by the presence of the transmitter chemical or some other substance generated by synaptic action. Typically, there is a mechanism which removes the transmitter chemical from the synaptic site after its message is conveyed so that a succession of messages does not lead to a build-up of transmitter chemical and a blurring of the instantaneous value of the messages. The action of this mechanism may be what produces the rapid exponential decay in short-term memory.

In any discussion of learning, it is important to keep in mind that learning is only a part of the story. In many creatures, even in some with very complex behavioral patterns, learning plays little or no role. In insects, fish, reptiles, amphibians, birds, and even to a large extent in mammals, the H, M, and G modules that produce behavior are genetically determined and only partially, if at all, modified by learning. Even in humans, the basic architecture of the brain, the major computational modules, and the wiring diagram of the neuronal pathways are fixed by the DNA code just as are the number of fingers, the position of the eyes, and the shape of the head. This suggests that, at most, learning makes microscopic differences in the detailed interconnections of the synapses. In no case does it drastically alter the basic structure and information flow of the brain. Thus, most of the basic computational functions in the behavior-generating systems may be prewired, particularly at the lower levels, with only minor structural modifications produced by learning.

In one sense, all behavior from instinct to human social and political customs is learned on an evolutionary time scale over many generations through the mechanism of natural selection. Behavior patterns that are successful tend to survive, and those that are unsuccessful die out. For individual creatures of instinct, all of the detailed interconnections that produce behavior are predetermined and fixed. For higher forms, at least some of the predetermined synaptic interconnection patterns are modifiable. Even in humans, there are basic prewired reflexes which form the basic neuronal substrate in which learning takes place. The learning process doesn't begin with a blank slate, but with a set of genetically prewired computing modules that are modifiable in some creatures.

In a hierarchy, learning must begin from the bottom up. In a newborn infant, the neuronal computation centers in the motor hierarchy are defined only by a few basic inborn reflexes, which themselves have developed in the context of the environment of the womb. Somehow a change occurs in the H, M, and G modules so that input commands can produce outputs strung together in such a way that skilled movements result.

Studies in child development indicate that simple motion primitives are learned first. Piaget has categorized the sequence of motor development in children into 11 stages over the first six years. Table I shows the sequential series of motor and perceptual skills that are acquired by a child in sequence as learning and maturation progress. At birth the child exhibits only reflexive grasping and arm-waving. Soon it develops the ability to intentionally control these. At about four months the child can track hand movements with the eyes and shortly thereafter can direct its hand to a target selected by the eyes. Soon thereafter the child learns to manipulate objects and distinguish between the changing shapes projected onto the retina by a rigid object as it is rotated or moved and the changes wrought by the mechanical defor- mation of a plastic object. Primitive movements, which are simple adaptations of prewired reflexes, are learned first. Then sequences of primitives are strung together into elemental movements. Strings of elemental movements are put together into simple skills and strings of simple skills become complex skills, etc. In the early years, instant reinforcement is important because the time constants of the lower levels of the behavioral hierarchy are short. As learning moves to the higher levels, delayed reinforcement is adequate.

A similar progression in language skills can be observed. The newborn infant is born with only the most basic verbal reflexes. At first speech primitives consisting of coos, gurgles, cries, and various phonetic sounds are learned. These are followed by strings of primitives formed into words and then strings of words combined into phrases. At each level, the M modules store sounds from the environment as T_R tra- jectories. Later the behavior-generating system learns to produce verbal outputs which mimic or duplicate these stored trajectories.

This sequence of events has also been demonstrated in birds. Marler, Tamura and Konishi have shown that a young white-crowned sparrow must hear the song of an adult at a particular time during its maturation in order to learn to sing. The young bird does not actually sing until a year after this learning experience. If the bird is deafened after hearing the adult song (i.e., after storage of the song in M) but before hearing itself sing (i.e., before transfer of the memory in M to the behavior in H), the result is the same as if the bird had been deafened at birth. However, once a bird has had an opportunity to compare its own song with the remembered song, it can continue to sing normally even if it is subsequently deafened.

Similarly in human children, the sound of adult speech is heard and remembered and at some future date is reproduced. Children are known to practice making sounds and to repeat phrases to themselves, testing the sounds and matching them to remembered experiences. By this means the child learns pronunciation and acquires not only words and idioms, but also dialects and accents.

This theory of learning assumes that there is some mechanism that has the capacity for measuring the degree of correspondence between the currently observed experience and the recalled memory. This is the function of the G modules, which compare the sensory data stream with the recalled expectations from the M modules. Since this function is a prerequisite to learning we can assume that the G functions are primarily prewired. However, it seems probable that the G functions are also subsequently modified by learning. This could occur by the mechanism of reinforcing the detection of certain features particularly advantageous for distinguishing between situations leading to reward and those leading to punishment.

To a very large extent the process of recognition and perception consists of creating the correct set of hypotheses in the behavior-generating hierarchy that addresses the M modules in a way that generates a set of expectations to match the current sensory data stream. The computation of match, or the filtering of data through a mask provided by the M modules, is a more or less standard type of computation that might well be genetically predetermined. Thus, learning can play some role in the ability of the G functions to extract features but not in the correlation of the **R** vectors with the **E** vectors.

CMAC AS A COMPUTER

The ability of CMAC to store and recall (and hence compute) a general class of multivariant mathematical functions of the form $\mathbf{P} = H(\mathbf{S})$ suggests that a relatively small cluster of neurons might also be able to calculate the type of mathematical functions required for multivariant servos, coordinate transformations, conditional branches, task-decomposition operators, and IF/THEN production rules. These are the types of functions discussed in Chapter 5 that were required for generating goal-directed behavior (i.e., the purposive strings of behavioral patterns such as running, jumping, flying, hunting, fleeing, fighting, and mating which are routinely accomplished with apparent ease by the tiniest rodents, birds, and even insects).

In the case of multivariant servos the **S** vector corresponds to commands plus feedback (i.e., $\mathbf{S} = \mathbf{C} + \mathbf{F}$). For coordinate transformations the **S** vector contains the arguments as well as the variables in the transformation matrix.

TABLE I

Age	Stage	Motor Ability in Human Children
Birth	1.	Purely reflexive grasping and arm-waving
	2.	Repeatable sequences of hand and arm movements
~ 4 months	3.	Eyes track hands
	4.	Hands controlled by eyes. Perceptual constancy of objects under rotation and translation
~ 1 year	5.	Ability to arrange objects in patterns
	6.	First attempts at symbolic representation (drawing pictures)
~ 2.5 years	7.	First ability to identify hidden objects by touch
	8.	Discrimination of topological forms by touch
~ 4 years	9.	Discrimination of Euclidian shapes by touch
	10.	Ability for systematic tactile exploration
~ 6 years	11.	Ability to take account for numbers, order, and distance in tactile input

Eleven distinctly separate hierarchical stages of sensory-motor development in human children between birth and about seven years of age (after Piaget and Inhelder).

Conditional Branching

For example, in order to compute conditional branches, one or more of the input variables in S can be used to select different regions in input space where entirely different functions are stored. Assume that in figure 6.12 a third variable s_3 had been included in the function being stored, with s_3 held constant at $s_3 = 0$ while storing the function $p = \sin x \sin y$. Following that, an entirely different function, say $p = 3x + 5y^2$, could be stored with s_3 held constant at $s_3 = 50$. Since every point in the input space for $s_3 = 0$ is outside the neighborhood of generalization of the input space for $s_3 = 50$, there would be no interference except for random hashing collisions. The stored function would then be

$$p = \sin x \sin y \quad \text{if } s_3 = 0$$
$$p = 3x + 5y^2 \quad \text{if } s_3 = 50$$

In the interval $0 < s_3 < 50$, the function would change smoothly from $p = \sin x \sin y$ to $p = 3x + 5y^2$. Additional functions could be stored for other values of s_3, or other conditional variables s_4, s_5, . . . might be used for additional branching capabilities.

If these conditional variables are part of a command vector, then each different input command can select a different subgoal generator. If they are part of the feedback, then different environmental conditions can trigger different behavioral patterns for accomplishing the subgoals.

Finite-State Automata

If some of the variables in the **P** output vector loop directly back to become part of the **S** input vector (as frequently happens in the cerebellum as well as in other parts of the brain), then CMAC becomes a type of finite-state automaton, string generator, or task-decomposition operator. For example, the CMAC in figure 6.22a behaves like the finite-state automaton in 6.22b. The loop-back inputs s_1 and s_2 define the state of the machine and s_3 is the input. The H function defines the state transition table. In general, it is possible to construct a CMAC equivalent of any finite-state automaton. Of course, CMAC can accept inputs and produce outputs which are non-binary. Furthermore, the outputs generalize. Thus, CMAC is a sort of "fuzzy-state automaton."

a)

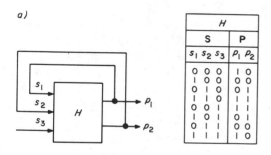

H				
S			P	
s_1	s_2	s_3	p_1	p_2
0	0	0	1	0
1	0	0	0	0
0	1	0	0	1
1	1	0	1	1
0	0	1	1	1
1	0	1	0	1
0	1	1	0	0
1	1	1	1	0

b)

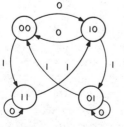

Figure 6.22: *A CMAC with feedback directly from output to input behaves like a finite-state automaton for binary inputs and outputs. It behaves like a "fuzzy-state automaton" for non-binary* **S** *and* **P** *variables.* (s_1, s_2) = *the state;* (p_1, p_2) = *the next-state.*

A CMAC with direct feedback from output to input demonstrates how a neural cluster can generate a string of outputs (subgoals) in response to a single input, or unchanging string of inputs. Additional variables added to **F** from an external source increase the dimensionality of the input space and can thus alter the output string (task decomposition) in response to environmental conditions.

The different possible feedback pathways to a CMAC control module cast light on a long-standing controversy in neurophysiology: are behavioral patterns generated by "stimulus-response chaining" (i.e., a sequence of actions in which feedback from sensory organs is required to step from one action to the next) or by "central patterning" (i.e., a sequence which is generated by internal means alone)? A CMAC hierarchy can include tight feedback loops from the output of one level back to its own input to generate central patterns, and longer internal loops from one level to another to cycle through a sequence of central patterns, as well as feedback from the environment to select or modify central patterns or their sequence in accordance with environmental conditions.

Computing Integrals

Direct feedback from output to input can also be used to compute the integral of a function. If an input carrying feedback from the output is simply added to the other inputs, the resultant function is the integral of the function computed on the non-feedback inputs. This is illustrated in figure 6.23. If the function $p^k = h(s_1^{k-1}, \ldots, s_N^{k-1})$ is computed by the module in figure 6.23a without feedback, then the function $q^k = h(s_1^{k-1}, \ldots, s_N^{k-1}) + q^{k-1}$ computed by the module in figure 6.23b is the integral of p. For example, if an h module computes the function $p = s_1 s_2$, then an h' module computing $q = s_1 s_2 + q$ computes the integral

$$q = \int_{-\infty}^{k} s_1 s_2$$

The ability to compute integrals is extremely important in detection and recognition of time-varying patterns. The integral over a time interval of a name vector will indicate the percentage of time that the pattern vector lies along the trajectory which maps into that name. Thus, for noisy data, the magnitude of the integral of a name vector over some time interval is a much more reliable recognition indicator than the instantaneous value of the name vector itself.

This type of integration is commonly used in electronic equipment such as radar or radio for the detection of weak signals buried in noise. The CMAC model with feedback from the output added to the input illustrates how such integration functions can be performed by a neurological computing module.

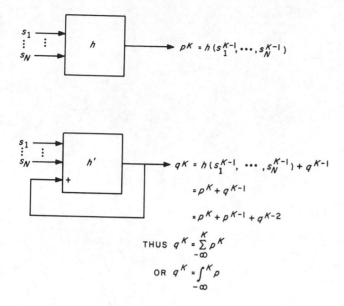

$$q^K = \int_{-\infty}^{K} p$$

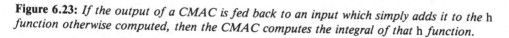

Figure 6.23: *If the output of a CMAC is fed back to an input which simply adds it to the* h *function otherwise computed, then the CMAC computes the integral of that* h *function.*

IF/THEN Productions

The ability of CMAC to compute simple arithmetic functions also suggests how CMAC might implement IF/THEN production rules. If the S vector (or the T_s trajectory) corresponds to a set of conditions making up an IF premise, then the P vector (or T_P trajectory) output is the THEN consequent. We have already shown how symbols can be represented as vectors and vice versa. Thus, the computation of an IF/THEN rule reduces to an arithmetic computation of the form $P = H(S)$.

The capability of CMAC to simulate a finite-state automaton, to execute the equivalent of a conditional branch, and to compute a broad class of multivariant arithmetic and integral functions implies that it is possible to construct a goal-seeking hierarchy of H, M, and G modules using nothing but CMACs. Conversely, it is possible to construct a hierarchy of computing modules, perhaps implemented on a network of microcomputers, which is the equivalent of a CMAC hierarchy. This has profound implications regarding the type of computing architecture which might be used to build a model of the brain for robot control. It suggests how we might structure control systems so as to give robots the skills and intellectual capabilities of biological organisms. We will return to these and other practical issues for robot-control systems in Chapter 9.

CHAPTER **7**

Modeling the Higher Functions

$\mathbf{W}$e have now shown how the Cerebellar Model Arithmetic Computer (CMAC) can compute functions, learn, recognize patterns, and decompose goals. We have also shown how a cross-coupled hierarchy of CMACs (see figure 5.24) can memorize trajectories, generate goal-directed purposive behavior, and store an internal model of the external world in the form of predicted sensory data. We will now attempt to show how this structure and its capabilities can give rise to perceptual and cognitive phenomena.

The fact that the mathematical details of the CMAC model were derived from the cerebellum, a portion of the brain particularly regular in structure and hence uniquely suitable for detailed neurophysiological analysis, does not mean that the results are inapplicable to other regions of the brain as well. The basic structure of a large output cell (sometimes called a principal, relay, or projection neuron) served by a cluster of local interneurons is quite typical throughout the brain. Such clusters commonly receive input from a large number of nonspecific neural fibers similar to the mossy fibers in the cerebellum. In many instances they also receive specific inputs which are more or less analogous to climbing fibers. As we might expect, there are many differences in size and shape of the corresponding cell types from one region of the brain to another. These reflect differences in types of computations being performed and information being processed, as well as differences in the evolutionary history of various regions in the brain. Nevertheless, there are clear regularities in organization and similarities in function from one region to another. This suggests that, at least to a first approximation, the basic processes are similar.

The implication is that the general mode of information processing defined by CMAC (the concept of a set of principal neurons together with their associated interneurons transforming an input vector $\mathbf{S}$ into an output vector $\mathbf{P}$ in accordance with a mathematically definable relationship H) can be useful in analyzing the properties of many different cortical regions and subcortical nuclei. This is particularly true since the accuracy, resolution, rate of learning, and degree of generalization of the CMAC *H* function can be chosen to mimic the neuronal characteristics of different areas in the brain.

It's an old idea that the central nervous system, which generates behavior in biological organisms, is hierarchically structured. The idea dates back considerably more than a century. The analogy is often made to a military command structure, with many hundreds of operational units and thousands, even millions, of individual soldiers coordinated in the execution of complex tasks or goals. In this analogy each computing center in the behavior-generating hierarchy is like a military command post, receiving commands from immediate superiors and issuing sequences of subcommands which carry out those commands to subordinates.

Feedback is provided to each level by a sensory-processing hierarchy that ascends parallel to the behavior-generating hierarchy, and that operates on a data stream derived from sensory units that monitor the external environment as well as from lower level command centers that report on the progress being made in carrying out their subcommands. Feedback is processed at many levels in this ascending hierarchy by intelligence analysis centers that extract data relevant to the command and control function being performed by the behavior-generating module at that level.

Each of these intelligence analysis centers makes predictions based on the results expected (i.e., casualties, rewards, sensory data patterns) because of actions taken. The intelligence centers then interpret the sensory data they receive in the context of these predictions. For example, in the military intelligence analogy, a loss of 60 men in an operation where losses had been predicted at 600 implies an unexpectedly easy success and perhaps indicates a weakness in the enemy position that should be further exploited. In the brain the observation of 60 nerve impulses on an axon where 600 had been anticipated may imply an unexpectedly weak branch in a tree which, if used for support, could result in a fatal fall.

The response of each command post (or data analysis center) in the hierarchy to its input depends on how it has been trained. Basic training teaches each soldier how to do things the "army way" (i.e., what each command means and how it should be carried out). Each operational unit in the military has a field manual that defines the proper or ideal response of that unit to every foreseeable battlefield situation. Each field manual is essentially a set of IF/THEN production rules or case statements, corresponding to a set of CMAC functions, $\mathbf{P} = H(\mathbf{S})$ or $\mathbf{Q} = G(\mathbf{D})$. At the lowest level in the military analogy these rules define the proper procedures for maintaining and operating weapons, as well as the proper behavioral patterns for surviving and carrying out assignments under battlefield conditions. At higher levels they define the proper tactics for executing various kinds of maneuvers. At the highest level, they define the proper strategy for deployment of resources and achievement of objectives.

In the case where each unit carries out its assignment "according to the book," the overall operation runs smoothly and the goal is achieved on schedule as expected. To the extent that various units do not follow their ideal trajectories, either because of improper training or because of unforeseen difficulties in the environment, the operation will deviate from the expected or planned schedule. Alternate tactics might be required. If a change in tactics still does not produce success, new strategies may be required. Of course, there is always the possibility that failure will occur, despite every effort. The goal will not be achieved or, worse yet, the organism may suffer a catastrophic setback.

There is considerable anatomical, neurophysiological, and behavioral evidence that the analogy between the brain and a military hierarchy is quite accurate. However, in saying this, it is important to keep in mind that the highly schematic hierarchy shown in figure 5.24 is a grossly oversimplified diagram of the vast interconnected hierarchical network—the brain. Figure 5.24 represents only a single chain of command from a single motor neuron up to a high-level command module. Every motor neuron in the nervous system can be thought of as being controlled by its own hierarchy which interweaves and overlaps extensively with the hierarchies of nearby synergistic motor neurons. Each sensory-motor system has its own set of overlapping hierarchies that become increasingly interrelated and interconnected with each other at the higher levels. Thus, the entire brain may have the topological shape of an inverted paraboloid as shown in figure 7.1.

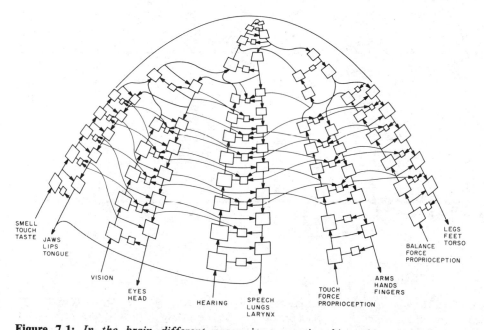

Figure 7.1: *In the brain different processing-generating hierarchies represent different sensory-motor systems. These become increasingly interrelated at the higher levels and eventually merge into a unified command and control structure. This enables a complex organism to coordinate its actions in pursuit of high-level goals.*

TRIUNE BRAIN HYPOTHESIS

There is, in fact, some evidence to suggest that the human brain is topologically similar to three (or more) concentric paraboloid hierarchies as illustrated in figure 7.2. Paul MacLean and others have hypothesized a triune brain wherein the inner

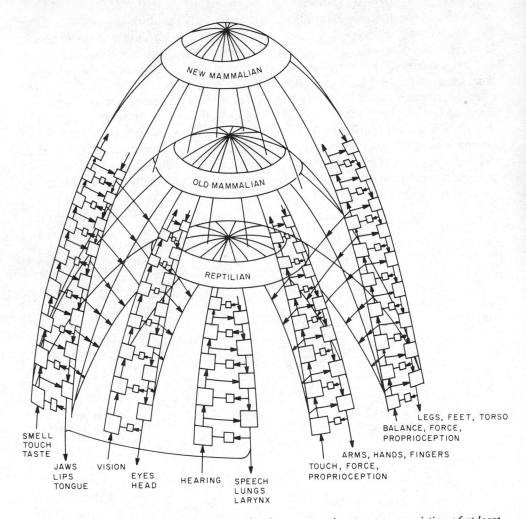

Figure 7.2: *The human brain is hypothesized to be a composite structure consisting of at least three layers: (1) a reptilian brain which provides basic reflexes and instinctive responses; (2) an old mammalian brain which is more sophisticated and capable of emotions and delayed responses; and (3) a new mammalian brain which can imagine, plan, and manipulate abstract symbols. The outer layers inhibit and modulate the more primitive tendencies of the inner layers.*

core is a primitive structure (i.e., the reptilian brain) which provides vital functions such as breathing and basic reflexive or instinctive responses such as eating, fighting, fleeing, and reproductive activities. Superimposed on this inner core is a second layer (i.e., the old mammalian brain) that is capable of more sophisticated sensory analysis and control. This second layer tends to inhibit the simple and direct responses of the first so they can be applied more selectively and responses can be delayed until opportune moments. This second brain thus provides the elements of planning and problem-solving, prediction, expectation, emotional evaluation, and delayed response to stimuli that have disappeared from direct observation. These are the characteristics of behavior which make possible the complex hunting strategies and social interactions of the mammals.

On top of this is yet a third layer (i.e., the new mammalian brain) which possesses the capacity to manipulate the other two layers in extremely subtle ways: to conceive elaborate plans, to imagine the unseen, to scheme and connive, to generate and recognize signs and symbols, to speak and understand what is spoken.

The outer layers employ much more sophisticated sensory analysis and control algorithms that detect greater subtleties and make more complex decisions than the inner more primitive layers are capable of performing. Under normal conditions the outer layers modify, modulate, and sometimes even reverse the sense of the more primitive responses of the inner layers. However, during periods of stress, the highly sophisticated outer layers may encounter computational overload and become confused or panicked. When this happens, the inner core hierarchy may be released from inhibition and execute one of the primitive survival procedures stored in it (i.e., fight, flee, or freeze). A similar takeover by the inner hierarchy can occur if the more delicate circuitry of the outer is disrupted by physical injury or other trauma. Thus the brain uses its redundancy to increase reliability in a hostile environment.

Of course, all three layers of the behavior-generating hierarchy come together at the bottom level in the motor neurons—the final common pathway.

MOTOR-GENERATING HIERARCHIES IN THE BRAIN

In the military hierarchy analogy, the motor neurons are the foot soldiers. They actually drive the muscles and glands to produce action. Their output firing rate defines the output trajectory of the behavior-generating hierarchy. A CMAC representing a spinal motor neuron and its associated interneurons receives commands C from higher motor centers as well as feedback F from stretch receptors and tendon organs via the dorsal roots. Additional components of the F vector come from other motor neurons reporting ongoing activity in related muscles. Components of the command vector to this lowest level come from the vestibular system, which provides inertial reference signals necessary for posture and balance. Other components of C come from the reticular formation, the red nucleus, and in primates, also directly from the motor cortex. A more detailed description of the actions of this lowest level motor computational center is contained in the section on the stretch reflex in Chapter 4. See particularly figures 4.6 through 4.9.

There is nothing analogous to climbing fibers for the motor neurons, but this is not surprising since there is evidence that little or no learning takes place at this first level in the behavior-generating hierarchy.

Much of the vestibular system input passes through, or is modulated by, the cerebellum, which receives feedback from joint position sensors, tendon tension sensors, and skin touch sensors. Thus, parts of the cerebellum, together with the primary motor cortex, the red nucleus, and the reticular formation represent a second level in the motor hierarchy.

The second level of the new mammalian motor hierarchy includes some neurons in the cortex. The motor cortex contribution to the second level has been called the transcortical servo-loop by Phillips. Evarts and Tanji have observed cells in the motor cortex whose response P to a stretch stimulus F can be altered (indeed completely reversed) by different command inputs C. As shown in figure 7.3, an experimental animal was trained to pull a lever upon feeling a jerk if a red light preceded the stimulus and push the lever if a green light preceded the stimulus. Both the command C (low firing rate = red, high = green) and the altered response P (pull if C = low, push if C = high) are observed. There is a measurable time delay which clearly separates the effect of feedback to the lowest level (10-20 milliseconds), feedback to the second level (30-50 milliseconds), and changes in command inputs to the second level (100-200 milliseconds).

Other experiments by Evarts and Thach have shown that neurons in the cerebellum, thalamus, and motor cortex alter their firing rates at various intervals prior to learned movements, and well in advance of any response feedback. This is the propagation of goals and subgoals down the motor hierarchy as the various levels receive commands and issue subcommands in preparation for the initiation of a task.

Further evidence that hierarchical structures exist and function as AND/OR task-decomposition operators in the generation and control of motor behavior can be found in almost any neurophysiological textbook. For example, brain stem transection experiments with animals and observations of injured humans where the spinal cord is severed at different levels have demonstrated a consistent hierarchical structuring of the sensory-motor system. If, as is shown in figure 7.4, the cord is severed from the brain along the line A-A, most of the basic motor patterns such as the flexor reflex and the reflexes that control the basic rhythm and patterns of locomotion remain intact. However, coordinated activation of these patterns to stand up and support the body against gravity requires that the regions below B-B be intact.

The stringing together of different postures to permit walking and turning movements requires the regions below C-C to be undamaged. In particular it is known that the rotational movements of the head and eyes are generated in the in-

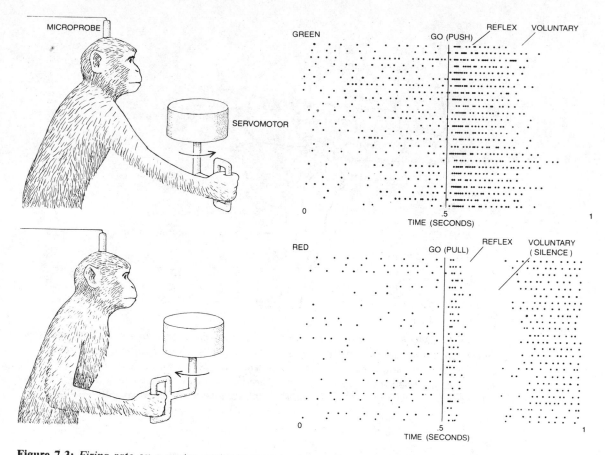

Figure 7.3: *Firing rate on a motor-cortex neuron in an experiment designed to examine the relation between voluntary and reflex responses. A red or green "get-set" light was turned on from 1-5 s before a "go" signal, a mechanical displacement of the handle from its neutral position. The change in firing rate in response to the get-set signals required about 200 ms to appear. Within about 10 ms of the "go" signal, a reflex response to the mechanical displacement can be seen. After about 40 ms, the voluntary response of push (increase firing) or pull (stop firing) can be seen to appear. The silence at the top far right and the activity at the bottom far right are due to the subject returning the handle to neutral after pushing (top) or pulling (bottom).* [From "Brain Mechanisms of Movement," by E. V. Evarts. Copyright © 1979 by Scientific American, Inc. All rights reserved.]

terstitial nucleus; the raising and lowering of the head in the prestitial nucleus; and the flexing movements of the head and body in the nucleus precommissuralis. Stimulation of the subthalamic nuclei can cause rhythmic motions including walking. A cat with its brain sectioned along C-C can walk almost normally. However, it cannot vary its walking patterns to avoid obstacles.

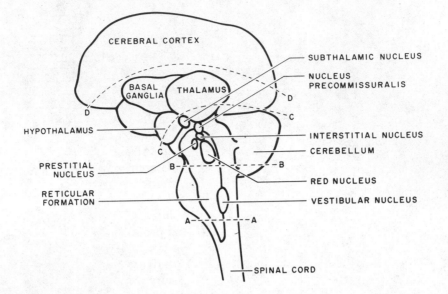

Figure 7.4: *The hierarchy of motor control that exists in the extrapyramidal motor system. Basic reflexes remain even if the brain stem is cut at A-A. Coordination of these reflexes for standing is possible if the cut is at B-B. The sequential coordination required for walking requires the area below C-C to be operable. Simple tasks can be executed if the region below D-D is intact. Lengthy tasks and complex goals require the cerebral cortex.*

Animals whose brains are cut along the line D-D can walk, avoid obstacles, eat, fight, and carry on normal sexual activities. However, they lack purposiveness. They cannot execute lengthy tasks or goals. Humans with brain disease in the basal ganglia might perform an apparently normal pattern of movements for a few seconds and then abruptly switch to a different pattern, and then another. One form of this disease is called St. Vitus' dance.

Higher levels of the behavior-generating hierarchy become increasingly difficult to identify and localize, but there is much to indicate that many additional levels exist in the cerebral cortex. For example, the motor cortex appears to be responsible for initiating commands for complex tasks. The ability to organize lengthy sequences of tasks, such as the ability to arrange words into a coherent thought or to recall the memory of a lengthy past experience, seems to reside in the posterior temporal lobe. Interactions between emotions and intentional behavior appear to take place in the mediobasal cortex, and long term plans and goals are believed to derive from activity in the frontal cortex. Hierarchies of different systems (i.e., vision, hearing, manipulation, and locomotion) merge together in the association areas.

SENSORY-PROCESSING HIERARCHIES IN THE BRAIN

It is a well-established fact that hierarchies of sensory-processing modules exist in the brain. In a famous series of experiments, Hubel and Wiesel demonstrated four clearly distinguishable hierarchical levels in the visual system. Similar sensory-processing hierarchies have been extensively studied in the auditory system and in the proprioceptive and kinesthetic pathways. Cross-coupling from these ascending hierarchies of sensory-processing modules to the motor-generating hierarchies provides the many different levels of sensory feedback information required at the various stages of the task or goal-decomposition process. At each level, output vectors from the previous level of the sensory-processing hierarchy provide inputs to the next higher level, as well as feedback to the same level of the behavior-generating hierarchy.

In the case of vision, the two-dimensional nature of input from the surface of the retina causes the computational modules in the visual processing system to be organized in sheets. This implies that a CMAC model of a typical level in the visual processing hierarchy would resemble the structure shown in figure 7.5. In this structure the sensory input D_1 might consist of a pattern of sensory variables E_1 defining

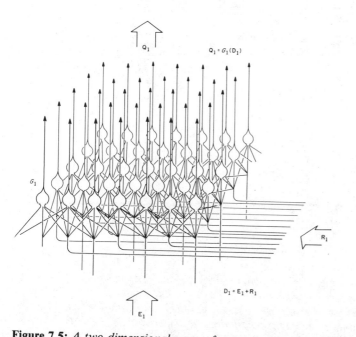

Q_1

$Q_1 = G_1(D_1)$

G_1

R_1

$D_1 = E_1 + R_1$

E_1

Figure 7.5: *A two-dimensional array of sensory-processing CMACs such as might exist in the visual system. The observed sensory image E_1 plus the prediction vector R_1 enters and is recognized by the operator G_1 as a pattern. The vector R_1 may select one of many filter functions or provide an expected image or map to be compared against the observed image.*

light intensity (perhaps in a particular color band) together with predicted variables $\mathbf{R}_1$ which select a particular filter function. The output $\mathbf{Q}_1 = G_1(\mathbf{D}_1)$ then might define a pattern of edges or line segments. This output forms part of the input $\mathbf{E}_2$ to the second level. Output from the second level $\mathbf{Q}_2 = G_2(\mathbf{D}_2)$, might define patterns of connected regions or segments.

Recent work by David Marr at the Massachusetts Institute of Technology and Jay Tennenbaum at SRI International suggests that the output vectors $\mathbf{Q}_i$ at various levels may define more than one type of feature. For example, a single level in the visual-processing system might contain a depth image (derived from stereo disparity, light gradients, local edge-interaction cues, etc.), a velocity image (derived from motion detectors), and an outline-drawing image (derived from edge detectors, line, and corner finders) in addition to brightness, color, and texture images of the visual field as shown in figure 7.6. These and many other kinds of information appear to

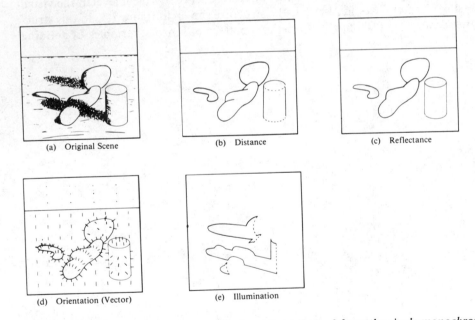

Figure 7.6: *A set of intrinsic images (b) through (e) derived from the single monochrome intensity image (a). The images are depicted as line drawings, but, in fact, contain values at every point. The solid lines in the intrinsic images represent discontinuities in the scene characteristic; the dashed lines represent discontinuities in its derivative. The distance image (b) gives the range along the line of sight to each visible point in the scene. The reflection image (c) gives the ratio of reflected light to illumination at every point. The orientation image (d) gives a vector representing the direction of the surface normal at every point. The illumination image (e) gives the amount of light falling on the scene at every point.*

exist in registration at several different levels of the visual-information-processing hierarchy—as shown in figure 7.7—so as to make possible the extremely sophisticated visual recognition tasks which our brains routinely perform. These different types of images interact, sometimes reinforcing each other to confirm a recognition and sometimes contradicting each other to reject one possible interpretation of the visual input in favor of another.

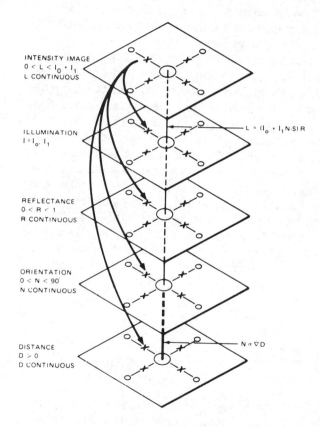

Figure 7.7: *The various intrinsic images can be developed at various hierarchical levels and brought into registration for sophisticated parallel computations related to image understanding.*

CROSS-COUPLING

Cross links from the descending hierarchies of motor-generating modules provide the many different levels of contextual and predictive information required at various stages of the pattern-recognition or sensory-analysis process. In the visual hierarchy, as well as in all other sensory-processing hierarchies, context variables $\mathbf{R}_i$ may define expected values of the $\mathbf{E}_i$ vectors. This implies that the addresses $\mathbf{P}_i$ and $\mathbf{X}_i$ have stored data from previous experiences when what is currently recalled as $\mathbf{R}_i$ was experienced as $\mathbf{E}_i$. In this case the recalled context $\mathbf{R}_i$ is essentially a stored image, or map, which is accessed by an associative address created by the behavior-generating hierarchy being in a state more or less similar to that which existed when the remembered experience (i.e., the map) was stored.

This implies that the sensory data processing hierarchy is a multilevel map (or template) matching process, and that in order to generate these maps the behavior-generating side of the cross-coupled hierarchy must be put into a state (or pulled along a trajectory) similar to that which existed when the template was recorded.

When this occurs, the interaction around the loop formed by the G_i, H_i, and M_i modules at each level is similar to a phase-lock loop, or a relaxation process. The data $\mathbf{E}_i$ enters the module G_i which recognizes it to be in a certain class $\mathbf{Q}_i$ with perhaps an error of $\mathbf{F}_i$. The recognition $\mathbf{Q}_i$ triggers an appropriate goal-decomposition (or subgoal selection) function in the H_{i+1} (or higher) modules which generates a command (or hypothesis) $\mathbf{C}_i$. This command, modified by the error $\mathbf{F}_i$, generates a subcommand (or subhypothesis) $\mathbf{P}_i$ and hence a predicted data vector $\mathbf{R}_i$. The prediction $\mathbf{R}_i$ may confirm the preliminary recognition $\mathbf{Q}_i$ and pull the context $\mathbf{P}_i$ into a more exact prediction via the feedback loop involving $\mathbf{F}_i$. Alternatively, the prediction $\mathbf{R}_i$ may cause G_i to alter or abandon the recognition $\mathbf{Q}_i$ in favor of another recognition $\mathbf{Q}_i'$.

LOOPS AND RHYTHMS

Obviously such looping interactions involve timing and phase relationships which may themselves have information content. Many sensory data patterns, especially in the auditory, visual, and kinesthetic pathways, are time dependent and involve some form of rhythmic or harmonic temporal patterns as well as spatial relationships.

As was discussed earlier, temporal patterns at various levels correspond to trajectories with different time rates of change, and hence (assuming approximately the same information content stored as trajectories at each level) different periods or complete rhythmical patterns. For example, at the lowest level of the auditory system, cochlear hair cells are excited by mechanical and electrical stimuli with frequencies ranging from about 20 Hz to 20,000 Hz. These sensory inputs thus have periodicities from 0.00005 to 0.05 seconds.

The highest frequency a nerve axon can transmit is about 500 Hz, but the brain handles higher frequencies in a manner somewhat reminiscent of the cerebellum's encoding of precise position. It encodes pieces of information about the phase of a wavefront on a number of different fibers. (See figure 3.27.) This means that by knowing which fibers are firing in which combinations at which instants, one can compute not only what is the fundamental pitch of the temporal pattern but what are all of its overtones. Thus, the CMAC G function at the lowest level (or really the loop comprised of the lowest level G, H, and M modules) can compute the Fourier transform, or the autocorrelation function, and presumably even the Bessel function describing the modes of vibration of the cochlear membrane.

Assume, for example, that the G, H, and M modules in figure 7.8 constitute a phase-lock loop such that the input PATTERN is a signal $f(t)$ and the PREDICTION is another signal $F(t - \tau)$. If the processing module G computes the integral

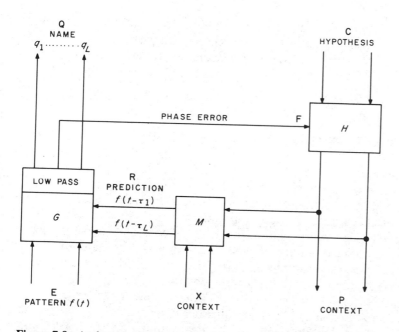

Figure 7.8: *A phase-lock loop consisting of a* G, H, *and* M *module. If the* H *and* M *modules produce a set of signals with nearly the same periodicity as the incoming signal* **E**, *the* G *function can compute a phase error signal* **F** *which pulls the* **R** *prediction into lock with the* **E** *observation. The* G *module can then also compute an autocorrelation function which gives a perception of pitch.*

of the product of the PATTERN · PREDICTION, then the output NAME is $\int f(t) \cdot f(t - \tau)$. When τ corresponds to 1/4 of the period of the input $f(t)$, the integral of the output will produce a phase ERROR signal which, when applied to the H module, can enable the PREDICTION signal $f(t - \tau)$ to track and lock onto the input PATTERN $f(t)$. If the loop consists of a multiplicity of pathways with different delays ($\tau > 0$), the output, when integrated, will produce an autocorrelation function

$$\phi_{ff}(\tau) = \lim_{T \to \infty} \frac{1}{2T} \int_{-T}^{T} f(t) \cdot f(t - \tau)\, dt$$

such that

$$Q = \begin{cases} q_1 = \phi_{ff}(\tau_1) \\ q_2 = \phi_{ff}(\tau_2) \\ \cdot \\ \cdot \\ \cdot \\ q_L = \phi_{ff}(\tau_L) \end{cases}$$

where $0 < \tau_1 < \tau_2 < \cdots < \tau_L$

It has been shown that such an autocorrelation function produces a perception of pitch which is in good agreement with psychophysical data. In figure 7.8 the presence of an output on element q_i would correspond to the perception of pitch at a frequency of $1/\tau_i$.

LOCKED LOOPS AND UNDERSTANDING

Figure 7.9 suggests how a hierarchy of phase locked loops might interact to recognize the variety of periodicities which provide the information content in spoken language and music. The coefficients q_i obtained from the lowest level loop form the input (together with other variables) to the second level.

If we assume that the sensory input to the first level consists of a pattern rich in information, such as music or speech, then as time progresses the trajectory of the input vector to the second level will also contain many periodicities. The principal difference from the standpoint of information theory is that the periodicity is now on the order of 0.05 seconds to 0.5 seconds. The trajectory input to the second level can, of course, be subjected to a quite similar mathematical analysis as were the trajectories of hair cell distortions and cochlear electrical stimulation which were input to the first level.

The principal difference is that at the second level and higher, information can be encoded for neural transmission by pulse frequency rather than pulse-phase modulation. Also, some of the mechanisms by which time integrals are computed

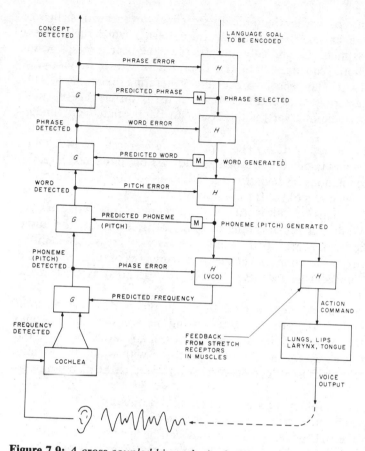

Figure 7.9: *A cross-coupled hierarchy in the hearing-speech system. The generating hierarchy decomposes language goals into strings of verbal output. When speech is being generated, the sensory-processing hierarchy provides feedback to control intensity and modulation. For listening only, the generating hierarchy provides hypotheses and predictions for use in detecting, recognizing, following, and understanding the sensory input.*

may be different. Nevertheless, processing by a CMAC *G* function can transform sections of the input trajectory into output vectors so as, in effect, to give them names. Characteristic patterns, or periodicities, at the second level are named notes when the sensory stimulus is music. When the stimulus is spoken language, they may be called phonemes.

The output of the second level forms part of the input to the third. The *G* function at the third level computes the names of strings of phonemes which it calls words, or strings of notes which it calls tunes. The *G* function at the fourth level computes names of strings of words which it calls sentences (or phrases), strings of tunes which it calls musical passages, etc. In music, the pattern in which the different periodicities match up as multiples and submultiples (i.e., the beat, notes, various voices, melodies, and chord sequences) comprise the inner structure, harmony, or "meaning." The ability of the sensory-processing generating hierarchy of the listener to lock onto the periodicities and harmonies at many different levels (and hence many different periodic intervals) is the ability to "appreciate" or "understand" the music.

Similarly, in speech the ability of the audio-processing hierarchy to lock on to periodicities at each level and to detect or recognize and pass on to the next level the information bearing modulations or deviations in those periodicities constitutes the ability to "understand" what is spoken. If the audio system locks on only at the first level, it detects phonetic sounds but not words. If it locks on the first two levels but no higher, it detects words but not meaningful phrases. If, however, the audio hierarchy locks on at the third, fourth, fifth, and higher levels, there is excited in the mind of the listener many of the same trajectories and sequences of interrelated and harmonious patterns (i.e., goals, hypotheses, sensory experiences) as exist in the mind of the speaker.

This suggests that we can define understanding to be the lock-on phenomenon that occurs at many levels in the processing-generating hierarchy of the one who understands. The depth of understanding depends on how many levels lock onto the sensory data stream, as well as on the degree of precision with which the various hypotheses generated at the different levels can track and predict the incoming sensory data stream.

In general, it is easier to follow a trajectory than to reproduce it. When observing a procedure, the generating hierarchy of the observer merely needs to produce hypotheses that are in the right vicinity so that they can be synchronized with the sensory input. Uncertainties at branch points in T_P do not matter greatly because errors are quickly corrected by comparing T_R with T_E.

On the other hand, reproducing a procedure requires that the H functions be capable of generating T_P trajectories that are precise over their entire length. They must not wander outside of the success envelope or miss any critical branch points. This is a much more exacting computational program. This suggests why a student might be able to follow the reasoning of a professor's lecture, but be unable to reproduce it on an exam. It explains why deep understanding requires drill and practice. Understanding is the product of an intimate interlocking interaction between the sensory-processing and behavior-generating hierarchies at many different levels.

If we define understanding to be the generation of hypotheses that can recall **R** vectors and T_R trajectories that track and predict the incoming sensory data, then a great number of phenomena related to perception become clear. For example, the spontaneous reversal of ambiguous figures, such as the wire-frame Necker cube, the staircase, or the face-goblet figure shown in figures 7.10 through 7.12, can be explained by assuming that each of the two possible interpretations corresponds to a hypothesis that produces **R** vector predictions matching the incoming sensory data. The fact that either hypothesis produces a lock-on makes it possible for the perception of the figure to flip from one interpretation to another. The fact that the two hypotheses are quite different forces the perceptual understanding to make one assumption or the other. The two hypotheses can't exist simultaneously.

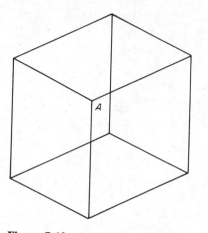

Figure 7.10: *A wire-frame cube is a classic example of perspective reversal. When gazed at steadily, the corner A alternates from outside to inside. Either hypothesis is equally valid, so whichever is chosen will be confirmed.*

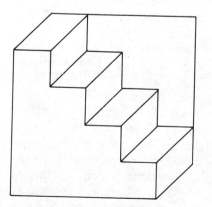

Figure 7.11: *An ambiguous staircase. The staircase appears to either sit on the floor or hang from the ceiling, depending on which internal mental hypothesis is chosen.*

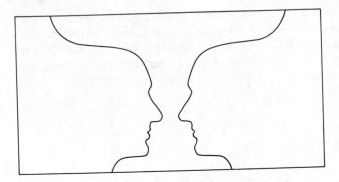

Figure 7.12: *This figure may be either a goblet or two faces staring at each other. Again, what is perceived depends upon what is hypothesized. Either of the two hypotheses will be confirmed by the sensory input.*

The creation of an expectation by a hypothesis is also what generates the subjective contours shown in figure 7.13. The edges that actually appear in the figures are sufficient to trigger the hypothesis of a surface to account for those edges. The lack of any contrary evidence to contradict that hypothesis allows it to stand. It is the hypothesis of a surface that generates the predicted edges that are perceived in the image but not contained in the sensory data. This phenomenon is sufficient to generate a perceived surface even in figure 7.13e where there are only nine isolated points to suggest a triangular surface lying over another triangle.

Incorrect hypotheses lead to illusions. For example, the Ponzo illusion of figure 7.14 arises from the fact that the depth cues produce a hypothesis of different distances in different parts of the picture. This hypothesis generates input to the sensory-processing system that adjusts perceived size in accordance with the hypothesized distance to the object in that part of the picture.

Subjective contours and optical illusions are classic examples of how we see what we expect to see. Our world model generates expectations based on hypotheses created in the task-decomposition hierarchy of our behavioral system. This ability is crucial to perception in many situations, especially where the sensory input has a low signal-to-noise ratio or is partially obscured. For example, in dimly lit scenes or where the object of interest is occluded by obstacles, pursuit behavior may be more dependent on the expected position of the target than on the observed position. In these cases, the predictions generated by the world model become the primary source of information for behavioral decision-making. Our actions become contingent upon the images of our world model. So long as the sensory input can provide an occasional data point that reinforces the expectation, behavior can proceed successfully despite the absence of continuous sensory observation.

Of course, our world model can often lead us astray. In a dark, empty house, a strange noise can elicit the expectation of a nonexistent burglar or ghost. On a dimly lit street, a moving shadow can call forth any one of a number of imaginary creatures that reside in our internal world model. In situations where sensory input is clear and unambiguous, direct observations correct erroneous expectations generated by the world model. This steers the hypotheses of the behavior-generating hierarchy to a correct interpretation of the external world. But when the sensory input is fragmentary or ambiguous, the uncontradicted incorrect predictions of the world model can produce many types of illusions.

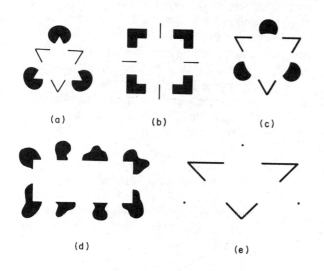

(a)   (b)   (c)

(d)   (e)

Figure 7.13: *Subjective contours are generated in the imagination of the viewer. The internal world model postulates simple geometrical shapes superimposed on each other to account for the otherwise complicated figures and unlikely coincidence of edge alignments. The internal expectations are inserted into the sensory data stream where they are perceived as if they originated in the sensory input.*

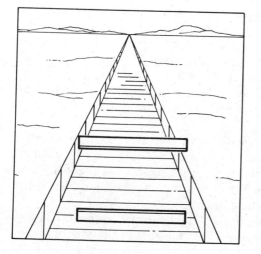

Figure 7.14: *Optical illusions such as this one arise because of depth cues that generate predictions of the relationship between the size of objects and the angles they subtend in the visual field. If two objects subtend the same angle, then the more distant one is expected to be larger.*

RHYTHM AND HARMONY

The cross-coupled hierarchy of figure 7.9 also goes far toward explaining the peculiar affinity of the ear for the rhythmic character of poetry and the numerical relationships involved in musical harmony. Poetic verse has a rhythmic meter which periodically terminates phrases with words that rhyme, i.e., that have the same ending sound. This corresponds to an interlocking harmonic periodicity at several different levels of the auditory-speech hierarchy. Great poetry has deep and rich harmonies that extend beyond the meter and word sounds to the higher levels where meaning and emotional responses are produced in the mind of the listener.

In music the most basic feature is the fundamental rhythm. The melody consists of a series of harmonically related notes played in phrases of a regularly recurring number of beats. If there are words, they usually are written in verse that matches the phrasing of the music. The number of interlocking rhythmic harmonies is a measure of the richness of the music. Most simple ballads have only a beat, one melody, and one verse. Polyphonic choral music might have many harmonically related melodies and many verses, all of which interlock in regularly recurring patterns. Symphonic music has an extremely complex array of instruments all playing different, but harmonically related, musical sequences.

The locked-loop concept may also explain the ability of the ear to ignore bursts of noise and to "flywheel" through auditory dropouts with apparent ease. It is a well-known phenomenon that sections of several tenths of a second can be cut out of a tape recording of speech or music without the listener being able to notice. The predictive capability of the cross-coupled hierarchy simply fills in the gaps, in many cases without the higher levels even noticing that anything is missing.

Cross-coupled hierarchies, of course, exist in all the sensory-motor systems, not just in the auditory-speech system. Thus, periodic patterns are intimately involved in all types of behavior.

Nature is full of periodicities: the pitch of a musical note, the beat of the heart, the rhythm of breathing. Many behavioral patterns such as walking, running, dancing, singing, speaking, and gesturing all have a distinctly rhythmic and sometimes strictly periodic character. All of life's activities are synchronized to the daily rhythms of daylight and darkness, as well as to the longer term cycles set by the phases of the moon and the seasons of the year. These are all regularly recurring patterns producing social as well as individual sensory-motor trajectories in the brain synchronized to these rhythms.

As a result there are rhythmically recurring addresses input to the associative memory modules in the internal world model. These produce rhythmically recurring expectations to be compared with rhythmically recurring sensory experiences. Thus, there exists a background of rhythmic patterns which permeate the entire processing-generating hierarchy of the whole brain.

One of the most important properties of regularly recurring temporal relationships is that they are predictable. This permits efficient learning and optimization of behavioral trajectories. If a sequence is recognized as repeating, then it is possible to predict the outcome. Unnecessary motions can be eliminated. Once we recognize the rhythm, we can anticipate when to leap to catch a prey, when to plant seed to grow a crop, when to release a spear to hit a target. Like wolves chasing a deer in a circle, we can position ourselves in an optimum place and wait for the goal to come to us. Behavior becomes much more successful and, hence, survival more likely.

Once we learn to recognize the recurrence of a pattern, we can begin to learn the meaning of deviations from the normal. The ability to predict implies the ability to detect the difference between what is predicted and what is observed. The information then lies in the error signal. Just as the modulation of a carrier contains the information in a radio signal, so the deviation of a sensory experience from the expected trajectory can contain the information in a neuronal signal. For example, in the summer we say "It's cold" if the temperature drops to 50 degrees Fahrenheit. But in the winter the same temperature would cause us to say "It's warm." The difference is in the expectation. Similarly, an unexpectedly high pitch in a voice can indicate excitement or agitation on the part of a speaker. The deviation in behavior of an individual from what is normally expected may indicate sickness or emotional distress.

Recognitions of gradual or small systematic deviations from the predictable lead to the learning of more sophisticated recognitions and predictions. For example, recognition of systematic deviations in the length of day or the position of the setting sun can lead to the prediction of the changing seasons and to behavioral decisions such as when to plant crops. Institutionalization of such observations can lead to the invention of calendars and the establishment of religions such those as practiced by the Mayans and the Druids. Recognition of the changing shape of the moon leads to the week and month. Recognition of the deviation between expectation and observation is a basis of sophisticated learning.

The difference between expectation and observation can also be used to modify the expectation. This enables us to perceive situations by modifying hypotheses in order to match expectations to observations. We can, in fact, define perception to be the act of finding a hypothesis that produces expectations matching observations.

Perception of a time sequential pattern implies the ability to predict the rest of the pattern once an initial recognition is accomplished. If the pattern recognizers in the sensory-processing hierarchy steer the control modules in the behavior-generating hierarchy so that a hypothesis is created that generates predictions to match the incoming flow of sensory data, then perception has occurred. Once the proper hypothesis is selected, the sensory data stream becomes predictable: it "makes sense."

In a phase locked loop, lock-on usually occurs with a positive snap, or "thunk." This is especially noticeable if the lock is preceded by an extended search. This corresponds to the Gestalt experience when we say "Aha!" or "I see!" Events become predictable and hence understandable.

When we can accurately predict our sensory input and are able to select behavioral patterns that consistently produce pleasing results, we are able to cope with our environment. It is thus not surprising that in a learning environment repetition is rewarding in and of itself. For example, children are fascinated by repetition. Ample evidence may be found in children's songs and games, and in the circumstances that accompany a child's familiar request, "Do it again, do it again." Adolescents tend to listen to the same recorded song or attend the same movie over and over until they have memorized every word and phrase. Even for adults in a potentially hostile world there is great survival advantage in being able to predict the results of future action. If the environment is periodic, this is much easier. Thus, any environment that exhibits a periodic character tends to be rewarding. For example, why are the rhythmic movements of dancing and marching to music so compelling? Isn't it the correlations and harmonic relationships that arise between trajectories in the behavior-generating and sensory-processing hierarchies? And why are daily routines and habits so comfortable, and the disruptions of an accustomed schedule so upsetting? Isn't it the secure feeling that comes from predictability and the lock-on that comes from a correspondence between the stored internal model and the observed sensory data stream?

Of course, we can't always accurately predict the future. Abrupt deviations from the predictable produce the sensation of surprise, which arouses attention and produces alerting signals. Events that are surprisingly pleasant are particularly rewarding, because they first alert and then reward beyond expectation. Pleasant surprises often make us laugh—a behavioral response.

The essence of humor seems to be pleasant surprise. The humorist can tell interesting stories that end with an unexpectedly clever twist—a double meaning or inverted logic. Risqué humor relies on the attention-alerting effect of skirting the limits of conventional morality.

On the other hand, unpleasant surprises evoke the emotional response of fear or anger. In a hostile environment, novel or unexpected events are fraught with danger. Deviations from the norm can result in disaster. The inability to predict, and hence to be surprised, constitutes a serious disadvantage. Without predictability, not only learning but survival itself is threatened. Continued or prolonged disruption of regular patterns, either in the internal rhythms or in external stimuli, destroys predictability, frustrates learning, and brings on punishing emotional stress that can produce neuroses.

THE ORIGIN OF LANGUAGE

The ability to generate and recognize regular sequences of pitch as phonemes, sequences of phonemes as words, and sequences of words as ideas is fundamental to the concept of language. Variation in these sequences gives the speaker the ability to encode information into messages. Recognition of these variations enables the listener to understand the messages.

This procedure gives a speaker the ability to transmit messages that can elicit specific patterns of activity in the mind of the listener. By this means the speaker can recruit help, enlist sympathy, give orders, and transmit all forms of sophisticated signals related to dominance, submission, and social interaction. Furthermore, by this mechanism he can induce into the highest levels of the sensory-processing hierarchy of the listener recalled memories of his own experience. He can tell tales, relate stories, and thereby provide others with second-hand information as to what strategies and goal decomposition rules he personally has found to be successful.

One of the most basic features of language is that it is a form of behavior. That seems an obvious thing to say, but evidently it is not. Many experts feel that because language is connected with the intellect (i.e., a higher function) it is quite divorced from mere motor behavior. However, there is no such thing as *mere* motor behavior. All behavior is the final output trajectory in the decomposition of high-level goals. The intellect is *not* something distinct from behavior. It is the deep structure of behavior. It is the set of nonterminal trajectories which generate and coordinate what finally results in the phenomena of purposive or intentional action.

Language is certainly like other behavior in that it results from the coordinated contractions of muscles in the chest, throat, and mouth. Like any other behavior such as walking, dancing, making a tool, or hunting for prey, language is both learned and goal directed.

As with all behavior, the purpose of language is to obtain reward, to avoid punishment, and to achieve success in the social dominance hierarchy. The unique feature of language behavior is that it allows communication between individuals to enlist help, to issue commands, to organize group behavior, and to receive feedback information from the sensory experiences of others.

WRITING

Written language very likely had its origins in goal-seeking activities. For example, the earliest writing in China began around 2000 B.C. as ideograms or symbols engraved on bones and shells for the purpose of asking questions of heaven. Each stroke or series of strokes asks a certain question or seeks guidance for a particular branch point in the behavioral trajectory of the life of the asker.

The earliest of all known writing is the Uruk tablets discovered in the Middle East and dated about 3100 B.C. This writing appears to be almost exclusively a mechanism for recording business transactions and land sales. These written symbols are now thought to be pictorial lists of tokens used for keeping track of merchandise or livestock. The tokens themselves first appeared 5000 years earlier during the beginning of the Neolithic period in Mesopotamia when human behavior patterns related to hunting and gathering were being replaced by others related to animal husbandry, agriculture, and the village market place.

This token method of accounting apparently served its purpose well, for the system remained virtually unchanged for about 5 millennia until the early Bronze Age when cities and city-states became the most advanced social organizations, and commerce grew into a large scale and complex enterprise. Then the requirements for more efficient accounting procedures led to the pictorial listing of tokens by writing on tablets—an early form of double-entry bookkeeping.

Once skill in this form of writing became widespread and commonly practiced, only a few additional symbols and some rules of syntax were required to express decrees, record dates, and relate accounts of significant events.

Thus, the language skill of writing evolved in small increments over many generations from the goal-directed manipulation of physical objects: first the objects themselves, then token objects, and finally images or symbols representing the tokens. The meaning of the symbols, as well as the rules of syntax, were obvious to anyone having an everyday familiarity with the manipulation rules for tokens. These in turn mimicked the rules for manipulation of the objects of merchandise. The manipulation of symbols in written language is a form of goal-seeking behavior which evolved from, and remains similar to, the manipulation of physical objects.

Skill in writing, as in any other complex goal-seeking activity, is acquired through painstaking training, endless practice, and numerous corrections of mistakes by a teacher. It is learned in stages, the lowest level primitives first (forming letters), then strings of primitives (words), then strings of strings (sentences), and so on. Only when the rules of spelling, grammar, and composition are more or less mastered can the scribe express or encode a thought (i.e, a high level trajectory) into a string of written symbols.

SPEECH

The origin of speech is less certain since it dates from a much earlier period. In fact, if we include the sounds of whales, animals, birds, and even insects as a form of speech, spoken language predates the origin of humanity itself. Surely any behavioral pattern which communicates a threat, signals submission, or expresses fear or acceptance is a form of language whether it be audible speech or sign language, or whether it be expressed by a mouse or a human. By this definition, some speech is very simple—a single facial expression, gesture, chirp, growl, or squeak for each emotional state encoded or intent expressed. Throughout the animal kingdom there exists a great variety of modes of expression and many different levels of complexity. Sounds such as the growls, whines, barks, and howls of the wolf express an extremely complex variety of social communications. One can easily feel caught up in a primitive community sing-along when listening to a recording of a wolf-pack chorus.

As we ascend the ladder of behavioral complexity, we find a corresponding increase in the ability to communicate complex messages. In most cases this appears to be not so much an increased vocal capacity as an increased complexity of deep structure underlying overt behavior. This implies that the ability to speak derives, first of all, from having something to say (i.e., from having internal trajectories of sufficient complexity that to attach facial expressions, gestures, and audible sounds to them results in complex and subtle messages).

Although there persists a sharp controversy over the language capacities of chimpanzees, chimps can be taught to encode words into sign language symbols. The pioneering work of Beatrice and Robert Gardner in teaching sign language to chimpanzees Washoe and Lucy has demonstrated that chimps can acquire and use a vocabulary of 100 to 200 words. Other chimps such as Lana at the Yerkes Primate Research Center have learned to express themselves in writing by using a specially designed computerized typewriter. All of these subhuman beings have demonstrated the ability to construct short sentences that request food and favors, ask and answer questions, make and deny assertions, and express observations about objects and events in the environment. Chimps in the wild have been observed uttering alarm calls that communicate the source of the danger: high "chutters" for pythons, slow-pitched staccato grunts for eagles, and a series of short tonal calls for leopards. The behavior of the other chimpanzees demonstrates that the message is understood. Thus, all the fundamental elements of language are present. A state of the world (a threat) is perceived by an individual. That individual encodes the perceived state of the world into a symbolic utterance. Another individual or group of individuals receives, decodes, and understands the language symbol, and takes appropriate action.

This process is nowhere near the richness of human language performance, but chimpanzee behavior is nowhere near human behavior in any domain. Compare human and chimpanzee behavior in hunting, fighting, using tools, building shelter, organizing society, or reasoning intellectually. The complex behavior-generating abilities of humans generate internal trajectories of sufficient complexity and subtlety that encoding them into words results in human language. The subtlety of human language simply reflects the subtlety of human behavior in general. The generation of natural human language implies a deep structure of behavior and thought that chimps simply do not possess. Chimp language is restricted to simple requests because that's all that goes on in the chimp brain: chimps do not have the computational structures of perception and motivation that are necessary to generate the highest level deep-structure trajectories of human language behavior. They cannot write papers or tell stories because they cannot generate thoughts of sufficient length and complexity. They cannot understand more than simple phrases because they do not have the computational hardware needed to generate hypotheses that can track and predict the data stream of an extended logical argument.

The distinction between human and animal language abilities lies in the sophistication of the deep structure mechanisms that generate both thought and behavior. Human language is vastly more rich and complex because of the additional levels in the human perceptual-behavioral hierarchy. Humans write papers on chimp language rather than vice versa because of the vastly more complex computational mechanisms that the human cerebral cortex allocates to the upper levels of perception, expectation, and behavior generation. Chimps can't behave or communicate at the human level because their brains don't have as much computational power dedicated to evaluating, planning, and acting as humans do.

Whether this is also true for the great whales is as yet unknown. The complexity of whale songs and the size of whale brains suggest that these creatures may possess intellectual and language capabilities comparable to humans.

STORYTELLING

The telling of tales and stories is a primitive and fundamental aspect of human language that has received relatively little attention from language researchers. Most work on language has centered on the rules of syntax and grammar and the informational structure of semantics. This would seem to be a classic case of failing to see the forest for the trees. Concentration on the mechanical details of vocabulary and sentence structure has largely obscured the more important capacity of the human mind to remember and relate tales of adventure and drama. In cultures where written language is unknown, storytellers are able to relate epic tales many hours long with the precision of a Broadway actor reciting a script. Persons familiar with such stories can detect the omission of a single word or the substitution of a single phrase.

In fact, the fundamental component of all literature is the story—the relating of the behavioral actions and experiences of a cast of characters. The storyteller creates in the mind of the listening audience a set of trajectories that approximate what would be felt and experienced if the listener were actually acting out the behavioral patterns of the characters in the story.

The close relationship of the story to behavior can best be understood by considering the nature of the many trajectories that comprise the deep structure of behavior. Consider once more the set of trajectories in figure 5.17. Each trajectory consists of a sequence of state vectors which can be put in one-to-one correspondence to a vocabulary of words. Thus, each trajectory defines a string of words that can be interpreted either as a program or as a story. If we choose to call it a program, each trajectory consists of a string of commands, or program statements, which are executed to generate behavior. However, we can just as easily interpret the string of words as a story. Each trajectory tells its own story. The low-level trajectories are very detailed stories, relating every movement of a particular muscle, or every behavioral primitive of a single limb. The high-level trajectories tell stories in a richer vocabulary, but with less detail. Trajectories in the behavior-generating hierarchy describe action. Trajectories in the sensory-processing hierarchy describe experiences and feelings. Trajectories in the world-model hierarchy describe hopes, expectations, and dreams. Thus, any behavioral sequence consists of hundreds of stories, all being related simultaneously with different levels of detail and describing different aspects of the behavior.

In the normal course of events, these trajectories (or stories) of the deep structure are played out in behavior, in experience, or in imagination. The translation of these trajectories into words gives rise to language. The narrator chooses a single string of words from the many available trajectories. Of course, the dramatic effect of his tale can be enhanced by skipping from one trajectory to another and from one level to another. He can drop down to a low-level trajectory to expand the details of the exciting parts of a story and then jump up to a high-level trajectory to skip quickly over boring or routine events. The storyteller can jump from a behavioral trajectory to an experience trajectory to an emotional trajectory to a belief trajectory. He can even jump back and forth between trajectories in different characters as he spins his tale.

The mind of the listener fills in the missing trajectories that the storyteller leaves out just as the vision system fills in the subjective contours of the missing parts of images such as are shown in figure 7.13. The storyteller's string of words generates hypotheses in the minds of the listening audience. These elicit memories and trigger the imagination to produce a full range of sensory and emotional experiences. Thus, the words of the storyteller pull the mind of the listener along the main experience trajectory of the story, and the imagination of the listener fills in the background.

PRIMITIVE HUMAN SPEECH

Among the most ancient forms of human speech that survive today are the tribal dances of the few remaining stone-age peoples. In such rites, information of vital subjects such as hunting (including the habits, ferocity and vulnerable areas of the prey), stalking, and using weapons are conveyed by dance, symbolic gestures, pantomime, songs, and shouts, as the hunters relate (indeed reenact) the exploits of the hunt. The storytellers replay the behavioral trajectories of their own hunting experience and attach verbal symbols and gestures to the portions which cannot be literally acted out.

Indeed, a great deal of human language behavior must have developed as a result of sitting around the fire relating tales of the day's adventures and making plans for tomorrow. Even in modern cultures, the majority of everyday speech consists of relating personal experiences. This is simply the straightforward encoding of behavior trajectories, or the recalled sensory experiences addressed by those behavioral trajectories, into a string of language tokens or symbols such as gestures, vocal cord, tongue, and lip manipulations. Thus, in the final analysis, all language is a form of goal-directed manipulation of tokens and symbols. The ultimate result is a manipulation of the minds and hence the actions of other members of the society.

Language is a tool by which a speaker can arouse or implant in the listener a great variety of behavioral goals, hypotheses, and belief structures. By the use of these means, a speaker can command, instruct, threaten, entertain, or chastise other persons in his group to his own benefit and for his own ends.

The implication for research in language understanding is that there is much to be learned from the relationship between language and other forms of behavior. How, for example, can behavioral goals and trajectories be encoded into strings of language symbols for making requests, issuing commands, and relating sensory experiences? How can patterns of trajectories be encoded and transmitted by one processing-generating hierarchy so as to be received and reconstructed by another?

Language generation and recognition depend upon many of the same mechanisms by which the rhythms, periodicities, and harmonic patterns of music, song, and poetry are recognized, tracked and predicted at many different levels.

The relatively simple and well-structured domains of music and pentameter may be particularly fertile, unexplored areas for research in language generation and understanding. The rhythmic character of the time-dependent interactions between stored models and sensory input should make the study of music recognition by computer an interesting and rewarding research topic. Coupled with the study of mechanisms for generating complex behavior in general, this provides a fresh new approach to the study of language.

MECHANISMS OF CHOICE

We turn now to the very highest levels in the sensory-processing, world-modeling, behavior-generating hierarchy. Up until this point, the hierarchies we have discussed have always had some higher level input. There must be a highest level: every hierarchy must have a top. In every brain, there must be some level at which the ultimate choices are made and from which the highest level goals are issued. For the purposes of this discussion, we will define the highest level H function in the behavior-generating hierarchy of the human brain as the WILL and the highest level G function in the sensory-processing hierarchy as the EMOTIONS. This is illustrated in figure 7.15.

Emotions

Emotions play a crucial role in the selection of behavior. We tend to practice what makes us feel comfortable and avoid what we dislike. Our behavior-generating hierarchy normally seeks to prolong, intensify, or repeat those behaviors that give us pleasure or make us feel happy or contented. We normally seek to terminate, diminish, or avoid those behavior patterns that cause us pain or arouse fear or disgust.

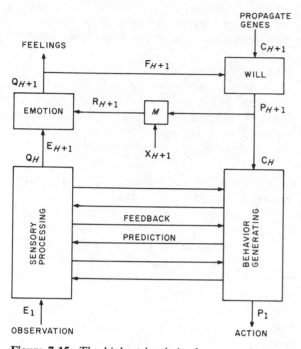

FEELINGS

PROPAGATE
GENES

Q_{H+1}

F_{H+1}

C_{H+1}

WILL

EMOTION

R_{H+1} M

P_{H+1}

E_{H+1}

Q_H

X_{H+1}

C_H

SENSORY PROCESSING

FEEDBACK

PREDICTION

BEHAVIOR GENERATING

E_1

OBSERVATION

P_1

ACTION

Figure 7.15: *The highest levels in the processing-generating hierarchy are the value-judging and goal-selecting mechanisms of the emotions and will. The emotions are the place where events, objects, and relationships are judged as lovable, disgusting, happy, sad, joyful, fearful, and so on. The will is where the decisions are made that commit an organism to a unified pattern of behavior directed toward a specific goal.*

In the past 25 years research has shown that the emotions are generated in localized areas, or computing centers, in the brain. For example, the posterior hypothalamus produces fear, the amygdala generates anger and rage, the insula computes feelings of contentment, and the septal regions produce joy and elation. The perifornical nucleus of the hypothalamus produces punishing pain, the septum pleasure, the anterior hypothalamus sexual arousal, and the pituitary computes the body's response to danger and stress. These emotional centers, along with many others, make up a complex of about 53 regions linked together by 35 major nerve bundles. This entire network is called the limbic system. Additional functions carried out in the limbic system are the regulation of hunger and thirst performed by the medial and lateral hypothalamus, the control of body rhythms such as sleep-awake cycles performed by the pineal gland, and the production of signals which consolidate (i.e., make permanent) the storage of sensory experiences in memory performed by the hippocampus. This last function allows the brain to be selective in its use of memory by facilitating the permanent storage of sensory experiences to which the emotional evaluators attach particular significance (e.g., close brushes with death, punishing experiences, etc.).

Input to the limbic system emotional centers consists of highly processed sensory data such as the names of recognized objects, events, relationships, and situations, such as the recognition of success in goal achievement, the perception of praise or hostility, or the recognition of gestures of dominance or submission transmitted by social peers. These inputs are accompanied by such modifier variables as confidence factors derived from the degree of correlation between predicted and observed sensory input.

Sensory processing at the level of the emotions is heavily influenced by contextual information derived from internal models and expectations at many different levels in the processing hierarchy. If a painful stimulus is perceived as being associated with a non–fear-producing source, we may attack the pain-causing agent. If, however, the perceived source of pain also induces fear, we may flee.

The evaluation of complex events such as social situations are even more dependent upon learned contextual interpretations. Consider, for example, the event diagramed in figure 7.16. Here the observation is that of a person talking to a flower. In some circles this would be perceived as deviant behavior. However, the emotional reaction would depend upon other perceptions such as the person talking to the flower is a) eccentric, b) retarded, or c) dangerously psychotic. These different qualifiers to the deviant classification can cause the emotions to output a) amusement, b) pity, or c) fear, respectively. Amusement input to the behavioral goal selecting module can lead to laughter, poking fun, or ridicule. Pity can evoke a behavioral pattern of sympathy. Fear can evoke an attempt to secure medical or psychiatric treatment or incarceration.

If, however, a person talking to a flower is recognized as perfectly normal, then the emotions will give no indication that the event is particuarly worthy of attention, or that there exists any need to deviate from whatever behavior is presently being executed.

In this model, the standards of normalcy and deviance are in the eye of the beholder, or at least in the expectations and beliefs stored in the processing-generating hierarchy. In many ways the emotional evaluators are even more dependent on internal beliefs than on externally observed facts. This is particularly true in the case where a person's belief structure discounts the reliability or moral worth of the physical senses, as is characteristic of philosophical constructs derived from gnosticism or asceticism.

Thus the emotions, just as any other sensory-processing module in the brain, simply compute G function on the D vector that they input to produce the Q vector that they output. Output from the emotional centers is known to be of two types: one consists of signals on nerve fibers; the other consists of hormones and chemical transmitters which convey their messages (Q vector values) via fluid transport mechanisms.

In simple creatures the emotional output vector can be restricted to a few components such as good–bad and pleasure–pain. In higher forms the emotional output is a highly multidimensional vector with many faceted components such as love, hate, jealousy, guilt, pride, and disgust. Part of this **Q** output may simply produce feelings (i.e., joy, sadness, excitement, and fear.). However, most of the **Q** output directly or indirectly provides **F** input to the highest level H function, the will.

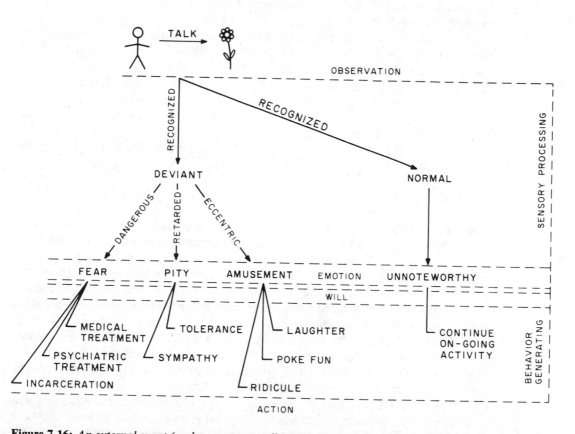

Figure 7.16: *An external event (such as a person talking to a flower) may be recognized as deviant or normal. If deviant, action may be selected appropriate to the emotional valuation of fear, pity, or amusement. If the event is recognized as normal and evaluated as unnoteworthy, no change in on-going activity is called for.*

Will

For centuries philosophers and theologians have debated the nature of the will. For the most part, this argument has centered on the question of whether humans have free will (i.e., the freedom to choose goals) or whether all choice is merely a reflexive or predestined response to the environment. Debates over free will revolve around the question of responsibility and guilt. The theology of sin and the legal questions of crime and punishment turn on the question of the individual's responsibility for his or her own personal behavior. If the individual is free to choose right from wrong, then when he chooses right he should be praised and when he chooses wrong he should be punished. If, however, the choice of the individual is predestined by God, or by fate, or is largely determined by the contingencies (i.e., the rewarding and punishing reinforcements of the environment), then the responsibility for the behavior of the individual is at least shared by, if not totally thrust upon, the external environment, be that society or the Divinity.

Most people would agree that the behavior of individuals is constrained by the range of role models made available to them as a result of the prevailing social structure and by accident of birth. To a large extent individual behavior is influenced by the amount and quality of the training received and by the degree of health, strength, intellect, and talent that a person is born with. Certainly, the really big events in life—whether there is war or peace, whether society is civilized or barbarous, whether one's parents are prosperous or poverty-stricken—are matters not much influenced by the will of the individual. These are the type of events that people ascribe to the will of God or to the fates.

The question of free will of an individual is on another scale. Free will implies an ability to choose from the variety of behavioral patterns available to the individual in the immediate environment. Free will involves many implicit assumptions about the rules of right and wrong, about motivation, about knowledge of what is possible, and about what the consequences of various actions might be.

If we define the will to be the highest level in the behavior-generating hierarchy, then the choices made are determined by the H function stored in this highest level module. Some may interpret this to mean that the choices made by the will are not free, because they are determined, even predestined, by the mathematical transformations of the H function. But the H function of the will merely embodies the rules of choice: *if* such and such is the state of the world, and *if* my emotions make me feel so and so, *then* I will do thus and thus. Certainly, the fact that there exists a computing module wherein resides an algorithm or set of rules for making these types of decisions does not negate the "freedom" of the decision. There are few restrictions on the set of rules that may be embodied in the H module of the will. The will receives input variables from literally hundreds of sources, including many from the emotions, as well as from internally generated chemicals and hormones. Since both emotions and hormone levels affect and are affected by what we call feelings and moods, the decisions made by the highest level H function are profoundly influenced by these variables.

Furthermore, the will has a great deal of control over what inputs it will entertain. This is evident in the fact that we tend to see what we want to see and hear what we want to hear. The emotions sit at the top of the sensory-processing hierarchy. Inputs to the emotions, and thus the emotional inputs to the will, are heavily influenced by the various processing and filtering functions that are selected by the behavioral choices of the H function of the will itself. In short, we can suppress inputs which are evaluated as immoral. Alternatively, we can execute behavioral actions which avoid temptation or which remove its input from our sensory channels.

Finally, the H function of the will, as well as the M functions of the world model, and the G functions of the entire sensory-processing hierarchy including the emotions can be altered as the result of learning and/or teaching. Thus, even though the decisions made by the H function of the will are theoretically deterministic and the resultant behavior patterns therefore predestined, the range of inputs is so large and the variability of the H function itself so wide that for all practical purposes the decisions made by the will are quite nondeterministic. They certainly seem so to the individual. The influence of emotional states, moods, and feelings are profound, and the H function itself has the capacity to change with experience. The H function is both culturally and individually determined. Thus, the model proposed here provides all the variability needed to satisfy the most ardent advocate of the doctrine of free will.

Yet there is a clear role played by the contingencies of the environment, by the reinforcements of reward and punishment, by the family, clan, and community, and by the national and religious heritage in the formation of the H function of the will; and not only of the will, but of the emotions, and the H, M, and G functions of the entire processing-generating hierarchy as well.

ORIGINS OF WILL AND EMOTION

What the G and H functions of the emotions and will are and where they originate is a matter of hot dispute. One recent theory proposed by sociobiology is that they are genetically determined, derived from information stored in the DNA molecule, as the result of millions of years of natural selection. This theory argues that innate behavior-selecting mechanisms have evolved so as to maximize the Darwinian fitness (the expected number of surviving offspring) of their possessors.

The incidence of behavior in many different species from insects to birds to mammals corresponds closely to mathematical predictions derived from genetics and game-theory analyses of strategies for maximizing the probability of gene propagation. Even cooperative or altruistic behavior such as that of the worker bee and ritualized behavior in animal contests and courtship can in many cases be explained by genetic arguments. However, the evidence for this theory is much stronger for insects than for higher forms, and the opinion that human emotions are transmitted genetically is not widely held.

A competing theory put forward by behaviorists is that in higher forms the evaluator functions of the emotion and the selector functions of the will are mostly learned, perhaps even imprinted, during the early years of development. Certainly many of the emotional evaluations and behavior-selection rules in the human brain are culturally determined, derived from religious teachings defining good and evil, or from social conventions defining duty, fairness, etiquette, and legality. As it says in Proverbs, "Train up a child in the way he should go, and when he is old, he will not depart from it." Fundamental rules of opinion and behavior are instilled in the young by parents, educators, and religious and state authorities. They are reinforced throughout life by peer group pressure, as well as by church and civil sanctions.

There are, of course, many persons who would disagree with both theories. Perhaps the most widespread opinion (which until recent years was virtually unchallenged) is that the human will and its emotional evaluator inputs are nonmechanistic in nature and therefore unknowable in some fundamental sense. Many would even claim that emotions and will are subject to, or controlled by, spiritual and supernatural forces. For example, the doctrine of original sin states that the highest level behavior-selecting mechanism, the human will, is basically defective because of the disobedience of Adam and Eve, and except for the intervention of divine grace is under the power of evil or Satanic forces. The literature surrounding the age-old controversy over free will versus predestination centers largely on the role of the divinity (or the stars or fates) in the determination of human behavior. Most cultures view the conscience (i.e., the emotional evaluator for right and wrong or good and evil) as a divine gift or manifestation of the indwelling of the spirit of God.

The emotions and will are a very basic (some would say primitive) and compelling part of our behavioral mechanism. Carl Sagan calls them the *Dragons of Eden*. Humans are often driven, sometimes beyond rational justification, to heroic feats of courage or physical endurance by the behavioral rules of duty or the emotions of love, pride, guilt, jealousy, and hate.

Whatever their origins, the G functions of our emotions and the H functions of the will can be modeled. They are rule based, and the rules are, for the most part, clearly defined. In many cases these rules are even written down as systems of moral philosophy, ethics, or rules of social behavior such as *Emily Post's Book of Etiquette*.

Nothing so complex need be modeled for the highest level G and H modules of a robot for many years. Nevertheless, every robot needs some sort of highest level evaluator and goal-selector function in order to exhibit any sort of autonomous behavior. At what point in the spectrum of multidimensional sophistication we choose to dignify an evaluator function with the term emotion or a goal-selection function with the term will, is not clear. What is clear is that simple approximations to the functions computed by the emotions and the will can be modeled by CMAC G and H functions operating on input vectors and computing output vectors. The degree of sophistication and complexity of the modeling is limited only by the ingenuity and resources of the modeler.

BELIEF AND FAITH

If the top level of the behavior-generating hierarchy is the will, and the top level of the sensory-processing hierarchy is the emotions, then the upper levels of the world model are the philosophical beliefs that shape our thoughts and control our behavior. A diagram of the types of beliefs contained at various levels of the world model is shown in figure 7.17. The memories and predictions of the world model at all levels are essentially beliefs, which are accumulated as a result of experience and modified by new types of experience. At the higher levels, however, the flow of information in the sensory-processing system is highly processed and abstract and may

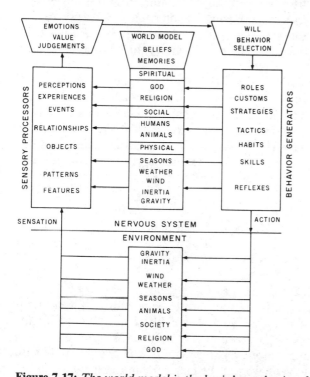

Figure 7.17: *The world model is the brain's mechanism for generating predictions and expectations for contemplated actions or recognized situations. At the lowest levels the world model generates expectations for simple actions and physical events. At a higher level, an internal model of peer group attitudes generates expectations for social behavior. At the highest levels, an internal model consisting of philosophical and religious beliefs generates expectations for consequences of moral and immoral behavior. Value judgments of what is good or bad are made by the emotions.*

come from a great variety of sensory sources. For example, higher level beliefs about many things are acquired from the experience and beliefs of others through the mechanism of language. Many beliefs are acquired from sayings, traditions, old wives' tales, legends, and myths. These are transmitted from parent to child and from authority figures such as chiefs, elders, and priests to the common people. In primitive tribal cultures, many of the beliefs concern gods, devils, ghosts, and spirits and consist of elaborate tales about what these disembodied creatures will do or feel in response to the behavioral choices of the individual or the society.

The fact that such higher level beliefs cannot be verified by comparison with direct sensory experience is often of little consequence. At these levels in the hierarchy of the brain, all sensory data is highly abstract and subject to filtering by expectations generated by the world model itself. Thus, the difference between information derived from a physical experience and a verbal description of such an experience is not large. Repeated listening to stories from authoritative sources such as textbooks or the Holy Scriptures and acting out solemn rituals such as scholastic examinations or religious ceremonies provide most of the experience needed to verify the predictions of the world model beliefs and solidify the conviction of their truth.

From a survival standpont it is quite immaterial whether the beliefs imbedded in the world model are true or false. It really doesn't matter much whether beliefs about demons, fairies, witches, and leprechauns have any correspondence to reality. All that is important is whether belief in such things gives the individual a basis for confidently selecting behavior that leads to happy and successful results, and for swiftly rejecting behavior that leads to punishment or disaster. For survival, it is only important that the resulting behavioral choices be, on the whole, beneficial to the individual and the society.

For learning and reinforcement, all that is necessary is that the predictions and expectations generated by the world model be *perceived* to be useful in selecting and guiding behavior that works to the advantage of the individual and society. If this is so, the world model will be reinforced. If not, then the contents of the world model will be modified or replaced.

It is important to realize that there is no way that the mind can ever really know the external world. The interface between neuronal activity and the physical environment is an impenetrable barrier. That boundary is like a mirror in which the mind sees the world as the reflection of its own internal beliefs. We can, of course, test our beliefs against observations. However, direct testing is possible only with those expectations stored at the lowest levels in the hierarchy that are related to immediate interactions with the physical and social environment. We construct the lower levels of our world model primarily through direct sensory experience. We test the expectation generated by those lower levels against everyday experiences: every time we throw a rock and observe its trajectory, we test our expectations concerning the effects of gravity and inertia. We compare our expectations concerning the wind and clouds and seasonal variations in the temperature and precipitation every time we observe the weather. A great deal of human conversation and thought is, in fact, dedicated to just such comparisons. We test our expectations concerning the behavior of animals and other humans every time we observe their habits or interact with them socially.

However, when we reach beyond everyday experience to philosophy and abstract scientific principles, it is not so easy to compare observation against belief. For example, how can we test our belief that the world is round? This is not directly observable except from outer space. How do we know that matter is made up of molecules and atoms and electrons and quarks? This is not observable by any direct measurement. In fact, most people don't have even the slightest notion of the evidence that substantiates these theories. They simply believe them on the authority of teachers and supposedly knowledgeable persons. Thus, modern science is itself a belief structure propagated not very differently from the myths of ancient religions. It is taught by a class of authoritative experts, who have much in common with priests and theologians.

Of course, scientific beliefs are not generally accepted unless a sufficiently large number of eminent scientists agree that the comparison between belief and observation can, in fact, be made and that under repeated trials the model always predicts exactly what is observed. This is the essence of the scientific method. It provides a systematic procedure for discovering and refining world model beliefs that accurately predict the results of behavioral experiments.

There will, however, always be some beliefs that can't be tested either by direct observation or by the scientific method. There will always be some questions that remain cloaked with mystery. There is always some point at which it becomes unclear whether what we are modeling is myth or reality. The belief model itself is always imaginary. Whether it has a counterpart in the external environment can't always be known for sure. It is here that faith enters. In the words of the apostle Paul, faith is "the conviction of things not seen"; it is the confidence we have that our model of the external world is a reliable guide for behavior. As we have said earlier, this is really all that is necessary.

Only two critical features are necessary for a set of IF/THEN rules embedded in the belief structure to be successful:

1. They must be easy to remember. This can most easily be accomplished by couching them in the form of compelling and exciting tales of adventure. Thus, it is not unusual for religious literature to be rich in stories of high adventure, with great heroes, great villains, and cosmic conflicts between the forces of good and evil.

2. The IF/THEN expectation generators must lead to socially advantageous behavior. In general, they must encourage hard work in the acquisition of food and shelter, and cooperation against enemies and the destructive force of nature.

As long as our beliefs lead us to behavioral choices that are successful in producing prosperity and happiness, that is all that counts. It really doesn't matter whether they are correct or even logically consistent. It is only when incorrect beliefs lead to behavioral choices that are unsuccessful or disastrous that they must be changed. Otherwise the individual or society that holds them will not survive in competition with others possessing more successful world models.

ACTING, OBSERVING, AND IMAGINING

The interdependency of the processing, generating, and world model hierarchies suggests at least three distinct modes of operation.

Acting—The Task-Execution Mode

In the task-execution mode the motor-generating hierarchy is committed to a goal, which it decomposes into subgoals, sub-subgoals, and finally into action primitives. In this mode the sensory-processing hierarchy is primarily engaged in providing feedback; first to aid in selecting the goal, then to steer the goal-decomposition process, and finally to direct the output drive signals to the muscles (or actuators) so as to follow a success trajectory.

Consider a simple, everyday goal such as the fixing of a leaking faucet. First, the sensory-processing system must recognize the fact that the faucet is leaking. This information is then evaluated by the emotions as something that needs attention. This evaluation is passed on to the will, where the rules of what ought to be done and under what circumstances reside. If there are no higher priority items vying for the attention of the will, then the goal <FIX FAUCET> may be selected. Once this occurs, the behavior-generating hierarchy will be committed to decompose this goal into a sequence of actions.

At each instant of time t_k the sensory-processing module at each hierarchical level extracts feedback vectors $\mathbf{F}_i^t$ required by the H behavior-generating modules at each level for goal decomposition. At the instant t_0 when the goal is selected, the feedback $\mathbf{F}_i^0$ at the various levels causes the selection of the initial subgoal decomposition $\mathbf{P}_i^0$. This determines the initial direction of the trajectories $\mathbf{T}_{P_i}$ on their way toward the goal state. As the task proceeds, the recognition of subgoal completions and/or unanticipated obstacles triggers the selection of the proper sequence of actions directed toward the goal achievement.

The entire set of trajectories $\mathbf{T}_{P_i}$ describes the sequence of internal states of the brain which underlie and give rise to the observable phenomena of purposive behavior. These are the deep structures of behavior. Only the output trajectory, the terminal or bottom level trajectory, is manifested as overt action. The extent to which the trajectories $\mathbf{T}_{P_i}$ are independent of feedback is the extent to which behavior is preprogrammed. The extent to which the feedback pulls the $\mathbf{T}_{P_i}$ trajectories along predictable paths to the goal state is the extent to which behavior is adaptive. For some goals, such as hunting for prey or searching for breeding territory, the selection of the goal merely triggers migratory searching behavior which continues until feedback indicates that the goal is near at hand. For such goals, behavior is indefinite and highly feedback dependent. For other goals, such as building a nest, making a tool, courting a mate, or defending a territory, behavior is more inner-directed, requiring only a few sensory cues for triggers.

In either case, while the brain is in the acting mode the sensory data flowing in the sensory-processing hierarchy is highly dependent on (if not directly caused by) the action itself. If the action is speech, the sensory-processing hierarchy is analyzing what is spoken and provides feedback for control of loudness, pitch, and modulation. If the action is physical motion, data from vision, proprioception, and touch sensors are all highly action dependent, and the sensory analysis is primarily directed toward servo-control of the action itself.

In the action mode, the M_i associative memory modules provide context in the form of predicted data to the sensory-processing modules in order to distinguish between sensory data caused by motion of the sensors and that caused by motion of the environment. What is predicted is whatever was stored on previous experiences when the same action was generated under similar circumstances. This allows the sensory-processing hierarchy to anticipate the sensory input and to detect more sophisticated patterns in the sensory data than would otherwise be possible.

Observing—The Sensory Analysis Mode

A second mode of operation of the crosscoupled hierarchy is the analysis of sensory data from external sources not primarily caused by action of the behavior-generating hierarchy. For example, when one listens to a concert, a speech, or a play, little action occurs in the muscles and motor neurons. The lower levels of behavior-generating hierarchies are quiescent, or set to a constant value, or given a command to execute an overlearned task which can be carried out without any assistance from the upper levels.

The sensory-processing hierarchies, however, are very busy. They are filtering and predicting, recognizing patterns and trajectories, locking on to rhythms and harmonious periodicities, and tracking targets of attention. Predictions generated by the M modules are clearly required for these types of analyses, whether or not the organism is engaged in physical activity. This suggests that the upper levels of the behavior-generating hierarchies (which are not currently required for generating behavior) might be used instead to generate hypotheses and subhypotheses which in turn produce context and predictions to aid the sensory-processing hierarchy in the recognition, analysis, and understanding of incoming sensory data.

At each level hypotheses which generate $\mathbf{T}_R$ predictions that match or track the $\mathbf{T}_E$ sensory data trajectories will be confirmed. If the hypothesized $\mathbf{T}_R$ trajectories are only close to the T_E observations, they can be pulled by error signal feedback T_F from the processing hierarchies. When a hypothesis is successful in generating predictions which match the sensory data stream, the loop at that level locks onto the sensory data. When lock-on is simultaneously achieved at many different levels, we can say that the processing-generating hierarchy "understands" the incoming data (i.e., it can follow and predict it at many different levels).

Attention

The directing or focusing of attention is essentially a purposive action whose goal is to optimize the quality of the sensory data. The basic elements of attention are orienting—positioning the body and sensory organs to facilitate the gathering of data—and focusing—blocking out extraneous or peripheral information so that the sensory-processing system can bring all of its capacities to bear on data that are relevant to the object of attention. The orienting element is simply a behavioral task or goal to acquire and track a target. The focusing element is a filtering problem that can be solved by a hypothesis or goal decomposition that evokes the appropriate masks or filter functions from the R_i modules so as to block out all but the relevant sensory input data. Figure 7.18 illustrates the filtering aspects of attention.

Thus, attending is a combination of observing and acting. It is primarily a sensory-analysis mode activity, strongly assisted from the task-execution mode.

Imagining—The Free-Running Mode

A third distinct mode of operation occurs when the upper levels of the processing-generating hierarchy are largely disconnected from both motor output and sensory input. In this mode high-level hypotheses T_{P_i} may be generated, and predicted sensory data T_{R_i} recalled. In the absence of sensory input from the external environment, these recalled trajectories make up all of the information flowing in the sensory-processing hierarchy. The processing modules G_i operate exclusively on the internally recalled R_i trajectories producing T_{Q_i} experiences and T_{F_i} feedback. The T_{S_i} trajectories act on the generating hierarchy to modify and steer the T_{S_i} trajectories creating new hypotheses T_{P_i}. The system is free-running, guided only by stored experiences M_i, learned interpretations G_i, and practiced skills H_i, for generating strings of hypotheses and decomposing goals and tasks. The upper levels of the cross-coupled hierarchy are, thus, imagining (i.e., generating and analyzing what would be expected if certain hypothesized goals and tasks were to be carried out).

Imagination is based on stored experiences and driven by hypothesized actions. It is constrained in large measure by the knowledge frames, world models, expected values, and belief structures (IF I do this, THEN such and so will happen) embedded in the upper levels of the cross-coupled processing-generating hierarchy.

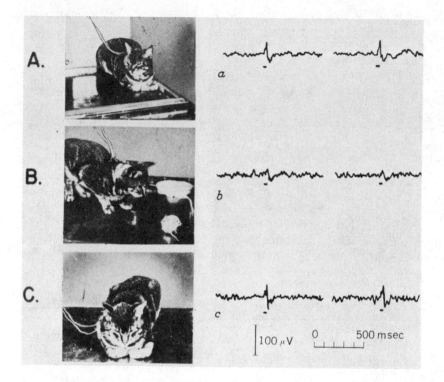

Figure 7.18: *Direct recording of click responses in the cochlear nucleus during three periods. (Top and bottom) Cat is relaxed, and the click responses are large. (Middle) The cat is visually attentive to the mice in the jar, and the click responses are diminished in amplitude. This illustrates the filtering of sensory input controlled by activity in the behavior-generating hierarchy.*

If we attempt to hypothesize some action X which lies outside of the neighborhood of generalization of prior experience, we get no recalled $\mathbf{R}_i$ vectors from memory M_i. In this case we say "we cannot imagine what X would be like."

One of the functions of the free-running mode is to remember or recall past experiences by hypothesizing the same goals as when the experience was recorded. Thus, in our imagination we can reach back and relive experiences, recall events, and remember facts and relationships from our past. Imagination, however, is not limited to duplication of past experiences. We can also rearrange sections of learned trajectories to create experiences in our minds that never occurred. We can string together trajectories in new combinations or insert new modifier variables in various hypothesis vectors. We can watch a bird fly and substitute a "self" variable in place of the bird to imagine ourselves soaring through the sky. We can listen to a story of adventure and imagine ourselves in the place of one of the characters. Imagination allows us to hypothesize untried actions and, on the basis of M functions learned during previous experiences, to predict the outcome.

Planning

Imagination gives us the ability to think about what we are going to do before committing ourselves to action. We can try out, or hypothesize prospective behavioral patterns, and predict the probable results. The emotions enable us to evaluate these predicted results as good or bad, desirable or undesirable.

Imagination and emotional evaluators together give us the capability to conduct a search over a space of potential goal decompositions and to find the best course of action. This type of search is called *planning*.

When we plan, we hypothesize various alternative behavior trajectories and attempt to select the one that takes us from our present state to the goal state by the most desirable route. Imagined scenarios that produce positive emotional outputs are flagged as candidate plans. Favorably evaluated scenarios or plans can be repeatedly rehearsed, reevaluated, and refined prior to initiation of behavior-producing action.

Imagined scenarios that produce negative evaluation outputs will be avoided if possible. In some situations it might not be possible to find a path from our present state to a goal state, or at least not one that produces a net positive evaluation. Repeated unsuccessful attempts to find a satisfactory, nonpunishing plan, particularly in situations recognized as critical to one's well-being, correspond to *worry*.

One of the central issues in the study of planning is the search strategy, or procedure, that dictates which of the many possible hypotheses should be evaluated first. In most cases, the search space is much too large to permit an exhaustive search of all possible plans, or even any substantial fraction of them. The set of rules for deciding which hypotheses to evaluate, and in which order, are called *heuristics*.

Heuristics are usually derived in an ad hoc way from experience, accident, analogy, or guesswork. Once discovered, they may be passed from one individual to another and from one generation to another by teaching.

Historically, artificial intelligence researchers have been fascinated by the subject of heuristics. At least a portion of this interest is a result of its recursive nature. A heuristic is a procedure for finding a procedure. When this recursion is embedded in a cross-coupled, processing-generating hierarchy with the rich complexity of the human brain, it becomes clear why the thoughts and plans of humans are filled with such exquisite subtleties and curious, sometimes insidious, reasoning. It also provides some insight into the remarkable phenomenon of self-consciousness (i.e., a computing structure with the capacity to observe, take note of, analyze, and, to some extent, even understand itself).

Much of the artificial intelligence research in planning and problem-solving has its origins and theoretical framework based on simple board games where there are a finite (although sometimes very large) number of possible moves. The discrete character of such games, together with the digital nature of computers, led naturally to the analysis of discrete trees, graphs, and search strategies for such structures.

Planning in a natural environment is much more complex than searching discrete trees and graphs. In the study of planning in the brain it is necessary to deal with the continuous time-dependent nature of real world variables and situations. States are not accurately represented as nodes in a graph or tree; they are more like points in a tensor field. Transitions between states are not lines or edges, but multidimensional trajectories, fuzzy and noisy at that. In a natural environment, the space of possible behaviors is infinite. It is clearly impossible to exhaustively search any significant portion of it. Furthermore, the real world is much too unpredictable and hostile, and wrong guesses are far too dangerous to make exploration practical outside of a few regions in which behavior patterns have had a historical record of success. Thus behavior, and hence imagination and planning, is confined to a relatively small range of possibilities, namely those behavioral and thought patterns that have been discovered to be successful through historical accident or painful trial and error. Both the potential behavioral patterns and the heuristics for selecting them are passed from one generation to another by parents, educators, and civil and religious customs.

Daydreaming or Fantasizing

The fact that the imagination can generate hypothetical scenarios with pleasurable emotional evaluations makes it inevitable that such scenarios will sometimes be rehearsed for their pleasure-producing effect alone. This is a procedure that can only be described as daydreaming or fantasizing.

When we daydream we allow our hypothesis generators to drift wherever our emotional evaluators pull them. Our imagination gravitates toward those trajectories that are emotionally most rewarding. Some of the most pleasurable scenarios we can image are physically impossible, impractical, or socially taboo. Most of us recognize these as fantasies and never attempt to carry them out. However, once a person adopts the intent to carry out a fantasy, it ceases to be a dream and becomes a plan.

Thus, planning and daydreaming are closely related activities, differing principally in that planning has a serious purpose and involves an intent to execute what is finally selected as the most desirable of the alternative hypotheses.

This model suggests that dreaming while sleeping is similar in many respects to daydreaming. The principal difference in night dreaming seems to be that the trajectories evoked are more spasmodic and random, and are not always under the control of the emotions and will.

CREATIVITY

The notion of planning or discovering procedures for achieving goals leads inevitably to the issue of creativity. If we assume that most of the H, G, and M functions in the processing-generating hierarchy are learned, then where is the creativity? Is creativity merely an illusion generated by the recursion of procedures for discovering procedures?

We as humans like to think of ourselves as creative. But what are we doing when we create something new? Typically, we borrow an idea from here, put it together with another from there, and give it a different name. We take a familiar behavioral trajectory, add a tiny variation, and claim that we have discovered something completely new—a new dance step, dress style, song, or idea. Seldom, however, are any of these more than the slightest deviation from a preexisting procedure or behavior trajectory. To quote Ecclesiastes: "There is nothing new under the sun."

True creativity, in the sense of the invention of an entirely new behavioral trajectory, is extremely rare, if it ever occurs at all. Furthermore, it is highly doubtful that a truly creative act would be recognized if it ever did occur. Our processing-generating hierarchies cannot lock onto sensory input patterns that are totally different from everything that is stored in them. We reject such inputs as meaningless noise, or as alien and possibly hostile. True creativity would be as incomprehensible as a book written in a foreign language or a theorem expressed in an unknown mathematical notation.

Yet, in one sense we are all creative in everything that we do, since no two behavioral trajectories are ever repeated exactly. However, the day-to-day variations in our ordinary behavior are not what we usually mean when we speak of creativity. We take pride in those moments of inspiration when something clicks, and we produce something inventive or creative beyond our daily endeavors.

If we analyze a list of the great creative ideas that have shaped human history, we find that even these have been little more than clever rearrangements of well-known preexisting patterns or procedures. For example, even in the great scientific discoveries such as Newton's laws of motion, Maxwell's electromagnetic equations, the discovery of electricity, or the invention of the steam engine, the creative act was more the product of hard work, careful procedures, and accident than any giant leap through logical space. In every case, the inventor was well trained in the skills of systematic thought related to the subject and had a deep understanding of the prior knowledge related to the subject matter. In every case, the creative genius was thoroughly immersed in the formal procedures and rules of the scientific method. And even then the insight came almost as if by accident. If anything, the genius lay in recognizing the implications of stumbling on a new hypothesis or a new sequence of ordering steps in a thought or terms in a set of equations.

This is not to discount the fact that we have a Gestalt experience of "Aha!" when we suddenly see something in a new way. There is a sudden surge of exhilaration that accompanies the moment of insight, i.e., the moment when a hypothesis is selected that generates a prediction matching the observed facts. The recognition of lock and the emotional evaluation that that particular lock-on is significant are the "Aha!" This, of course, is as much a part of the act of genius as the selection of the successful hypothesis.

There were millions of persons in James Watt's day who had observed the motion of a lid on a boiling kettle. There may even have been many who connected the heat of the flame with the mechanical motion. However, it was only Watt who recognized the implications of what he saw and who hypothesized the construction of a machine to do industrial work. In fact, Watt's contribution to the steam engine was not in the design of the cylinder and pistons but in the concept of injecting a spray of cold water into the steam-filled cylinder to create a vacuum on the return stroke.

This was an act of creative genius. But what went on in the mind of the genius? First was the recognition, then the hypothesis, and then the hard work of turning the moment of insight into a piece of working machinery. There was no great leap through uncharted regions of thought space. There was at most a tiny evolutionary step, an almost accidental superposition of the recalled memory of a piston on the observed image of a moving kettle lid. Watt could make this superposition because he already had imbedded in the H, M, and G functions of his mind the learned skills of making and working with pistons and cylinders.

The implication is that we need no elaborate mechanisms to account for creativity beyond what we have already set forth for explaining goal-seeking behavior. What is truly remarkable about the creative person is the ability to select hypotheses, to recall realistic expectations, and to accurately process and evaluate these expectations according to a set of logical rules. These are the mechanisms required for sophisticated goal-directed behavior. Nothing more, other than habits of careful investigation and observation and a fortunate choice of attentional goals, is needed to account for even the greatest acts of creative genius.

Consider the fact that it took the human race many millenia to learn to start a fire, to grow a crop, to build a wheel, to write a story, to ride a horse. Even the Greeks did not know how to build an arch. Yet these are all simple procedures that any child can understand and more or less master. Surely our ancestors as adults were as intelligent and creative as today's children. Why did they fail for hundreds of years to discover these simple yet highly useful procedures?

Because they had no one to teach them. A modern child knows about wheels because he is taught. He plays with toys that have wheels. He rides in vehicles with wheels. If a modern child grew up in a culture where he never saw a wheel, he would never think of one, nor would his children, or his grandchildren, any more than his ancestors did for thousands of years before him.

This is not to say that there is not a creative aspect to genius, whether it be artistic or scientific genius. We reserve our highest acclaim for the person who discovers or devises something new. There are many artisans for every creative genius. Even so, the creation of a new art form, or even a new scientific concept, is seldom appreciated unless the details are worked out. The acclaim to genius is heavily dependent on how skillfully the work is performed, how useful or entertaining it is, and how well it harmonizes with the prevailing knowledge base and belief structure of the peer group.

The reason we value creativity so highly is because it is so rare and so highly advantageous. It is rare precisely because there are no mechanisms for creativity in the brain. There are only mechanisms for sophisticated behavior. Creativity is so advantageous because once a new and useful procedure like navigating a ship, making steel, or flying an airplane is discovered, it can easily be taught to others. We all possess the most remarkable mechanisms for learning and executing complex behavior. Once a new invention is developed, it can be taught in schools and a whole society can benefit from the results.

Thus, we learn to solve problems, to invent, and to be creative in much the same way as we learn any other goal-directed behavior pattern such as hunting, dancing, speaking, or behaving in a manner that is acceptable to and approved by our peers: we learn from a teacher. The beauty and the sense of awe and wonder we experience when confronted by work of creative genius derives much more from the skill and precision with which it is executed than from the novelty of the creation.

If there are no specific mechanisms in the brain for creativity, then it would seem foolish to attempt to design creative robots. This is certainly true at least until our robots become as skilled and dexterous and adept at complex sensory-interactive goal-directed behavior as the lower mammals.

If we design systems with sufficient skill in executing tasks and seeking goals, and sufficient sophistication in sensory analysis and context sensitive recall, and if we teach these systems procedures for selecting behavior patterns that are appropriate to the situation, then they will appear to be both intelligent and creative. But there will never be any particular part of such a device to which one can point and say "Here is the intelligence," or "Here is the creativity." Skills and knowledge will be distributed as functional operators throughout the entire hierarchy. To the degree that we are successful, intelligence and creativity will be evidenced in the procedures that are generated by such systems.

Above all, we should not expect our robots to be more clever than ourselves, at least not for many decades. In particular we should not expect our machines to program themselves or to discover for themselves how to do what we do not know how to teach them. We teach our children for years. It will take at least as much effort to teach our machines.

We must show our robots what each task is and how to do it. We must lead them through in explicit detail and teach them the correct response for almost every situation. This is how industrial robots are programmed today at the very lowest levels, and this is, for the most part, how children are taught in school. It is the way that most of us learned everything we know, and there is no reason to suspect that robots will be programmed very differently. Surely it is as unreasonable to expect a robot to program itself as it is to expect a child to educate himself. We should not expect our robots to discover new solutions to unsolved problems or to do anything that we, in all the thousands of generations we have been on this earth, have not learned how to do ourselves.

This does not mean that once we have trained our robots to a certain level of competence they can't learn many things on their own. We can certainly write programs to take the routine and the tedium out of teaching robots. Many different laboratories are developing high-level robot programming languages. We already know something about how to represent in computers knowledge about mathematics, physics, chemistry, geology, and even medical diagnosis. We know how to program complex control systems and to model complicated processes, and we are rapidly learning how to do it better, more quickly, and more reliably. Soon, perhaps, it will even be possible to translate knowledge from natural language into robot language so that we will be able to teach our robots from textbooks or tape recordings more quickly and easily than humans. We can even imagine robots learning by browsing through libraries or reading scientific papers.

But it is a mistake to attempt to build creative robots. We are not even sure what a creative human is, and we certainly have no idea what makes a person creative, aside from contact with other creative humans—or time alone to think. Is it both? Or neither?

We should first learn how to build skilled robots—skilled in manipulation, in coping with an uncertain or even hostile environment, in hunting and escaping, in making and using tools, in encoding behavior and knowledge into language, in understanding music and speech, in imagining, and in planning. Once we have accomplished these objectives, then perhaps we will understand how to convert such skills into creativity. Or perhaps we will understand that robots with such skills already possess the creativity and the wisdom that springs naturally from the knowledge of the skills themselves.

CHAPTER **8**

Robots

We come finally to the subject of robotics. From this point on, we shall attempt to apply our knowledge of how the brain produces goal-directed behavior in biological organisms to the problem of how computers can be made to produce similar behavior in mechanical machines.

Man's fascination with machines that move under their own power and with internal control is at least as old as recorded history. As early as 3000 B.C., the Egyptians are said to have built water clocks and articulated figures, some of which served as oracles. The ancient Greeks, Ethiopians, and Chinese constructed a great variety of statues and figures that acted out sequences of motions powered by falling water or steam. Hero of Alexandria amused Greek audiences around 100 B.C. with plays in several acts performed entirely by puppets driven by weights hung on twisted cords. Much later, a great number of timepieces were contrived that performed elaborate scenarios on striking the hour. Some of these clocks still exist today. In Piazza San Marco in Venice there is a clock tower, built in 1496, with two enormous bronze figures on top that strike a bell with hammers on the hour. See figure 8.1. The clock itself not only tells the time but indicates the position of the sun and moon in the zodiac. In the Frauenkirche in Nuremberg, there is a famous clock built in 1509. On the hour, a whole troupe of figures appears in procession, ringing bells, playing instruments, and summoning passersby to worship.

During the latter half of the 18th century, a number of Swiss craftsmen, most notably Pierre and Henri-Louis Jaquet-Droz, constructed a number of lifelike automata that could write, draw pictures, and play musical instruments. The Scribe, shown in figure 8.2, was built in 1770. It is an elegantly dressed figure of a child that writes with a quill pen that it dips in ink and moves over the paper with graceful strokes. This amazing android is controlled by an elaborate set of precision cams driven by a spring-powered clock escapement, shown in figure 8.3. A similar automaton, known as the Draughtsman, was built three years later. It has a repertoire of four drawings, one of which is shown in figure 8.4. The action patterns for these drawings are stored on three interchangeable sets of twelve cams. During pauses between drawings, while the cams are changing their positions, the puppet blows the dust off his drawing paper using a bellows placed in his head for this purpose. The Musician, shown in figure 8.5, actually plays a miniature organ. The fingers strike the keys in the proper sequence to produce the notes. The breast rises and falls in simulated breathing, the body and head sway in rhythm with the music, and the eyes glance about in a natural way. The Scribe, Draughtsman, and Musician still exist in working condition in the Musée d'Art et d'Histoire in Neuchâtel, Switzerland, where they are operated occasionally. A similar picture-drawing automaton, the Philadelphia Doll constructed by Henri Maillardet in 1811, can be seen at the Franklin Institute in Philadelphia.

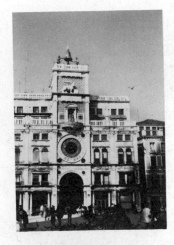

Figure 8.1: *Clock tower in Piazza San Marco, Venice, Italy, built in 1496. On the top can be seen two giant figures with hammers that strike the bell on the hour. Below is the figure of a Winged Lion, the symbol of the city of Venice. The clock itself not only tells the time, but indicates the position of the sun and moon in the zodiac.*

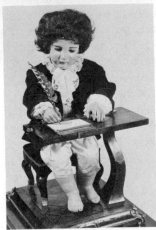

Figure 8.2: *The Scribe, a lifelike automaton built in Switzerland by Pierre and Henri-Louis Jaquet-Droz. When the Scribe writes, his eyes follow the tracing of each letter and his attitude is attentive.*

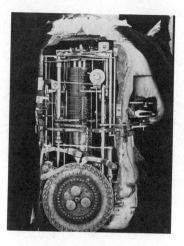

Figure 8.3: *The mechanism that drives the Scribe. Cams that control the movement of the hands in forming letters can be seen arranged in a stack in the upper and middle parts of the mechanism. There are three cams for each letter, one for each of the three degrees of freedom of the puppet's hand. Each turn of the stack forms a single letter. The disk at the lower part of the mechanism selects the vertical position of the stack and, hence, the letters to be formed. There are also sets of cams for various other actions to be performed: begin a new line, dip the pen in the ink, etc. The 40 positions on the lower disk are the program. The setting of the levers on this disk select the specific letters or actions to be performed at each step in the program. The mechanism can be programmed to execute any desired text of up to 40 letters and actions.*

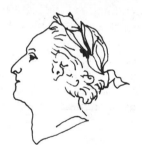

Figure 8.4: *A portrait of Louis XV executed by the Jaquet-Droz Draughtsman. The Draughtsman is a twin of the Scribe. It also has three sets of cams for producing three-axis motions. There are 36 cams in all, producing drawings with up to 12 parts each.*

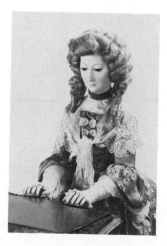

Figure 8.5: *The Musician, a Jaquet-Droz puppet that plays a miniature organ. The mechanism that raises and lowers the fingers is a drum embedded with studs similar to those used in a music box. There are ten rows of studs, one for each finger. A set of cams moves the arms back and forth to bring the fingers into position over the proper keys. Another mechanism makes the chest rise and fall at regular intervals to simulate breathing. The eyes, head, and torso are also driven in coordination with the hands and arms to produce life-like movements.*

THE FRANKENSTEIN MOTIF

The fascination, awe, and sometimes fear that surround the subject of robotics center on the notion of creating artificial life. The potentially threatening and uncontrollable consequences of this possibility have been the theme of many books and movies. One of the first and most influential works in this area was Mary Shelley's *Frankenstein*, published in England in 1817. Only a year before the book appeared, Mary Shelley had visited Neuchâtel where the Jaquet-Droz automata were then, as now, on display. The theme of *Frankenstein* is the danger of artificial life run amuck. Dr. Frankenstein, a well-intentioned scientist, creates an uncontrollable monster with superhuman strength and a defective intellect.

The word "robot" was coined a century later, in 1921, by Czechoslovakian playwright Karel Capek in his play *R.U.R. (Rossum's Universal Robots)*. Robot derives from the Czech word for "worker." Capek's *R.U.R.* echoes the Frankenstein theme through a melodramatic plot involving a brilliant scientist named Rossum who manufactures a line of robots designed to save mankind from work. Rossum's robot project is marvelously successful in the beginning, but the plot turns sinister when the robots are used in war to kill humans. Eventually, after the robots are given emotions and feelings by an irresponsible scientist in the Rossum laboratory, disaster strikes. The mechanically perfect robots no longer tolerate being treated as slaves by imperfect humans. A rebellion ensues and soon all human life is exterminated. Figure 8.6 shows the last human survivor, a clerk in Rossum's laboratory, meeting his end. Variations on these motifs have dominated science fiction and movie literature on robots for decades.

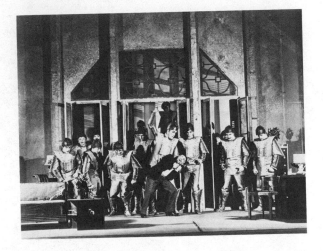

Figure 8.6: *A scene from the play* R.U.R. *where rebellious worker robots turn on their human creators and kill them. At the end of the play all human life is exterminated.*

Two notable exceptions to this trend are stories by Isaac Asimov and the recent series of motion pictures spawned by *Star Wars*. In *Star Wars*, robots are depicted as lovable friends and loyal companions to humans. In Asimov's stories, robots are constructed and programmed with the idealism of Asimov's Three Laws of Robotics which state:

1. A robot may not injure a human being or, through inaction, allow a human to be harmed.
2. A robot must obey orders given by humans except when that conflicts with the First Law.
3. A robot must protect its own existence unless that conflicts with the First or Second Laws.

ROBOT REALITY

In the real world, mankind is by no means in physical danger from rebellions by neurotic robots and is unlikely to be so for at least several centuries, if ever. The reality of modern computer science, artificial intelligence, and robotics is that machines have extremely primitive motor and intellectual capacities. Despite the highly publicized advances in modern computer science and control theory, the sensory-perception, decision-making, and intellectual capabilities of robots are far inferior to humans and will remain so for many years to come. The only exception to this is in certain narrowly restricted or highly structured domains such as board games or bodies of knowledge that can be expressed as formal mathematical statements. So, too, the mechanical dexterity and sophistication of sensory interaction in real robots are far inferior to that of the human body or, for that matter, of insects. The images of robots projected to the public by television shows such as *Million Dollar Man* and *Bionic Woman* are pure fiction. Most of the robots that frequent the movie sets are nothing more than humans dressed up in robot suits (figure 8.7), and the robot figures appearing in amusement parks and public exhibitions are either controlled by totally prerecorded programs or are cleverly disguised remote control devices that owe their intellectual capacities to a concealed human operator.

If it were possible to build a robot that were as intelligent and as skilled in moving about, carrying, and building things as an ant, then it would be possible for robots to perform incredible feats of construction. Consider what ants can build. Watch an ant hill and see what ants can do. Ants can carry loads much bigger than they are, run over the most difficult terrain, hang upside down, climb straight up a tree trunk or stalk of grass, and do so for hours, at a furious pace. An ant can cover a distance equal to its body length in a fraction of a second, which is about 60 miles an hour for a robot the size of a small car. We only have to contrast this behavioral

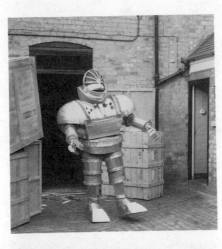

Figure 8.7: *A scene from the popular BBC television series* Dr. Who. *In such productions, the robot is usually a human actor dressed up in a robot costume.*

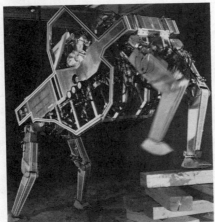

Figure 8.8: *The experimental walking truck built by the General Electric Company for the U.S. Army in 1969. This project was a failure because of the unanticipated computational difficulty of simultaneously controlling all of the degrees of freedom in the four legs. It proved beyond the capability of a human operator to control this vehicle under most conditions. This failure dramatically demonstrated the sophistication that control systems must have to produce successful walking behavior in legged mechanisms.*

dexterity with the clumsy lumberings of the walking truck shown in figure 8.8 to understand how far we are far from creating a robot with the physical skills of an ant.

Some might even contend that it will never be possible to create a robot as marvelous as an ant. In some ways this is undoubtedly true, at least not for a hundred years, or perhaps a thousand. The truly interesting question is, "What is possible in five years, in ten, in twenty, in fifty—the remaining years of our lives?"

Clearly it is possible to build vehicles that move about at many times the comparative speed of insects, whether they walk, fly, or swim. We know how to build and fuel efficient power plants and how to build transmission systems to transport and modulate the power.

What we do not know is how to build the sensory-interactive control systems necessary to direct that power to accomplish goals and execute skilled tasks in an unstructured, uncooperative, and even hostile environment. Furthermore, we cannot yet build the mechanical structures inexpensively. The cheapest computer-controlled industrial robot with five servoed degrees of freedom, one parallel jaw gripper, and a crude sense of touch and vision costs about $60,000, and it cannot lift one-tenth of its own weight.

Yet the problem is much more fundamental than merely the cost of mechanical hardware. The software does not exist at any price that could control a six-legged walking machine with two arms and a full set of force, touch, and vision senses in the performance of tasks like building a brick fireplace, laying a hardwood floor, installing a bathtub, or painting the front of a house.

Nevertheless, in spite of the present profound inadequacies in robot sensory-motor skills, robot technology will very soon play a major economic, scientific, and military role in human affairs. As crude as they are, industrial robots are already beginning to make a significant contribution to several manufacturing processes such as spray painting, unloading die-casting and injection-molding machines, tending presses, spot welding automobile bodies, handling materials, and arc welding. These are important and expensive operations in the manufacture of many valuable articles such as automobiles, tractors, trucks, and earth-moving equipment. Much of the computer and control technology that was and is being developed in artificial intelligence and robot laboratories is crucial to the performance of modern missile guidance systems, particularly in the smart bomb and cruise missile systems, and soon will undoubtedly be incorporated into many other weapons and electronics warfare systems as well.

Over the next two centuries, many, if not most, jobs in factories and offices will be performed by a robot labor force. Robots will surely play a major role in planetary exploration and in the exploitation of the two-thirds of the Earth's surface covered by oceans. Robots will eventually appear in the household, although the cost of general-purpose mechanical servants will probably limit their use for several decades.

At present, robot technology has two major branches, one technological and the other scientific. In the development of practical industrial robots the primary criteria are reliability and cost-effectiveness. In the scientific study of robotics, (often conducted under the heading of artificial intelligence) the emphasis is on exploring fundamental questions of sensory perception, motor control, and intelligent behavior.

INDUSTRIAL ROBOTS

Most of the industrial robots used in factories throughout the world exhibit few of the characteristics that the average person would associate with the term "robot." Many are "pick-and-place" machines that are capable of only the simplest kinds of motion. These machines have little or no ability to sense conditions in their environment. When they are switched on, they simply execute a preprogrammed sequence of operations. The limits of motion of each joint of the machine are fixed by mechanical "stops," and each detail of movement must be guided by means of an electric or pneumatic impulse originating at a plugboard control panel.

Figure 8.9 shows a popular variety of a pick-and-place robot. Programming of this machine is accomplished by connecting pieces of plastic tubing to the appropriate nipples on the pneumatic control unit shown in figure 8.10. The bottom part of the control unit is a sequencer which provides pressure and vacuum to a set of nipples in a timed sequence. The upper part of the control unit contains a set of nipples which activate each of the joint actuators. Connections made between the various nipples determine which joints are actuated, and in which direction, at each step. Whenever a new program is needed, the programming connections are relocated and the mechanical stops repositioned to set up a new sequence of movements.

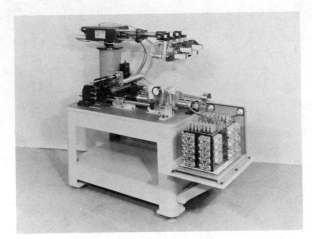

Figure 8.9: *Pick-and-place manipulators are the simplest of present-day industrial robots. This table-mounted version, made by Auto-Place, Inc., of Troy, Michigan, is powered by air. Six double-action air cylinders enable the robot to slide back and forth, lift, rotate, reach, grasp, and turn objects over. The sequence of operations is programmed by means of the sequencing module shown at the right of the table.*

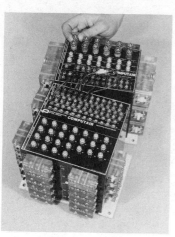

Figure 8.10: *A pneumatic control unit for the Auto-Place robot. Programming is accomplished by connecting pieces of plastic tubing from the actuator cylinders to the appropriate nipples on the pneumatic sequencer.*

This type of robot-programming technique represents the absolute minimum of sophistication. Many people feel that such a machine should not even be dignified by the name robot. Nevertheless, the basic elements of robotics are present: the machine is programmable, it is automatic, and it can perform a wide variety of manipulatory tasks.

A more sophisticated level of control can be achieved by adding servomechanisms that can command the position of each degree of freedom to assume any value. The Unimate robot shown in figure 8.11 was one of the earliest servo-controlled robots and is still a highly successful model. The addition of servo-control calls for feedback from sensors such a potentiometers, encoders, or resolvers which measure the position of each joint. The measured positions are compared with commanded positions, and any differences are corrected by signals sent to the appropriate joint actuators.

There are several ways to program a servo-controlled manipulator. Conceptually, the simplest is a potentiometer board, similar to the plugboard system. The positions of the joints at each step are determined by values set on the potentiometers rather than by mechanical stops. This technique was used by early models of the robot shown in figure 8.12.

The capability of robots actuated by servomechanisms is greatly enhanced by the addition of an electronic memory for storing programs and digital control circuitry. Such a robot is programmed by leading it through the desired sequence of positions. A human tutor uses a hand-held control box, shown in figure 8.13, with a rate-control button that enables him to control each of the robot's joints. The human programmer uses such a control box to guide the robot to the desired positions for each program step. By pushing a button the programmer can record the position of each point in the robot's program.

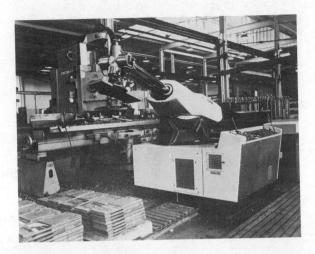

Figure 8.11: *A Unimate 2000 robot picking up a metal plate to be loaded into a machine tool shown in the background. This robot is controlled by a program stored in a digital electronic memory. Each point in the robot's program consists of six binary numbers specifying the location of the six degrees of freedom of the robot gripper.*

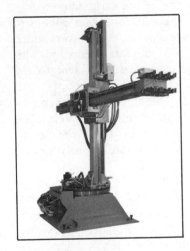

Figure 8.12: *The Versatran Model FA robot. The Versatran line, formerly manufactured by AMF, is now produced by Prab Conveyors, Inc. Points in this robot's program can be specified by potentiometers or can be stored in digital memory.*

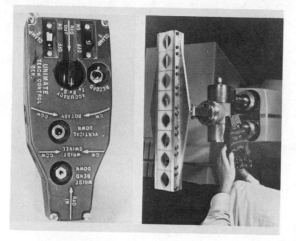

Figure 8.13: *The hand controller used to program the Unimate robot. This device has rate-control buttons for moving each joint in one direction or the other. The operator uses these buttons to drive the robot to the desired position for each program point. He then pushes the record button to store the six values which specify the positions of the six axes at that point.*

When the program is played back, the control system simply commands each joint to move to the positions recorded for each step. Once the robot goes into operation on the production line it repeats the recorded program over and over again, moving from one recorded point to the next according to a fixed timing cycle, either on completion of the last step or in response to an interlock signal from external machinery. This type of robot is called a "point-to-point" robot because the exact path of the robot is defined only at a few selected points. Most point-to-point robots have programs of only a few hundred steps. Figure 8.14 shows a schematic diagram of the record and play-back circuitry.

An electronic memory enables a robot to store several programs and to select one or another depending on different input commands or on feedback from external sensors. For example, robots that spot weld automobile bodies can be programmed to handle a variety of automobile models intermixed on an assembly line. A coded signal indicating which body model is positioned in front of the robot is used to select the appropriate entry point in the robot's program memory.

If smooth, continuous motion is required, a magnetic tape capable of storing many thousands of closely spaced steps can be used for a control system. Continuous-path programs allow the robot to move smoothly through space along a completely defined trajectory. This is most often used for paint spraying. Figure 8.15 shows a continuous-path, paint-spraying robot. Typically, the continuous-path robot is led through its task by a human who performs the job once. This path is recorded on tape and replayed each time the robot is called upon to perform the same job.

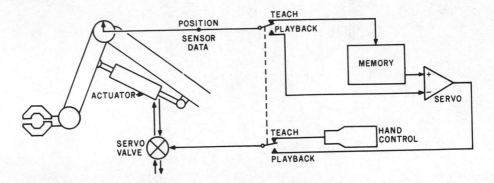

Figure 8.14: *Programming an industrial robot is usually done by using a hand control unit to teach the robot by guiding it through a sequence of positions which are recorded in memory. Once the teach operation is completed, the control system is switched to the playback mode. The robot then repeats the recorded sequence of operations automatically.*

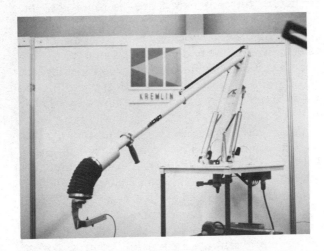

Figure 8.15: *An Italian-made paint-spraying robot. The wrist of this robot is controlled by cables and can flex both side-to-side and up-and-down like an elephant's trunk. This enables the spray nozzle on the tip to paint hard-to-reach spots.*

The addition of a computer with arithmetic and logic capabilities makes it possible to implement higher levels of control. With a computer it is possible to program the robot to move its hand in straight lines, or along other geometric paths, between the recorded points. This is illustrated in figure 8.16. The computer allows the programmer to specify points via a keyboard as well as by leading the robot through the task. Figure 8.17 shows a man programming a Cincinnati Milicron T³ robot. In figure 8.18 the author enters programming instructions to a "Scheinman arm" laboratory research robot through a keyboard. With this, robot motions can be specified in various coordinate systems. The robot can be commanded to move in a Cartesian coordinate system defined relative to a work table (x,y,z) or relative to a tool in the robot's hand (x', y', z'), as shown in figure 8.19. If the coordinate system is fixed relative to the work table, it is easy to deal with parts arranged in regular arrays. If the coordinate system is defined relative to a point on a moving conveyor belt, as shown in figure 8.20, the robot can work with parts on the moving belt. If the coordinate system is defined relative to a set of features (e.g., corners and edges) of the part itself, the robot can be commanded to orient itself relative to a part, to insert a tool or a part into a hole, or even to execute the type of motion required to turn a crank or twist a nut with a wrench. A computer also allows the robot's motions to be smoothly coordinated and to execute smooth accelerations and decelerations to maximize the speed with which heavy objects can be manipulated.

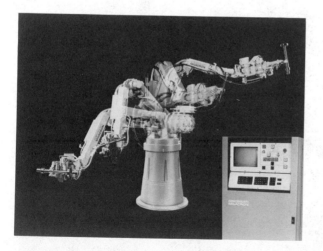

Figure 8.16: *A Cincinnati Milicron T³ robot with its computer control unit and display console. This robot can be programmed to move its gripper in straight lines from point to point. The computer calculates the velocities and accelerations needed for each joint to produce coordinated motions.*

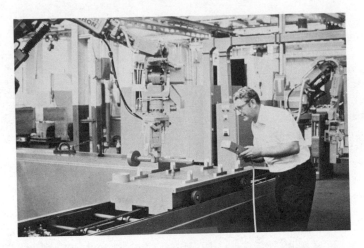

Figure 8.17: *Even computer-controlled robots are typically programmed by the teach method. Specific points in space where parts are to be placed, welds are to be made, or other operations are to be performed are specified by leading the robot to the points and pressing a "record" button. A computer control system makes this programming task easier by allowing the programmer to move the robot hand along axes defined in the coordinate systems of the work space or the fingertips or tool point of the robot itself. This robot stores the program points in x,y,z coordinates and gripper orientation.*

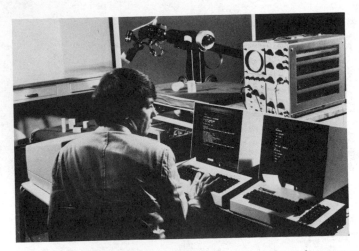

Figure 8.18: *Programming of a laboratory robot through a computer terminal. Data specifying points in space where operations are to be performed may be defined by Computer-Aided-Design (CAD) data bases or from sensors such as video cameras and touch detectors. Programming by teaching may still be used for some elemental moves, but automatic optimization programs will refine these preliminary trajectories into graceful, efficient motions.*

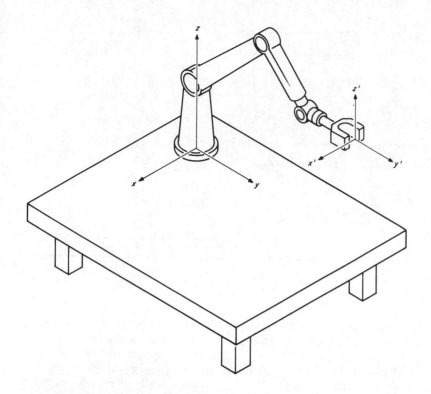

Figure 8.19: *Two coordinate systems. One, the x,y,z system is defined with the table top as the x-y plane, the origin at the center of the robot pedestal, and the x axis aligned parallel to one edge of the table. A second coordinate system, the x,′ y,′ z′ system, is defined with the y′ axis along the direction the finger tips are pointing, the x′ axis parallel to the line joining the two fingertips, and the origin at the tip of the fingers (or at the tip of a tool held in the fingers). A computer can allow robot motions to be specified as vectors in either of these two coordinate systems.*

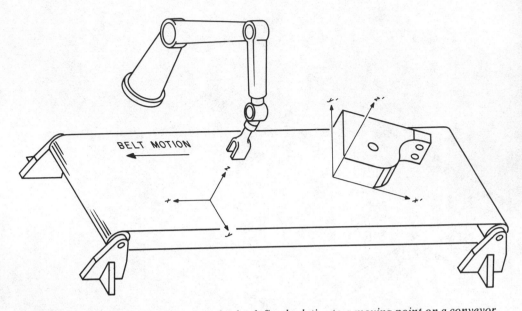

BELT MOTION

Figure 8.20: *Coordinate systems may also be defined relative to a moving point on a conveyor belt or relative to an object to be handled. Here the x,y,z system is defined with the x-y plane in the plane of the belt, the x axis along the direction of the belt's motion, and the origin fixed at a specific point on the belt. The x,′ y,′ z′ system is defined with the origin at one vertex of an object that the robot will pick up. The x,′ y,′ and z′ axes are defined along the edges emanating from that vertex.*

ROBOT SENSES

The great majority of industrial robots, even those with computers, have little or no sensory capabilities. Feedback is limited to information about joint position, combined with a few interlock and timing signals. Most robots can function only in environments where the objects to be manipulated are precisely located in the proper position for the robot to grasp.

For many industrial applications, this level of performance is quite adequate. Until recently, the majority of robot applications consisted of taking parts out of die-casting and injection-molding machines as shown in figure 8.21. In this task, the parts produced are always in exactly the same position in the mold so that the robot needs no sensory capability to find the part or compensate for misalignments. Another principal application is the spot welding of automobile bodies, shown in figure 8.22. Here, the car bodies are positioned and clamped so that each body is always exactly in the same place as the one before. Thus, the robot needs no sensory capability to find where to place the welds.

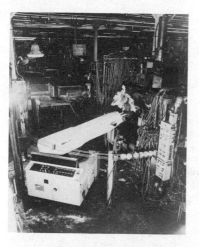

Figure 8.21: *A Unimate robot unloading a die-casting machine. This was one of the earliest industrial applications of robots and still represents a large fraction of all robot installations. In this task, the part to be grasped is always in exactly the same position, so the robot needs no sophisticated sensory or computer control capability. This type of work is tedious heavy labor for human workers, and the work environment is filled with hot, foul-smelling fumes. Thus, few workers employed in tending injection-molding machines mind being replaced by robots, as long as they are given comparable jobs elsewhere.*

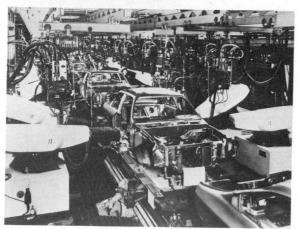

Figure 8.22: *Unimate 2000 robots spot welding automobile bodies on a General Motors Vega line. Spot welding is one of the largest applications of industrial robots today.*

Only since the advent of robots with computers has it become possible for robot spot welders to operate on moving auto bodies, shown in figure 8.23. In this application, an encoder is attached to the moving line to indicate to the robot how fast the car body is moving. An optical sensor indicates when each car moves into the work area so that the robot can begin its programmed routine. The robot's computer then transforms the coordinate system of the program to follow the conveyor line.

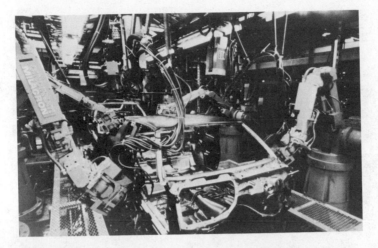

Figure 8.23: *Cincinnati Milicron robots spot welding automobile bodies on a moving line at the General Motors Assembly Division in Lakewood, Georgia. Four T³ robots place 200 spot welds on each of 48 car bodies per hour as they move past on a conveyor. This robot is programmed in a coordinate system fixed in the auto body, and the computer offsets that program as the auto body moves past the robot. The ability to work on moving objects makes it possible to use a much simpler and less expensive transfer mechanism for moving the car bodies past the robots.*

Over the last decade, robot spot welding has become a significant factor in automotive production. Over 50 percent of all the automobiles built today are welded by robots.

Of course, in the industrial world, the question of whether to use sensory capabilities such as vision is purely one of economics. There are three possible approaches:

1. Maintain knowledge of the exact position and orientation of parts throughout the manufacturing process.
2. Reacquire this information at each work station in the manufacturing process through conventional positioning and feeding mechanisms.
3. Use TV cameras and complex video-processing systems to search for and find parts that are not precisely positioned.

Which is cheaper and easier? In most cases, the answer is either method number one or two. Robot sensors, particularly vision sensors, are expensive and the processing of sensory data can be extremely complex. Typically, powerful computers and sophisticated software are required, and often programs must be specially written for each specific application. Thus, although robot vision is an interesting and challenging field with great promise for the future, it is still almostly entirely confined to the research laboratory. The exception to this is the industrial applications where vision is used for inspection tasks, such as to verify whether bottles are filled, labels are correctly placed, etc. Nevertheless, robot vision research is progressing rapidly. Computing power is becoming less expensive, and robot control systems are being designed to use visual information in directing the robot in its task

Robot Assembly

Even the relatively difficult task of robot assembly can often be accomplished with little or no sensing of events in the environment. For example, engineers at the Kawasaki laboratories in Japan have shown that robots can put together complex assemblies of motors and gearboxes with no more than high-precision position feedback, cleverly designed grippers, and fixtures for holding parts that flex by a slight amount when the parts are brought together. Other experiments have shown that a small amount of vibration or jiggling, together with properly designed tapers and bevels, can accommodate for slight misalignments and prevent jamming when two pieces with close tolerances are assembled.

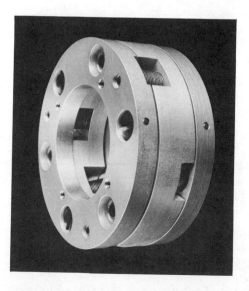

Figure 8.24: *A commercial Remote Center Compliance (RCC) device. This device, when mounted between the robot wrist and gripper, compensates for misalignments and thus can minimize assembly forces and the possibility of jamming.*

Paul C. Watson, Samuel Drake, and Sergio N. Simunovic, working at the Draper Laboratories in Cambridge, Mass., developed a unique device called a Remote Center Compliance (RCC) device, shown in figure 8.24. The RCC device mounted in the robot wrist allows parts to be fitted together without jamming, regardless of slight misalignments. With use of the RCC, bearings and shafts can be reliably inserted into holes with very small clearance.

Daniel E. Whitney and James L. Nevins, also at the Draper Labs, demonstrated the RCC on the robot in figure 8.25 in the assembly of a commercial automobile alternator. In this demonstration, the robot had a tool changer that allowed it to use a number of different grippers and power tools to accomplish various portions of the assembly task. The program sequence by which the alternator was assembled and the tools used in the assembly are shown in figure 8.26.

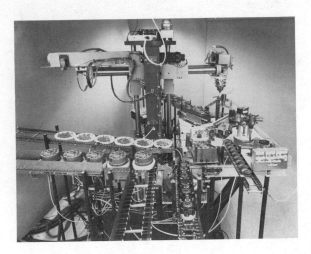

Figure 8.25: *An experimental robot assembly project at the C. S. Draper Laboratory. Automobile alternators were assembled from a number of subassemblies shown entering the robot work station via conveyor feeders. This robot has a number of different gripping devices which can be changed automatically. A circular rack of interchangeable tools and grippers is visible just below and to the right of the robot wrist. This assembly task requires six different tools to assemble the seventeen different parts fed by gravity from twelve feeders. The assembly is performed on two different fixtures, one for the main assembly, the other for a subassembly.*

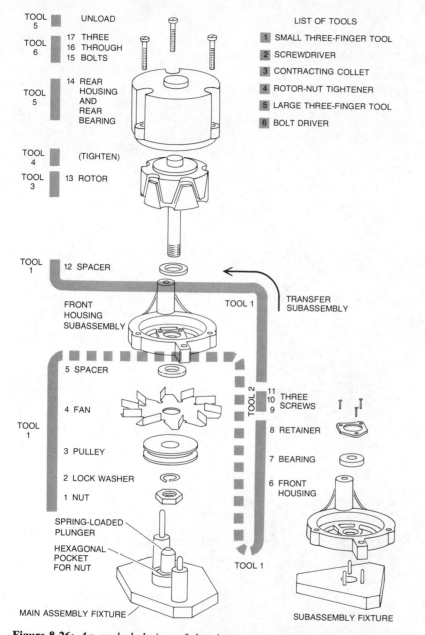

Figure 8.26: *An exploded view of the alternator being assembled in figure 8.25 shows the sequence in which its parts are put together by the robot and identifies the tools that perform each subtask. Time and motion studies indicate that alternators could be assembled in a factory by a robot similar to this one in approximately one minute and five seconds.* [*From "Computer-controlled Assembly," by J. L. Nevins and D. E. Whitney. Copyright © 1978 by Scientific American, Inc. All rights reserved.*]

Other research laboratories have also experimented with robot assembly. Experiments at Stanford University as well as in a number of other labs have used vision to acquire parts that are not precisely positioned. In one of the first robot assembly experiments ever performed, that of the water pump shown in figure 8.27a, the robot used a TV camera to locate the various parts. Figure 8.27b shows the TV image seen by the robot eye. Similar assembly research has been performed in Artificial Intelligence Laboratories at MIT, Edinburg University, S.R.I. International, and in a number of industrial laboratories including IBM, Westinghouse, and General Electric.

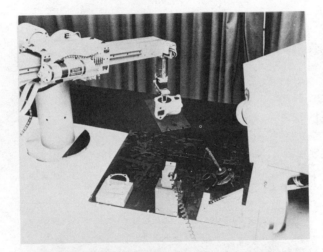

Figure 8.27a: *An assembly experiment performed in the AI Lab at Stanford. The TV camera at the right views and identifies various components such as the housing, gasket, and rotor assembly of a water pump. The vision system then calculates the position and orientation of each component so that the robot arm can perform the assembly operation. The object at the bottom center of the figure is an electric bolt-runner that the robot picks up and uses to screw the assembly together.*

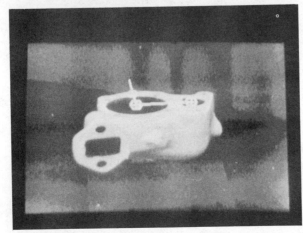

Figure 8.27b: *A display of the Stanford University robot-vision system automatically recognizing and locating the positions of two holes in the water pump housing.*

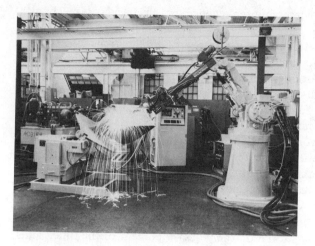

Figure 8.28: *A Cincinnati Milicron computer-controlled T^3 industrial robot performing an arc-welding task. The work is presented to the robot by a two-axis automatic positioning table which is controlled by the same computer as the robot. Behind the robot is the computer control cabinet and the welding power supply. Mounted high on the arm are a spool of welding wire and a wire-feeder mechanism.*

In recent months there have been a number of new robot companies formed. For the most part these new ventures are targeted for assembly. Many large corporations such as General Motors, Texas Instruments, International Harvester, Volkswagon, Fiat, Renault, Hitachi, and General Numeric are entering the robot research arena, hoping to use robots in their manufacturing operations.

It is important to note that despite extensive research, robot assembly has yet to prove itself to be economically practical in more than a very few applications. There are a number of reasons for this. First of all, robots are very expensive—almost as expensive as special-purpose assembly machines. There are only a few jobs where the number of items to be assembled is too few to justify a special-purpose, high-speed assembly machine, yet is numerous enough to justify the cost of the robot and the tooling required for robot assembly.

A second reason is that robots are slow and clumsy compared either with a special-purpose assembly machine or with a human worker. The human is incredibly dexterous and adaptable to many different jobs. Human hands and fingers can literally fly over the work, handle limp goods, and work in cramped quarters with little difficulty.

Third, a human comes equipped with a vision system that far surpasses any robot vision system likely to be marketed in this century. The human also has a fantastic sense of touch discrimination. He or she can take verbal instructions from speakers of many dialects, can employ sophisticated reasoning powers, can notice defects in parts or products, and can take corrective action that is far beyond the capacities of the best robot.

Finally, the human works relatively cheaply, can be hired one week and fired the next, can be easily moved from one job to another, and can be supervised by a person with no special skills in computer science or electrical or mechanical engineering.

Yet robots are very cost-effective in a number of applications. Besides the injection-molding, die-casting, and spot-welding applications, robots have demonstrated their abilities in forging, materials handling, machine tool loading, investment casting, arc welding, and inspection. The cost of purchasing and maintaining a robot on the job is about $5.00 per hour. In many applications, this is half or even a third of the cost of human labor.

Industrial robots usually work no faster than humans can in the same job. But they do work more steadily, without coffee or lunch breaks, or trips to the rest room. This can be very significant. For example, in arc welding, a very tedious, hot, smoky job, the human must wear a face mask and heavy protective clothing. A human welder has difficulty in keeping the welding torch applied to the work for more than about 30 percent of the time. However, a robot arc welder, such as shown in figure 8.28, can usually keep its torch on the work 90 percent of the time. Thus, even though the robot can weld no faster than a human, it produces about three times as much output per shift. If the robot works for one third the wages, the productivity gain for only one shift is about 900 percent. When the same robot can work two, three, or even four (Saturdays and Sundays) shifts per week, the economic payoff is that much greater.

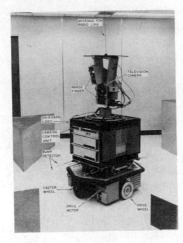

Figure 8.29: *Shakey, the S.R.I. robot designed as a research tool for studying artificial intelligence issues in vision, navigation, planning, and problem-solving. Shakey was controlled by a PDP-10 computer through a radio link. It carried a TV camera, an optical range finder, and touch sensors so that it could know when it had bumped into something. Its vision system could detect the dark baseboards around the walls and could discriminate the shapes of various rectangular and triangular boxes in the room.*

Sensory Interaction

Despite the enormous economic potential, present-day robots are simply incapable of performing most industrial jobs. The principal impediment is that they lack the sensory capabilities to enable them to compensate for unstructured conditions in the work environment. In most arc-welding applications, for example, it is necessary for the welder to work in a number of different positions. To do this he must be able to see where the weld is to be made and to adjust the welding process to the slight differences in the conditions of the work. Similarly in assembly, machine tool loading, and materials handling, the acquisition of parts often requires an ability to measure where the parts are. The robot's program must be adjusted to take into account the difference between ideal and actual conditions.

As vision research progresses, as cheaper cameras and computers are designed and manufactured (prices on both are falling dramatically), and as software is developed, robots will eventually be able to see, and rather well, especially under controlled conditions. Within the 1980s, industrial robots will be equipped with many different kinds of sensors that will enable them to measure the state of the environment. Control systems will be designed to act and react to the sensory information in a successful goal-seeking manner. Sensors will be designed to measure the three-dimensional space around the robot and to recognize and measure the position and orientation of objects and relationships between the objects in that space. Sensory-processing systems will be able to analyze and interpret the raw sensory data and compare it against an internal model of the external world to detect errors, omissions, and unexpected events. Finally, there will be a control system that can accept high-level commands and break down those commands into effective behavior within the context of the conditions reported by the sensory-processing system.

To be economically practical, the software for all these capabilities must fit in a small minicomputer, or a network of microcomputers, and it must run fast enough so that the robot can react to sensory data within a small fraction of a second. Finally, the entire robot system, including the sensors, computers, mechanical structure, and power system, must cost less than what is normally paid to human labor for the same work.

Given these very stringent requirements, it is almost surprising that robots are practical at all. Yet, the progress in industrial robotics is rapid, and robots are being successfully used in a growing number of applications. As the number and sophistication of their sensory capabilities increases and the cost of computing power continues to decline, the number of potential applications will grow. As that happens, robots will become an increasingly important economic factor, and more and more money will become available for research and development.

A good strategy for the would-be roboticist would be to start from the present state-of-the-art as practiced in industrial robotics and gradually expand the sensory and control capabilities until the more difficult tasks become tractable. In fact, this strategy has been pursued successfully by a number of robotics research laboratories. For example, the robotics group at S.R.I. International, directed for a number of years by Charles Rosen and afterward by David Nitzan, began their robotics work as an outgrowth of the Shakey project. Shakey, shown in figures 8.29 and 8.30, was an early robot, conceived as a demonstration project for the Advanced Research Projects Agency (ARPA) artificial intelligence program. Shakey could be given a task such as finding a box of a given size, shape, and color and moving it to a designated position. Shakey was able to search for the box in various rooms, cope with obstacles, and plan a suitable course of action. In some situations, the performance required the implementation of a preliminary action before the principal goal could be achieved. In one instance, illustrated in figure 8.30, Shakey figured out that by moving a ramp a few feet it could climb up on a platform where the box had been placed.

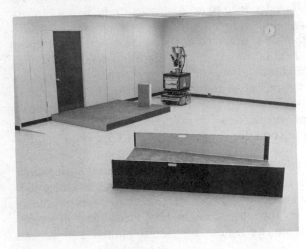

Figure 8.30: *Shakey was able to find its way around a suite of several rooms connected by a number of doorways. It could detect which pathways were clear and which were blocked and plan an optimum pathway on command. It was even able to accept a task such as "push the box off the platform." This was accomplished by developing a strategy of pushing the ramp to the platform so that it could climb up and push the box off.*

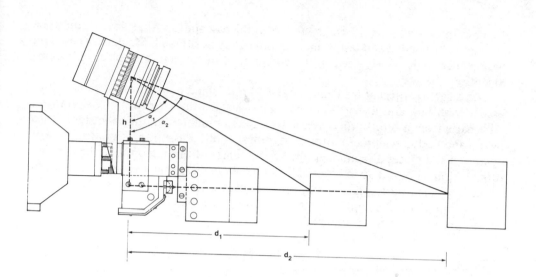

Figure 8.31: *A side view of the vision system used on the National Bureau of Standards research robot. A strobographic flash unit projects a plane of light into the region in front of the robot fingertips. A camera mounted on the robot wrist measures the apparent position of the light reflected from an object and computes the position and orientation of the reflecting surface. If the camera sees a bright mark at angle α_1, the reflecting object must be located at distance d_1. If the bright mark is seen at angle α_2, the reflecting object is at distance d_2. The known value of h makes the distance calculation a simple problem in trigonometry.*

When the Shakey project ended, the S.R.I. robotics group turned their attention to the problems of industrial automation. They established an industrial affiliates program, whereby any company desiring to get expert advice and share in state-of-the-art research in industrial robotics could become a partner in research.

The S.R.I. research program has produced a number of significant contributions to the field. One of the most notable of these is a robot vision system which includes a TV camera, a computer interface, a microcomputer, and a software package with a number of binary image processing capabilities. The S.R.I. vision system converts the TV image to a binary (black-white) image and computes a number of features on the resulting image regions. For example, the system computes the area and perimeter of connected regions, their set inclusion relationships, their degree of elongation along various axes, and their position and orientation in the visual field. This vision system, used in a number of industrial applications, is now marketed commercially. S.R.I. has also explored other industrial applications in parts acquisition, welding, three-dimensional vision, and force and touch sensing.

Artificial intelligence techniques have also been applied to a number of industrial applications at MIT. Professor Berthold Horn developed a method for aligning integrated circuit chips under a microscope so that leads could be automatically bonded and test probes automatically positioned. Machinery based on these principles is widely used in the commercial manufacture of electronic components.

A research project at the University of Rhode Island under the direction of Professors John Birk and Robert Kelly has demonstrated the use of robot vision to acquire parts from a bin. In this case, a TV camera mounted on the robot looks into the bin and finds a region of uniform brightness. This, it assumes, is a flat surface of a part. Then it places a vacuum gripper in the center of this region, lifts the part out of the bin, and holds it up in front of a second TV camera that analyzes the shape of the now isolated part. This determines the orientation of the part relative to the robot gripper, and the control system uses this information to place the part in a desired position in a work fixture.

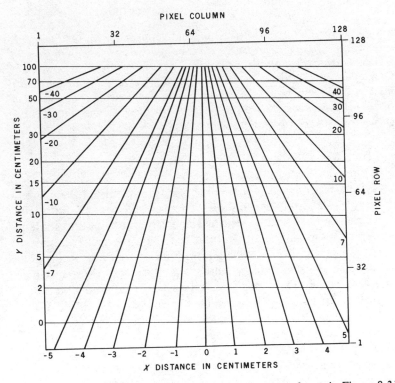

Figure 8.32: *A calibration chart for the vision system shown in Figure 8.31. The pixel row and column of any illuminated point in the TV image can be immediately converted to x,y position in a coordinate system defined in the robot fingertips. The x-axis passes through the two fingertips and the y-axis points in the same direction as the fingers. The plane of the projected light is coincident with the x-y plane so that the z coordinate of every illuminated point is zero.*

At the National Bureau of Standards a vision system designed by the author uses a plane of light to determine the position and orientation of parts on a table. As shown in figure 8.31, light from a slit projector mounted on the robot's wrist is projected into the region in front of the fingertips. When this light strikes an object it makes a bright line which is observed by the TV camera also mounted on the robot's wrist. The geometrical relationship between the projector, the camera, and the bright line allows the vision system to compute the position of the object relative to the fingertips. Figure 8.32 shows a calibration chart that the computer uses to transform from row and pixel number of a spot on the bright line to x and y position in the coordinate system of the fingertips. The shape of the line is a depth profile of the object. The slope of any segment of this line indicates the orientation of the corresponding portion of the front surface of the part relative to the fingers. This information is then used by the control system to move the robot hand to reach out and grasp an object, as shown in figure 8.33. This robot can operate on a random pile of blocks and cylinders and sort them into a regular array. It can also measure the shape of a casting, find the edge of a window frame, detect the crack between a pair of bricks, or measure the angle between two pieces of steel. This is the most basic type of sensory information required to perform tasks in the factory and on the construction site.

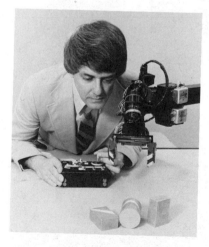

Figure 8.33: *The NBS experimental robot approaching a cylindrical object. The bright streak across the cylinder and table top is produced by the plane of the light projector. The image of this streak of light is processed by the vision system to measure the three-dimensional position and orientation of the object and to assist in recognizing the type of object being viewed. This projection technique makes it possible to directly measure the three-dimensional shape of the object regardless of its reflectance properties or the nature of the background.*

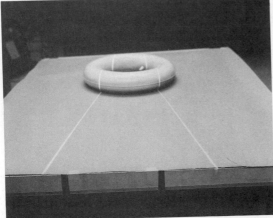

8.34a.

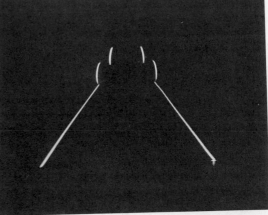

8.34e.

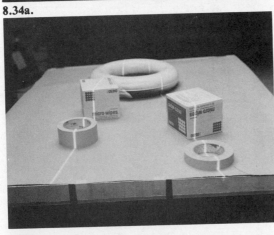

8.34b.

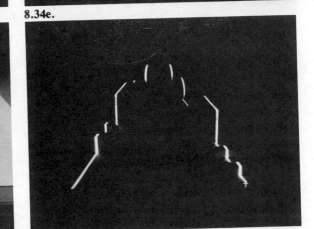

8.34f.

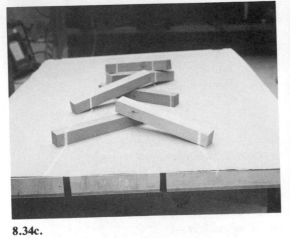

8.34c.

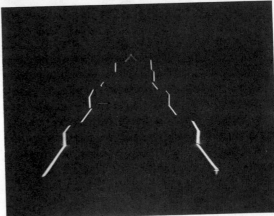

8.34g.

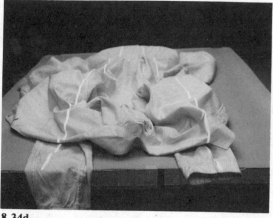

8.34d.

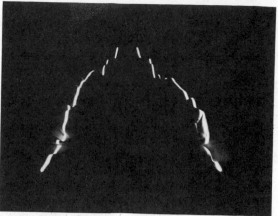

8.34h.

Figure 8.34: *A series of pictures made at the Jet Propulsion Laboratory by projecting a pair of vertical planes of light onto objects on a table top. The pictures shown in (e), (f), (g), and (h) are thresholded versions of (a), (b), (c), and (d) respectively. If the thresholded images are scanned from left to right, the distances of the bright pixels from the edges of the frame are directly proportional to the distances of the illuminated points from the camera. Thus, the distance to, and height of, any object illuminated by either of the lines of light can be calculated by simple trigonometry or from a look-up table. The planes of light can be scanned back and forth to build up a depth map of the entire region in front of the camera.*

A similar use of structured lighting at NASA's Jet Propulsion Laboratory (JPL) in Pasadena, California, illustrates the power of this technique to simplify the measurement of depth information. Figure 8.34 shows a set of experiments by Alan Johnston. JPL scientists have also built a stereo vision system that can measure the distance to an object, determine its shape, and track a moving object. These systems make it possible for a robot arm to reach out and grasp an object like a rock or, presumably, capture an animal like a toad. This JPL project is directed toward building a robot vehicle capable of exploring the surface of the moon and planets.

CONCLUSIONS

Robotics has come a long way from the great clock tower in Piazza San Marco. The technologies of electronics, computers, and servomechanisms have made enormous strides in recent years; the technologies of semiconductor sensors, memories, and microcomputers are still in their ascendancy. Yet paradoxically, the actual state of the art in robotics falls far short of the popular imagination. For years, science fiction robots have been the heroes and villains of countless spellbinding tales. The fictional robot is as familiar to most Americans as Superman or Wonder Woman. Unfortunately, it is just as unreal. Industrial robots costing $50,000 apiece seem pedestrian compared to the popular image of walking, talking, mechanical humanoids with superhuman skills and strength. Today only the superhuman strength is a reality.

But tomorrow will be different. We have only just learned to build good numerically controlled machines. Only in the past ten years have computers become inexpensive enough to dedicate a single computer to a robot. It will soon be practical to use five or ten powerful computers for controlling a single robot. Microcomputer technology is making this not only conceivable, but simple and inexpensive. Already computers for robot-control systems cost only a fraction of what the mechanical hardware costs.

The technology of robotics has come to the edge of a historical breakthrough. Within this decade industrial robots will begin to play a major role in the process of industrial manufacturing. By the turn of the century, robots will have fundamentally altered the entire industrial process. In the long term, this cannot but profoundly affect the course of human civilization.

CHAPTER **9**

Hierarchical Robot-Control Systems

As long as a robot program is reasonably simple and the sensory interaction is confined to a few conditional branches, the structure of the control system is not critical. However, once the control system begins to interact in a sophisticated way with the sensory data, to modify trajectories, to institute alternative strategies, and to substitute goals and subgoal decompositions in response to changing conditions sensed in the environment, then the structure of the relationship between the sensory and control systems becomes crucial.

Control programs grow exponentially in complexity with the number of sensors and with the number of branch points in the program. Once there are more than a few sensors, each producing data that can affect the selection of a number of optional behavior trajectories, control programs written on a single level can become enormously complex to write and virtually impossible to debug.

At this point the problem of controlling a sensory-interactive robot becomes similar to that of controlling any complex system such as an army, a government, a business, or a biological organism. Introducing the type of hierarchical command and control structure that has historically proven successful in controlling such systems then becomes necessary. The secret of a hierarchical control system is that it can be partitioned to limit the complexity of any module to manageable limits regardless of the complexity of the entire structure.

Figure 9.1 illustrates the basic logical and temporal relationships in a hierarchical computing structure. On the left is an organizational hierarchy wherein computing modules are arranged in layers like command posts in a military organization. Each chain of command can be represented by a computational hierarchy, as shown in the center of figure 9.1. The input commands to each of the levels trace trajectories through state space, creating a behavioral hierarchy as shown on the right of figure 9.1. The lowest level trajectories of the behavioral hierarchy correspond to observable output behavior. All the other trajectories constitute the deep structure of behavior.

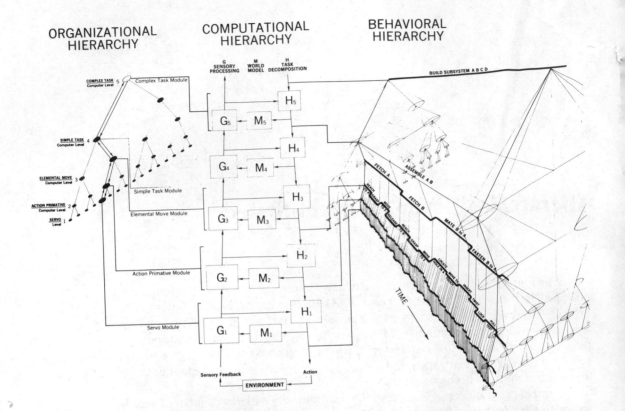

ORGANIZATIONAL HIERARCHY

COMPUTATIONAL HIERARCHY

BEHAVIORAL HIERARCHY

Figure 9.1: *Relationships in hierarchical structures. On the left is an organizational hierarchy consisting of a tree of command centers, each of which possesses one supervisor and several subordinates. Commands from above come from only one source but may be modified by contextual information sources, including lower, equal, or higher level computing centers.*

Each actuator at the lowest level is driven by a chain of command centers, or a computational hierarchy, as shown in the center. The computational hierarchy consists of a cross-coupled triple of task-decomposition modules, sensory-processing modules, and world-model modules. Each task-decomposition module is serviced by a sensory-processing module that extracts the information from the sensory data stream needed to make intelligent behavioral decisions at that level. Each sensory-processing module is provided with a continuous stream of expectations and predictions generated by a world-model module at that level. Each world-model module receives inputs describing the actions, plans, and hypotheses generated in the decomposition module at that level.

The sensory-processing modules compare the information from the world-model modules with the sensory input being observed. The difference between predictions and observations alters hypotheses or actions. Correlations between prediction and observation confirm hypotheses and reinforce actions.

Commands can be represented as vectors and sequences of commands as trajectories in a behavioral hierarchy, shown on the right. The string of commands comprising each trajectory in the behavioral hierarchy represents a path through a program (or state diagram describing the computational activity) in the various task-decomposition modules.

PROGRAMMING A HIERARCHICAL CONTROL SYSTEM

The simplest form of a robot program is a linear string of low-level position, velocity, or force commands. Such commands are typically of the form GO-TO<POINT>, GO-AT<VELOCITY>, or EXERT<FORCE>. These are the type of program statements that are generated by a human teacher who uses a control box to lead the robot through a set of recorded points. A program of this type can be represented as a sequence of states in a Petri diagram, shown in figure 9.2. Each node in the diagram corresponds to a command, or program statement. The edges between the nodes correspond to the conditions that cause the program to step from one command to the next. In the absence of sensory input, the conditions for stepping from one command to another may simply be the transition of a clock or an indication that the robot has reached the point where it was commanded to go. This may be derived from noting that the servo-error signals are all less than some threshold.

Slightly more sophisticated programming may use sensory interlocks that synchronize the sequence timing to that of other devices or processes. In some cases, these external sensory signals can be used to execute conditional branches. This gives rise to the type of state graph illustrated in figure 9.3. Conditional branching enables a robot to select one of several different programs depending upon sensed conditions in the environment. Thus, the robot can modify its behavior in response to external conditions and events.

More sophisticated yet are robots that can offset recorded points and trajectories by an amount determined by sensors. This enables a robot to track moving objects and operate on or manipulate parts that are not previously aligned to a known reference. When this is represented graphically, the state nodes corresponding to program commands may lie anywhere within extended regions of state space. The extent of these regions corresponds to the range of the sensed variables. The dimensionality of the state space corresponds to the number of command and sensory input variables that enter that particular computing module.

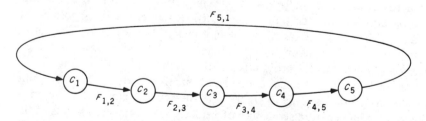

Figure 9.2: *A state-space graph representing a simple robot program. Each state C_i corresponds to a single instruction or primitive action in the robot's program. F_{ij} represents the logical conditions required for the state transition from C_i to C_j. The state transition corresponds to the program counter stepping from one instruction to the next.*

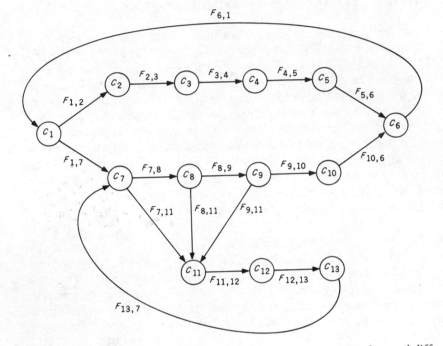

Figure 9.3: *Conditional branching enables a robot to select one of several different state trajectories (or program pathways) depending on sensed conditions.*

As the length and complexity of branching in robot programs increases, it becomes tedious to write them as linear strings of instructions in a single computer program. Furthermore, it soon becomes evident to anyone actually writing such programs that the same, or highly similar, substrings occur repeatedly. The obvious solution to this is to define macros, or subroutines, that generate the often-used substrings. Of course, it is always possible to partition any particular task program into a set of macros as shown in figure 9.4. If one can define a set of macros that can partition all programs within a certain class of tasks, it then becomes possible to write programs for that class of tasks completely in terms of macros. The set of macros then becomes an instruction set for a higher level programming language. Strings of macros represent robot programs written in the higher level language.

This implies that in a hierarchical control system, there exists a programming language at each level. For example in figure 9.1, the set of elemental-move commands are macros which generate sequences of velocity and force commands at the primitive action level. Given a set of such macros, together with the variables which define the destination of the resulting trajectories, one can express the robot program completely in terms of the elemental moves. Thus, the set of elemental moves comprises a robot programming language at the second hierarchical level.

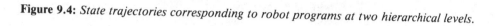

STATE TRAJECTORY = PROGRAM AT MACRO LEVEL

T_C MACRO

T_C PRIMITIVE

STATE TRAJECTORY = PROGRAM AT PRIMITIVE ACTION LEVEL

Figure 9.4: *State trajectories corresponding to robot programs at two hierarchical levels.*

For example, the command set shown in figure 9.5 comprising the programming language VAL (supplied with the Unimate PUMA robot) is essentially a set of elemental-move commands.

Of course, strings of macro statements at the elemental move level can themselves be partitioned into consistently recurring groups to form second-level macros. These correspond to VAL subroutines. A well-designed set of such subroutines can become statements in a programming language at the simple task level. Similarly, recurring groups of simple task commands can be defined as third level macros, or complex task commands. In principle, this process can be repeated any number of times to create a hierarchy wherein modules at each level contain a library of programs, written in a programming language peculiar to that level. Each statement at a particular level consists of an input command which, in the context of the feedback at that level, generates a sequence of subcommands to the next lower level. At the very top is a single command, or task name, which is decomposed through a succession of hierarchical levels, until at the lowest level a string of action primitives produces the forces and motions to accomplish the top-level goal.

The number of macros required at each level depends upon the breadth and degree of generality of the robot skill mix. In a restricted domain such as manufacturing, the number of skills is limited. Time and motion studies of human workers and robots in manufacturing indicate that the number of different types of elemental moves required to perform routine mechanical manufacturing tasks is not large. There is a reasonably small set of different types of action at the elemental move level, such as reach, grasp, lift, transport, position, insert, twist, push, pull, and release. A list of modifier variables, derived in part from feedback, can specify where to reach, when to grasp, how far to twist, and how hard to push.

Program Instructions

In these commands, "location" refers to "precision point",
"transformation", or "compound transformation".

APPRO	APPRO <location>[1], <distance>
APPROS	APPROS <location>[1], <distance>
CLOSE	CLOSE <distance>
CLOSEI	CLOSEI <distance>
DEL	DELAY <time>
DEP	DEPART <distance>
DRA	DRAW [<dX>],[<dY>],[<dZ>]
DRI	DRIVE <jt>,<change>,<time>
GO	GO <location>[1]
GR	GRASP <distance>,[<label>]
MOVE	MOVE <location>[1]
MOVEI	MOVEI [<jt 1>],...,[<jt n>],[<hand>],[<speed>]
MOVES	MOVES <location>[1]
OPEN	OPEN <distance>
OPENI	OPENI <distance>
READ	READY
REL	RELAX

AB	ABOVE
BE	BELOW
FL	FLIP
LE	LEFTY
NOF	NOFLIP
RI	RIGHTY

FR	FRAME <trans> = <trans 1>,<trans 2>,<trans 3>
H	HERE <trans 1>[,<trans 2>] ... [,<trans n>]
	or HERE <precision point>
INV	INVERSE <trans> = <trans 1>[:<t 2>] ... [:<t n>]
SET	SET <trans> = <trans 1>[:<t 2>] ... [:<t n>]
	or SET <precision point> = <precision point>
SETI	SETI <i,var 1> = <i,var 2> [<operation> <i,var 3>]
SH	SHIFT <transformation> BY [<dx>],[<dy>],[<dz>]
TO	TOOL [<transformation>]
TYPEI	TYPEI <i,var>

```
GOS         GOSUB <program>
GOT         GOTO <label>
IF          IF <i,var 1> <relationship> <i,var 2> THEN <label>
IFS         IFSIG [<channel>],[<channel>],
                  [<channel>],[<channel>] THEN <label>
IG          IGNORE <channel> [ALWAYS]
PA          PAUSE <string>
REACT       REACT <channel>,[<program>] [ALWAYS]
REACTI      REACTI <channel>,[<program>] [ALWAYS]
RET         RETURN [<skip count>]
SI          SIGNAL <channel 1>[,<channel 2>,...,<channel 8>]
ST          STOP
W           WAIT <channel>


CO          COARSE [ALWAYS]
FI          FINE [ALWAYS]
INTOF       INTOFF [ALWAYS]
INTON       INTON [ALWAYS]
NON         NONULL [ALWAYS]
NU          NULL [ALWAYS]
SP          SPEED <value> [ALWAYS]


REM         REMARK [<string>]
TYPE        TYPE [<string>]
```

Figure 9.5: *The instruction set for the VAL robot programming language. This is the language provided with the Unimation PUMA robot.*

THE STATE-MACHINE HIERARCHY

From one perspective, the type of hierarchical structure described above is nothing more than good top-down structured program design applied to robot tasks. Each macro represents a relatively short sequence of instructions and a limited and well-structured set of branches. Programs at each level tend to be readable, understandable, and easy to debug and test for correctness.

However, if the computing modules in the hierarchy are constructed as state machines (i.e., finite-state automata), the implications extend considerably beyond mere programming convenience. In this case, each computing module is an autonomous process which, at each instant in time, reads its input and computes an output. This means that sensory data can interact with the task-decomposition process at any level at any time, altering it and so making the system responsive in real time to events in the environment.

The sophisticated real-time use of sensory measurement information for coping with uncertainty and recovering from errors requires that sensory data be able to interact with the control system at many different levels with many different constraints on speed and timing. For example, as shown in figure 9.6, joint position, velocity, and sometimes force measurements are required at the lowest level in the hierarchy for servo feedback. This data requires very little processing, but must be supplied with time delays of only a few milliseconds. Visual depth, proximity data,

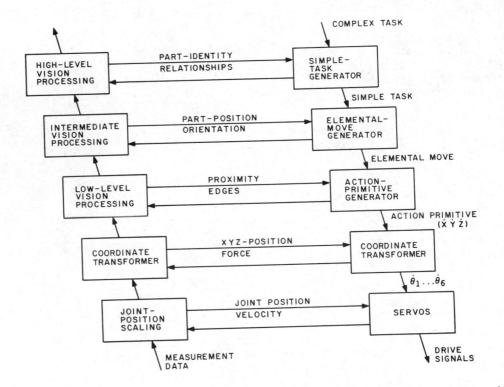

Figure 9.6: *A cross-coupled sensory-control hierarchy. The links from left to right provide feedback for controlling behavior. The links from right to left provide context and expectations for processing sensory data. This figure illustrates the type of feedback information provided to the task-decomposition hierarchy at each level. In this diagram the lowest level of the hierarchy of figure 9.1 has been split into two levels: one for coordinate transformations between work space (or end effector space) and joint space; the other for servo-computations on the joint positions and velocities.*

and information related to edges and surfaces are needed at the primitive action level of the hierarchy to compute offsets for gripping points. This data requires a modest amount of processing and must be supplied within a few tenths of a second. Recognition of part position and orientation requires more processing and is needed at the elemental move level where time constraints are on the order of seconds. Recognition of parts and/or relationships between parts that may take several seconds is required for conditional branching at the simple task level.

Attempting to deal with this full range of sensory feedback in all of its possible combinations at a single level leads to extremely complex and inefficient programs. An obvious strategy might be to use structured programming with layers of subroutines. But using conventional macros and subroutines does not help in the case of complex sensory interaction, because of the hopeless complication of multiple interrupt servicing at many levels of subroutine calls simultaneously. Interrupt-driven sensory interaction has the additional disadvantage of making complex programs very difficult to debug.

This suggests that conventional programming approaches to sensory-interactive robot-control systems are fatally flawed. Only if the various modules in the control hierarchy are treated like state machines does it become simple to write and debug programs for sensory-interactive behavior.

THE SENSORY HIERARCHY

Sophisticated analysis of measurement data, particularly vision data, is inherently a hierarchical process. If the vision-control system is partitioned into a hierarchy, the various levels of feedback information can be introduced to the appropriate control levels in a simple, straightforward way. As described in earlier chapters, each level of the sensory hierarchy consists of a G module containing a library of sensory-processing algorithms. These sensory-processing modules extract from the sensory data stream the information necessary for the control decisions being made in the H modules at the same level. Each G module receives two sets of inputs: the first, a set of sensory experience variables $\mathbf{E}$ which may be an image; and the second, a set of recalled expectation variables $\mathbf{R}$ which also may be an image. At higher levels, both the $\mathbf{E}$ and $\mathbf{R}$ vectors may be abstract data structures representing edges, connected regions, corners, holes, patterns, dimensions, or names of objects and relationships. The $\mathbf{R}$ input may also contain information that indicates which sensory-processing algorithms should be applied to the sensory input. The output of the G module is a $\mathbf{Q}$ vector that contains information indicating the amount and possibly the direction of the error between the sensory input and the recalled expectation. The $\mathbf{Q}$ vector can also contain the name of recognized features of the sensory input, information regarding the degree of correlation between observed input and the expectation, and confidence factors associated with the recognized features.

It is important to keep in mind that sensory measurements are made in the coordinate system of the sensors and that this is quite different from the coordinate system of the joints of the robot. If the sensory data is simply used to execute conditional branches in the program, the coordinate system of the sensor is immaterial. However, if the sensory data is used to modify the position, force, or velocity of the robot's behavior trajectory, then it is necessary to transform the measurement vector from the coordinate system of the sensor to the coordinate system of the joints. For example, if a force sensor in the robot fingers measures a force along some vector relative to the fingertips, a coordinate transformation is necessary before the control system can cause joints of the robot to move so that the hand travels in a known direction relative to the sensed force. This is accomplished in the coordinate transformation module of figure 9.6.

In order for a robot to respond to sensory data while it is in the process of acting, such as while pursuing a non-cooperative target, the coordinate transformation calculations must be performed continuously with computation delays of no more than a few milliseconds. In the case of a robot with an articulated arm, like the ones shown in figures 8.23 through 8.29, this involves solving a set of six equations with six unknowns. Since these transformations occur at a very low level in the hierarchy, they must be performed every few milliseconds. This requires an enormous amount of high speed computations. The coordinate transformation computations for a single six-axis arm can easily keep a small minicomputer fully occupied. The mathematics of these transformations are contained in a number of papers referenced in the bibliography.

USE OF THE WORLD MODEL

The type of feedback information typically required by the control system depends upon what task is being performed. Also the type of sensory data received often depends upon the actions being executed by the control system. Thus, the processing of sensory data must be done within the context of the actions generated by the control system. As conditions change, different sensors, different resolutions, and different processing algorithms could be needed. The speed requirements of real-time control do not permit all resolutions and all processing algorithms to be applied all the time. Thus, a real-time allocation of measurement and processing resources must be done.

Furthermore, sensory data often must be compared with expectations and hypotheses in order to detect missing objects or events, or to detect deviations from desired trajectories. Thus, the control system must have the capacity to tell the sensory system what to expect and when to expect it. This requires that there be links from the control hierarchy to the sensory-processing hierarchy as well as the other way around.

Thus, each level of the hierarachy contains a set of M modules that generate the expectations for the sensory-processing G modules. Input to the M modules consists of **P** vectors from the behavior-generating H modules together with **X** vectors from various other computing modules that indicate the state of various pertinent variables from other regions of the processing-generating hierarchy. The M modules contain memories of previous experiences, maps, templates, and other data structures. The entire set of M modules comprises an internal model of the external world. The M modules provide answers to the question: if I do such and such, what will happen? As the task execution proceeds, the M modules of the world model produce sequences of expected data to the sensory-processing modules at each level.

Under ideal conditions these expected values will accurately predict the observed data. In other situations, the processing modules at each level will detect deviations between predictions and observations and produce error signals. These become the **F** vectors that modify the task decomposition at each level to maintain the robot performance within the limits of a success envelope.

In general, any deviation from the ideal task performance will be detected at the lowest level first. If the lowest level H function is capable of coping with that error, then no higher level action need be taken. However, if the error persists or grows in spite of the action of the lowest level H function, then it will be detected at the next higher level where a different task decomposition may be selected. By this means it becomes possible to implement very sophisticated multilevel error-correction procedures in a relatively straightforward manner.

The G and M modules can be represented as state machines just like the H modules. Each module reads its input and its own state at time t, computes its output and its next state, and waits for the next input at $t + 1$. Thus the interfaces between the modules are well-defined, and the programs embodied in each module are short and structured.

SOFTWARE DESIGN

The design of a software system that can implement the multilevel branching of the cross-coupled, processing-generating hierarchy is conceptually straightforward. At each level of the generating hierarchy, the H function represents a table, or list, of states and state mappings, one of which is selected by every possible combination of input vectors **C** + **F**. At each time tick k, the input **C** + **F** constitutes an address, or pointer, to a node which contains either the output **P** itself or a procedure for computing **P**. This is illustrated in figure 9.7.

Theoretically, all H, M, and G modules can be implemented by program statements of the form IF < state, input >/THEN < output, next-state >. This is equivalent to $\mathbf{P} = H(\mathbf{S})$. It is a canonical form for represented knowledge, rules of behavior, and algorithms for perception.

One method of implementing the H, M, and G modules is by a state-table as shown in figure 9.8. Here the simple task < FETCH(X) > is defined. The left-hand

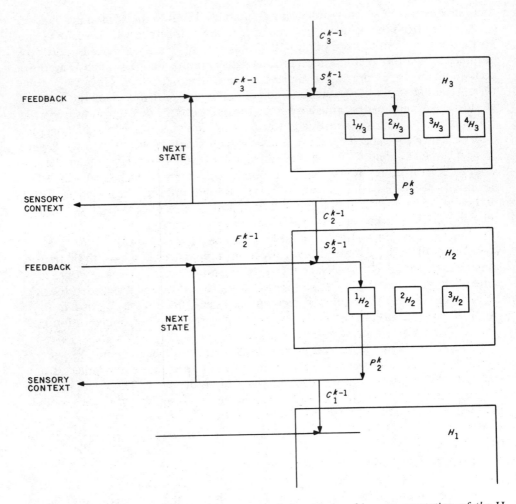

Figure 9.7: *A software architecture diagram of the state-machine representation of the* H *modules in the task-decomposition hierarchy. The input* $\mathbf{S}_i^{k-1} = \mathbf{C}_i^{k-1} + \mathbf{F}_i^{k-1}$ *constitutes an address, or pointer, to a node that contains either the output* $\mathbf{P}_i^k$ *itself or a procedure for computing* $\mathbf{P}_i^k$.

side of the table consists of a command vector **C** and a feedback vector **F**. The **C** vector consists of a command FETCH and an argument X. The **F** vector consists of a state defined by the previous output plus feedback consisting of processed sensory data from the external environment as well as information from lower-level modules. The right-hand side of the state-table defines (or points to procedures that define) a **P** vector that consists of an output command to lower-level H modules, the next state information to be used internally, and sensory context information to be

$\mathbf{C}^{k-1}$	$\mathbf{F}^{k-1}$		$\mathbf{P}^k$		
Command (Argument)	State	Feedback	Output	Next State	Sensory Context
FETCH(X)	0	—	SEARCH FOR(X)	1	g_1
FETCH(X)	1	Dist(X) = ?	SEARCH FOR(X)	1	g_1
FETCH(X)	1	Search fail	STOP REPORT FETCH-FAIL	0	g_0
FETCH(X)	1	Dist(X) > a	GO TO (Pos(X))	1	g_1
FETCH(X)	1	Dist(X) ≤ 0	ORIENT ON(X)	2	g_2
FETCH(X)	2	Orient(X) > 0	ORIENT ON(X)	2	g_2
FETCH(X)	2	Orient(X) ≤ 0	GRASP(X)	3	g_3
FETCH(X)	3	Touch < T	GRASP(X)	3	g_3
FETCH(X)	3	Touch ≥ T	GO TO JIG(X)	4	g_4
FETCH(X)	4	Dist(JIG) > 0	GO TO JIG(X)	4	g_4
FETCH(X)	4	Dist(JIG) = 0	INSERT(X)	5	g_5
FETCH(X)	5	Force < 0	INSERT(X)	5	g_5
FETCH(X)	5	Force > 0, Insert done	RELEASE	6	g_6
FETCH(X)	6	Releasing	RELEASE	6	g_6
FETCH(X)	6	Release done	STOP Report FETCH-DONE	0	g_6
FETCH(X)	—	Subtask fail	STOP Report FETCH-Fail	0	g_0

Figure 9.8: *A state-table representation of the task-decomposition function at the simple task level. A state-table such as this is one method of implementing the function* $\mathbf{P} = H(\mathbf{S})$.

sent to M modules. The sensory context information addresses the M module that retrieves an $\mathbf{R}$ vector to be sent to the G module. In this example, when the sensory context output is g_2, the sensory-processing module is instructed by the M module to use the G function that computes the orientation of X. The M module may also be instructed to generate an expected value for Orientation(X). The feedback information then indicates whether Orientation(X)≤0, or Orientation(X)>0. When the sensory context output is g_1, the G function which computes the distance to X is evoked.

Figure 9.9 illustrates an entire library of procedures in an H module and the state-table for accessing them. At each clock tick k, the left-hand side of the state-table is searched for an entry corresponding to the input $\mathbf{C} + \mathbf{F}$. If an entry is found, the pointer is set to that location, and the first node in the right side of the state-table is used as a pointer to a procedure that computes an output $\mathbf{P} = H(\mathbf{S})$. If no entry can be found, the pointer is set to an error condition and a procedure is evoked to output the appropriate failure activities. In most cases, a failure condition will output a $<STOP>$ command to the H module below and a failure flag to the H module above.

Each entry in the state-table represents an IF/THEN rule, or production. With this construction, it becomes possible to define behavior of arbitrary complexity. An ideal task performance can be defined in terms of the list of events that take place during the ideal performance. Deviations from the ideal can be incorporated by simply adding the deviant conditions to the left-hand side of the state-table and the appropriate action to be taken to the right-hand side. Any conditions not explicitly covered by the table result in a failure routine being executed.

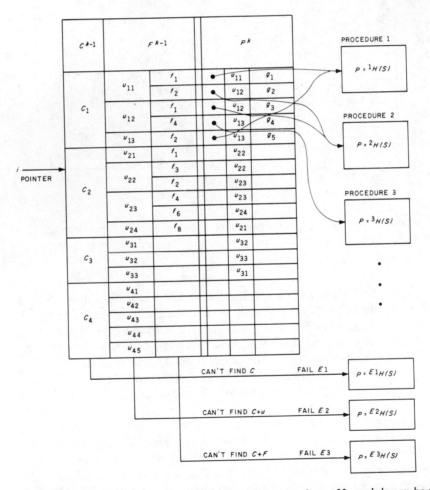

Figure 9.9: *The entire library of procedures that comprise an* H *module can be represented as an extended state-table. This extended table is simply the union of all the state-tables that represent all of the tasks that can be decomposed by the* H *module.*

CMAC CONTROL SYSTEMS

This state-table representation of an *H* module is of the same form as the computations performed by CMAC. It is thus theoretically possible to implement such a hierarchical control system using only CMAC modules. However, this has not yet been done in a practical application. In the work to date, it has always been more convenient to implement the state-machine properties of an *H*, *M*, or *G* module by more conventional methods. Implementation of a hierarchical robot-control system using CMAC modules is a research topic that remains to be explored.

CMAC is a neurological model that illustrates how the brain uses memory recall to compute most of its mathematical functions. CMAC demonstrates how the computations performed by any single layer of neurological tissue are equivalent to those performed by a state-machine. The CMAC hierarchical model demonstrates how a properly structured network of state-machines can produce sensory-interactive goal-directed behavior of arbitrary complexity. Unfortunately, CMAC suffers from the practical problem that multidimensional functions require enormous amounts of memory to compute by table look-up, even when the CMAC mapping algorithms are used. Furthermore, CMAC must be trained, and there are many difficult problems of learning in multilayered interconnected networks.

In the brain, mechanisms have evolved to deal with these problems. For example, the brain has no difficulty in growing synapses (the memory elements of the brain) by the billions. The total number of synapses in the brain is astronomical. Just a single output cell, such as would be modeled by a single CMAC, may have as many as 200,000 weights. A layer of such cells, possibly required for one level of processing of a visual image, might consist of a million cells, with a hundred trillion weights. If only four bits of computer memory are required for each weight, the amount of computer memory required to mimic the brain's mechanism for computing by table look-up obviously far exceeds the bounds of practicality.

Yet a single microcomputer using algorithmic procedures can often accomplish in only a little more time the same amount of image processing that a layer of visual cortex performs. Some simple kinds of processing, such as computing areas of connected regions or detecting edges, lines, or corners, can be done in less than a second. An array of ten or a hundred microcomputers could perform the same processing job in a few milliseconds, or as quickly as the brain can. Single-chip array processors of this size will certainly exist long before programmable memories with trillions of bits are available. Thus, modern microelectronic technology can provide the computing power to duplicate the performance of a CMAC module without duplicating the enormous memory capacity required to compute by memory recall. The state-machine performance of several *H*, *M*, or *G* modules can often be accomplished by a single microcomputer.

The fact that it is possible to construct the equivalent of a CMAC hierarchy out of microcomputers using conventional sequential algorithms and programming code has prompted researchers to pursue the algorithmic procedure method first. Once the capabilities of hierarchical control systems are fully demonstrated by these methods, one may return to the CMAC model to understand more about structuring robot sensory-interactive control systems.

In the design of practical robot-control systems (as opposed to brain modeling research), it is recommended that the state-machine architecture of the CMAC hierarchy be used, with each of the computing modules implemented by algorithmic or production rule programming methods whenever that is simpler. Just as the Wright brothers observed the aerodynamic properties of birds in flight, but used propellers instead of flapping wings to power their aircraft, so we can observe the hierarchical structure of the brain and the state-machine properties of neurological tissue and yet use microcomputers and algorithmic programming procedures to implement our state-machine hierarchy for robot-control systems.

A MICROCOMPUTER NETWORK IMPLEMENTATION

At the National Bureau of Standards, Anthony Barbera and M. L. Fitzgerald have constructed a state-machine hierarchical control system for a robot in a network of microcomputers. This system maps the logical structure of figure 9.6 into the physical structure of figure 9.10. The coordinate transformations of figure 9.6 are implemented in one of the microcomputers of figure 9.10. The elemental move trajectory planning is implemented in a second microcomputer of figure 9.10. The processing of visual data is accomplished in a third microcomputer, and the processing of force and touch data in a fourth microcomputer. A fifth microcomputer provides communication with a minicomputer with additional modules of the control hierarchy. Researchers anticipate that these will eventually be embedded in a sixth microcomputer.

Communication from one module to another is accomplished through a common memory "mail drop" system. No two microcomputers communicate directly with each other. This means that common memory contains a location assigned to every element in the input and output vectors of every module in the hierarchy. No location in common memory is written into by more than one computing module, but any number of modules may read from any location.

Time is sliced into 28-millisecond increments as shown in figure 9.11. At the beginning of each increment, each logical module reads its set of input values from the appropriate locations in common memory. It then computes its set of output values which it writes back into the common memory before the 28-millisecond interval ends. Any of the logical modules which do not complete their computations before the end of the 28-millisecond interval write extrapolated estimates of their output accompanied by a flag indicating that the date is extrapolated. The process then repeats.

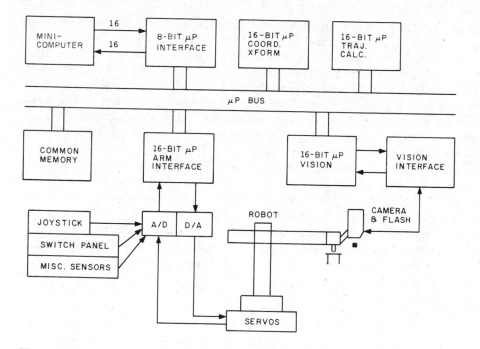

Figure 9.10: *A microcomputer network developed at the National Bureau of Standards for implementing a hierarchical robot control system.*

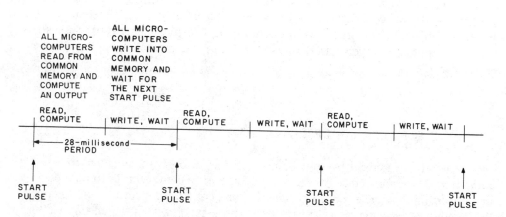

Figure 9.11: *A timing diagram of the activity in the microcomputer network shown in figure 9.10.*

Each logical module is thus a state-machine whose outputs depend only on its present inputs and its present internal state. None of the logical modules admit any interrupts. Each starts its read cycle on a clock signal, computes and writes its output, and waits for the next clock signal. Thus, each logical module is a state-machine with the IF/THEN or $P = H(S)$ properties of a CMAC function.

The common memory "mail drop" communication system has a number of advantages and disadvantages. One disadvantage is that it takes two data transfers to get information from one module to another. However, this is offset by the simplicity of the communication protocol. No modules talk to each other so there is no handshaking required. In each 28-millisecond time slice, all modules read from common memory before any are allowed to write their outputs back in.

The use of common-memory data transfer means that the addition of each new state variable requires only a definition of where the newcomer is to be located in common memory. This information is needed only by the module that generates it so that it knows where to write, and by the modules that read the information so that they know where to look. None of the other modules need know, or care, when such a change is implemented. Thus, new microcomputers can easily be added, logical modules can be shifted from one microcomputer to another, new functions can be added, and even new sensor systems can be introduced with little or no effect on the rest of the system. As long as the bus has surplus capacity, the physical structure of the system can be reconfigured with no changes required in the software resident in the logical modules not directly involved in the change.

Furthermore, the common memory always contains a readily accessible map of the current state of the system. This makes it easy for a system monitor to trace the history of any or all of the state variables, to set break points, and to reason backwards to the source of program errors or faulty logic.

The read-compute-write-wait cycle, with each module a state-machine, makes it possible to stop the process at any point, to single step through a task, and to observe the performance of the control system in detail. This is extremely important for program development and verification in a sophisticated, real-time, sensory-interactive system in which many processes are going on in parallel at many different hierarchical levels.

SINGLE COMPUTER IMPLEMENTATION

A hierarchical control system can, of course, also be implemented in a single computer. The architecture of the microcomputer network can be simulated in a single progam that cycles once per time tick and can be stopped, or single stepped. The single program may consist of a set of processes, each of which in their turn is allowed to read input variables from a block of common memory, perform some functional operation on those input variables, and hold their outputs in temporary storage until all the processes have completed their read cycle. Then each of the processes is allowed to write its output variables into common memory. The program then cycles back to the beginning and restarts. Any process that cannot finish its computation in a single cycle can hold temporary results until its next turn in the next cycle. When it finally does complete its computation, it writes its output during the allotted time slot and waits for the next read period. This is a programming technique that is often used in process-control, systems-simulation, and multitask modeling.

Thus, there are many ways to implement the hierarchical control structure described above. It can be done with a large main-frame computer, a powerful minicomputer, a network of microcomputers, or even by a network of CMACs. The modular, state-machine approach separates the H, M, or G functions into simple, understandable blocks of code which can be written, debugged, and optimized independently. The modules have a simple canonical form that makes them understandable and the code readable. It forces a partitioning of the problem into manageable chunks, which can be independently analyzed, reduced to algorithms, and then reassembled into a complex intelligent system. This provides a systematic approach to the synthesis of intelligent behavior. It can start with the simple tasks that are within the capacity of present-day robots, gradually adding new modules to increase the computing power and sensory capability of the system. Each additional sensory module increases the sophistication of the sensory interaction, and each new control module adds a new motor skill. Each new memory or sensory-processing module increases the perceptual capacities. Most important, each new level in the hierarchy produces a quantum jump in the intelligence of the system. This modular approach thus provides the beginnings of an evolutionary framework for upgrading the simple behavioral patterns of the pick-and-place robot to eventually approach the intellectually sophisticated and enormously complex behavioral patterns produced by the human brain.

FUTURE DEVELOPMENTS

It seems likely that it will soon be possible to design a cross-coupled, processing-generating hierarchy, similar to that suggested in figure 7.2, consisting of hundreds, even thousands, of microcomputers. The technology of large-scale integration is headed in this direction, with large systems now being contemplated for the control of entire factories. The hierarchical sensory-control structure makes it possible for many different computing modules, each doing its limited assigned task, to be integrated into a coordinated system so that parts, tools, and materials all arrive at the right place at the right time. The correct operations can then be performed, the results inspected, the finished work dispatched to the next work area, and a report made to the next higher level in the hierarchy. The same type of hierarchical control system suggested here for robots can be extended to integrate robots, machine tools, materials transport systems, inventory control, safety, and inspection systems into a sensory-interactive, goal-seeking hierarchical computing structure for a totally automatic factory.

Of course, it is at the higher levels that the implementation of the hierarchy in small modular state-machine computational modules has not yet been proven feasible. This is still an open issue about which one can only speculate at this time.

CHAPTER **10**

Artificial Intelligence

The goal of work in artificial intelligence is to build machines that perform tasks that normally require human intelligence. This approach completely leapfrogs the entire insect and animal kingdom, and strikes at the peak of creation, human intelligence. The audacity of the attempt is mind-boggling. It leaps straight from the inanimate computer to the most complex expression of the biological world, the intellect of the human brain. Yet the results have not been entirely unsuccessful. A great deal has been learned about planning, problem-solving, language and speech understanding, perception of visual images, representation of knowledge, and the mathematical formalisms that describe these processes.

It is beyond the scope of this book to review the enormous literature in the field of artificial intelligence. This is an extensive and active research area for which there are a number of excellent textbooks and introductory surveys. Some of these are contained in the bibliography to this book. There are, however, a few selected topics in artificial intelligence (AI) that are relevant to the hierarchical control concepts we have outlined.

PLANNING AND PROBLEM-SOLVING

Planning and problem-solving are two of the central topics in artificial intelligence. The principal issue in these areas is the search for, and optimization of, a success trajectory through the space of all possible states of the world. Since this is obviously an infinite space, the first step is to limit the problem domain to some subset of all possible states of the world. One way to do this is to select a finite problem. A game like tick-tack-toe has a relatively small number of possible states, and the entire state space can be exhaustively searched rather easily. Figure 10.1 shows part of the graph that completely describes the space of all possible states in the game of tick-tack-toe. On the other hand, a game like chess has a space of all possible states that is so large that it could not be exhaustively searched by the fastest computer in the world during the life span of the universe.

Problems in the real world often have an infinite space of possible states, yet many of these are obviously solvable. Real-world problems are routinely solved by persons of modest intellect and training. In fact, real problems of enormous complexity such as hunting for food, escaping from danger, winning a sexual partner, or rearing offspring are regularly solved, not only by humans, but also by animals and insects. Many everyday problems are apparently nowhere near as subtle or difficult as board games like chess. For example, the simple everyday problem described in Chapter 1 of buying a record at the shopping center clearly involves an infinite space of possible states. Each step taken could be performed by a continuum of muscle contraction forces. The problem could be solved in a wheelchair, on a bicycle, or even by rolling one's body along the ground. An interesting feature of human problem-solving is that we rarely think of all the possible alternatives—we just do the simplest thing without much thought.

The traditional artificial intelligence approach to computerized problem-solving is to define a set of states (i.e., configurations of the world) and rules for transforming one state into another. In a board game, there is usually an initial state (or set of states) from which the game begins and a final state (or set of states) that signals the end. The rules of the game are the rules for moving pieces that transform the game from one state to the next. One can construct a graph, such as shown in figure 10.1, that represents all possible trajectories through the state space of the game. Any single playing of the game is represented by a single trajectory through this graph.

Much AI (artificial intelligence) research has concentrated on the question of finding a winning trajectory. This is usually accomplished by defining an evaluation function, which computes some scalar value of goodness, or advantageousness, of any state. From any current position, or state, all possible states that can be reached by a given number of legal moves are evaluated for goodness, and the path leading to the state with the best evaluation is chosen for the next move. The evaluation function used in AI corresponds to the emotions in the biological brain. Both are used by their respective systems to select optimum behavioral trajectories.

Research in AI has also focused on methods for finding effective evaluation functions. Some efforts have attempted to devise evaluation functions that learn from mistakes and thus improve their performance. The checker-playing program of A. L. Samuel is an early and notable example of this strategy. Other research areas have attempted to apply different evaluation functions under different board conditions, such as opening, mid-game, and end-game phases. This is a simple form of hierarchical decomposition.

Still other strategies have concentrated on the order of the search (i.e., which states to evaluate and in which order). It is clear from figure 10.1 that a great majority of the possible moves are strategically poor and are apparently not even considered by human tick-tack-toe players. How does one find the good moves and avoid the bad? For example, should one evaluate all possible single moves from the current position, or should one follow promising pathways through several moves before evaluating the next possible move from the current position? There is a computational cost associated with each evaluation and a finite amount of computation that can be performed between each move. Thus, the program that uses its computational resources most efficiently is most likely to be successful.

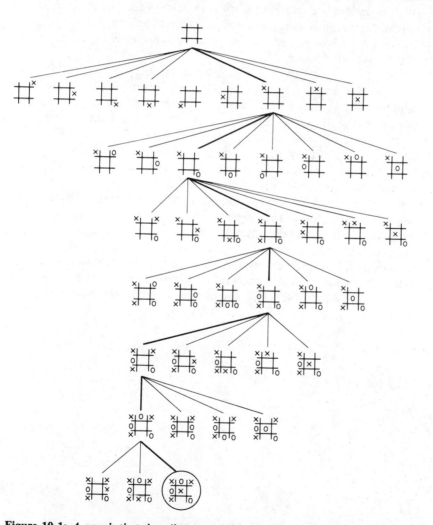

Figure 10.1: *A graph that describes part of the space of all possible states of the game tick-tack-toe. The dark trace indicates the sequence of moves actually made during one playing of the game. Strategies for searching such graphs to find trajectories leading to winning states is a classic topic in artifical intelligence research.*

Perhaps the major difference between human and machine approaches to problem-solving is that the brain performs many parallel operations while computers do not easily represent parallel processes in search strategies. This is particularly true for computers programmed in LISP, the principal programming tool of AI research. Thus, much effort has been expended on making early decisions about which moves are unpromising so that the decision tree can be pruned.

Procedures for deciding which search strategies and which evaluation functions to apply in which situations are called heuristics. Heuristics are essentially a set of rules that reside one hierarchical level above the move selection and evaluation functions of the search procedure. A heuristic is a strategy for selecting rules, i.e., a higher level rule for selecting lower level rules.

Attempts have been made to duplicate human problem-solving strategies. Perhaps the best known example is the General Problem Solver (GPS) developed by Allen Newell and Herbert A. Simon. Newell and Simon recorded the human thought processes reported by students as they struggled with problems in abstract mathematics. From these observations they developed for GPS a technique called means-ends analysis. Simply stated, this consists of observing the goal state, comparing it with the existing state, and then searching for a transformation rule that can change the existing state into a form closer to the goal state.

This process implies an ability to measure the state-space distance between the existing state and the goal state and to associate a transformation with each possible difference condition. In complex problems, the number of possible difference conditions can be astronomically large.

Attempts to deal with this led eventually to the concept of problem reduction using AND/OR graphs. The basic notion here is a hierarchical decomposition of a single difficult (or high-level) problem into a sequence of simpler subproblems. If all

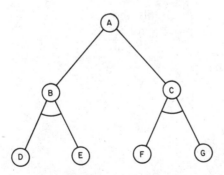

Figure 10.2: *An AND/OR graph. Nodes B and C are OR nodes under A. Nodes D and E are AND nodes under B. F and G are AND nodes under C. AND nodes are indicated by an arc joining them.*

of the subproblems need to be solved in order to solve the higher level problem, the decomposition is represented by an AND node. If only one of several subproblems needs to be solved in order to solve the higher level problem, the decomposition is represented by an OR node. Figure 10.2 shows a simple AND/OR graph. Node A represents a problem that can be solved by solving either subproblem B or C. Sub-problem B can be solved by solving both sub-subproblems D and E. The strategy is to repeatedly decompose problems into subproblems until finally at the bottom of the AND/OR graph there are a sequence of primitive subproblems for which there exist transformation rules corresponding to one-step solutions.

AND/OR graphs were first used by James Slagle in a program called SAINT that solved freshman calculus problems in symbolic integration. Soon afterward, this technique was used by Rigney and Towne for analyzing the structure of serial action schedules for industrial tasks. It has subsequently been used for many different types of problem-solving, including task decomposition for robots. The task-decomposition hierarchies discussed extensively in Chapters 5 through 7 are essentially AND/OR graphs with time and feedback inputs explicitly represented. The trajectories shown in figure 5.17 correspond to a string of AND nodes that decompose the complex task <ASSEMBLE AB>. Figure 5.21 corresponds to a set of alternative OR nodes that are selected under different external conditions.

PRODUCTION SYSTEMS

Some of the most remarkably successful artificial intelligence programs are those based on production rules. The word "production" is derived from the work of Post in the 1930s in which he devised a system of rules (he called them productions) for manipulating symbols. Post Productions form the theoretical basis for mathematical linguistics and for the symbol manipulation performed in computer assemblers, compilers, and interpreters.

The principal idea is that there exists a set of symbols and a set of rules for transforming one string of symbols into another string of symbols. A set of symbols (that is divided into non-terminal symbols, terminal symbols, and a starting symbol) together with a set of production rules for transforming strings of symbols, is called a grammar and is shown in figure 10.3. A grammar generates a language, which is the entire set of strings that can be generated from all possible ways of applying the rules in the grammar. The application of these transformational grammars to natural language research is most closely associated with the work of the linguist Noam Chomsky.

The transformational rules of a grammar are analogous to functions. Particular strings in the language correspond to states. Each rule can be represented in the form of IF<string1>/THEN<string2>; <string1> is called the premise, <string2> the consequent. The premise can be any string. It can be a string of conditions related to the spectrum of organic molecules, and the consequent a probability that the molecule producing the spectrum has a particular structure. The premise can be a set of symptoms and results of blood tests and the consequent a probability that a certain infectious disease is present.

One of the first successful production-based systems is a program called DEN-DRAL. The DENDRAL system works out the structure of molecules from chemical formulas and mass spectrograms. First a set of production rules is applied to the mass spectrogram to create lists of required and forbidden chemical substructures. These rules are of the form:

IF there is
a high peak at mass/charge point 71, and
a high peak at mass/charge point 43, and
a high peak at mass/charge point 86, and
any peak at mass/charge point 58,
THEN
there must be an N-PROPYL-KETONE3 substructure.

DENDRAL contains about 10 such production rules for any given category of chemical compounds. The application of these rules to the mass spectrogram reduces the number of possible chemical structures from several hundreds or thousands to several tens. Once this is done, a second set of production rules operates on the remaining candidate compounds to predict what the mass spectrogram would look like if that particular compound were the experimental one. Then each of the predicted spectrograms is compared with the observed spectrogram, and the best match is determined. There are about 100 production rules in this second set.

Grammar G

Symbols:

S = Sentence
NP = Noun Phrase
VP = Verb Phrase
V = Verb
N = Noun
PP = Prepositional Phrase
P = Preposition

Rules:

S → NP VP
VP → V NP
VP → V NP PP
PP → P NP
P → to
V → gave
NP → N
NP → the N
N → Sam
N → John
N → apple

Figure 10.3a: *A grammar consisting of a set of symbols and a set of rules for transforming symbols into other symbols.*

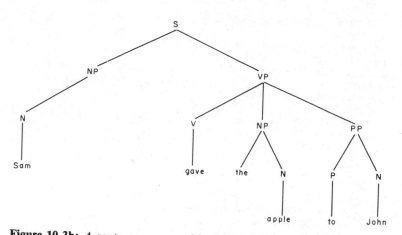

Figure 10.3b: *A sentence generated by the grammar of part (a).*

The DENDRAL program has been tested extensively and found to perform about as well as an experienced chemist on the particular type of compounds covered by the set of rules in the program. The success of the DENDRAL program has led to further research and the development of several other programs with names such as meta-DENDRAL, CONGEN, and SECS.

A similar program called MYCIN was developed to deal with the diagnosis of bacterial infections. MYCIN currently contains about 500 production rules of the following type:

> IF
> the infection type is primary-bacteremia, and
> the suggested entry point is the gastrointestinal tract, and
> the site of the culture is one of the sterile sites,
> THEN
> there is probability (*p*) that the organism is bacteroides.

Each rule returns a probability. MYCIN applies all 500 rules to the set of symptoms and then combines the resulting probabilities in an AND/OR tree to select the most likely type of infection.

One of the interesting features of this type of system is the canonical form of the knowledge. Each rule is a modular chunk of knowledge that is applied whenever the appropriate premise is present. It is the type of reasoning that humans are used to, and the form of the knowledge makes it particularly easy to translate from natural language into the productions rules and vice versa. The program includes a language translator so that it can be used interactively by doctors who are not computer scientists. A typical MYCIN print-out is shown in figure 10.4.

```
**HOW DO YOU USE THE TYPE OF THE INFECTION?

The following rules use:
    the type of the infection
154, 578, 574, 572, 570, 565, 564, 559, 557, 553, 551, 549, 547, 545, 543,
    541, 539, 537, 535, 533, 531, 529, 523, 520, 519, 517, 515, 513, 511,
    507, 300, 289, 288, 287, 280, 174, 167

Would you like a summary of all the parameters concluded by these rules?
**NO
Which of the rules do you wish to see?
**280


RULE 280
IF:       1) The infection which requires therapy is meningitis, and
          2) The type of the infection is fungal, and
          3) Organisms were not seen on the stain of the culture, and
          4) The patient is not a compromised host, and
          5) The patient has been to an area that is endemic for
             coccidiomycoses, and
          6) The race of the patient is one of: black asian indian, and
          7) The cryptococcal antigen in the csf was not positive


THEN:     There is suggestive evidence (.5) that cryptococcus is not one of
          the organisms (other than those seen on cultures or smears) which
          might be causing the infection.


Author:   YU
Justification:   Dark-skinned races, especially Filipino, Asian, and Black
(in that order) have an increased susceptibility to coccidiomycoses
meningitis.
Literature:   Stevens, D. A. et al. Miconazole in Coccidiomycosis. Am J Med,
60:191-202, Feb 1976.
```

Figure 10.4: *A record of a dialogue between the MYCIN program and a user. The inputs typed by the human are preceded by the prompt characters* **.

By looking at a trace of which productions were used in which order, the program can answer why a certain question was asked or how a certain conclusion was derived. For example, the following type of exchange is typical:

Doctor: *How do you know that the culture was taken from a sterile source?*
Mycin: *Rule001 and Rule022 gave suggestive evidence.*
Doctor: *How was Rule001 triggered?*
Mycin: *It was known that the site is one for which sterility depends on method. The method is one of the recognized ones for the site, and it is not known if care was taken; therefore there is strongly suggestive evidence that the culture was taken from a sterile source.*

If the doctor disagrees with MYCIN's conclusion, he can walk back from the conclusion through the AND/OR tree examining each production rule invoked to see where his reasoning differs from that of the program. This may lead to the modification of some rule or to the addition of a new rule. This is a classic case of learning from a teacher.

The performance of the MYCIN program has been tested against the performance of specialists with varying degrees of expertise. The results of two series of tests on 80 patients in one case and 10 patients in another showed the MYCIN program scoring higher than any of the human prescribers. The scoring was done by a panel of eight prominent specialists of infectious diseases at institutions not connected with the MYCIN project.

MYCIN has not yet been used in clinical settings. To be practical for everyday use it must be extended to cover all the major infections likely to be found in a hospital. This implies that additional hierarchical levels of production rules are needed to select the set of lower level rules that apply to the particular type of infection encountered.

The ability of production rule-based systems to perform expertly in a wide variety of fields, from organic chemistry to diagnostic medicine to geology, is well-documented. Production rules are exactly the type of functional operators required at the upper levels of a hierarchical processing-control system. At these levels of the hierarchy where this type of behavioral decision needs to be made, the requirements for speed are not demanding. Computation times of several seconds, or even minutes, are acceptable. Even the most sophisticated production-based systems have a reasonably small set of production rules (i.e., less than a thousand). Such a system can easily return a decision, or recommend an action, in a few seconds even if implemented on a microcomputer.

Thus, the application of rule-based expert systems to the high-level, goal-decomposition modules of a hierarchical control system for an intelligent robot or an automatic factory is a likely prospect within the next decade. Before the turn of the century this type of production-based system may be capable of performing all of the day-to-day operating decisions required in most factories and offices.

LANGUAGE UNDERSTANDING

One of the most difficult topics in artificial intelligence is language understanding. An early goal of work in this area was automatic translation. In the late 1950s and early 1960s, compilers and assemblers were very successfully translating one computer language into another. It thus seemed reasonable to suppose that similar, albeit more complex, programs could be written to handle the translation of natural language. Of course, it was not expected that the full range of natural language would yield immediately. Shakespeare into Russian might take some time, but surely translation of scientific papers on a restricted domain of topics from Russian into English would be relatively straightforward. Unfortunately, the translation of natural language turned out to be much more difficult to automate than anyone suspected.

Much time and money were expended only to find out that a reasonable translation of a text from one language to another requires a lot more than a dictionary and a simple grammar. Unless understanding occurs as an intermediate state between two language encodings, unexpected and even bizarre results are obtained. For example, "The spirit is willing, but the flesh is weak" may get translated into "The wine is good, but the meat is bad." It is necessary for the translator to understand the meaning of the subject matter of the discourse. The words to be translated must be understood in terms of historical events—actions, reactions, observations, experiences, and relationships of objects and actors in the physical or mental world. Only then can these entities be recoded into the language strings of the "foreign" language.

As a result of the failure of language translation projects, research was redirected toward language understanding, since it had become clear that this was a precursor to translation.

Language understanding is itself a difficult problem, but some significant progress has been made and some important insights have been achieved. Language understanding draws heavily on the work in question answering, which is a data-base retrieval problem, as well as on semantic nets, which is a data-base structure and entry problem. The test of a language-understanding system is usually some form of dialogue between a human and a computer program. This dialogue may include some graphic input or output via light pen or graphics display. Conceivably it could also include the behavioral response of a robot to commands or advice given by a human.

Understanding is, of course, multileveled, occurring at a number of different hierarchical levels. For example, understanding the word <STOP> is straightforward. It involves simply recognizing a string of symbols or characters or detecting a particular spoken word. Evidence that the command has been understood occurs when the receiving entity terminates whatever activity was on-going. On the other hand, understanding the Gettysburg Address requires not only the recognition of a particular string of words, but also prior knowledge of history and a complex model of human emotion, including the concepts of nobility, sacrifice, war, and death. Furthermore, evidence indicating that the Gettysburg Address has been understood must itself be extremely complex.

One of the most impressive and still most influential works in the field of language understanding is that of Terry Winograd, completed at MIT in 1971. This system works in the restricted domain of a simulated robot arm operating on a set of simulated objects in a simulated world. The discourse is in the form of a human instructing the robot arm to manipulate the objects in the world. Figure 10.5 shows a computer graphics display of the objects and the robot arm in the simulated world.

PICK UP A BIG RED BLOCK

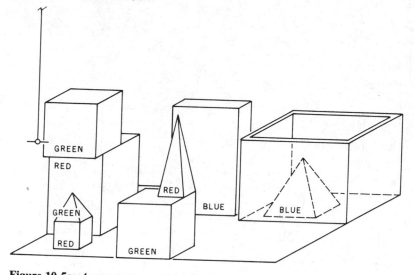

Figure 10.5a: *A computer graphics display of the "blocks world" that is the subject of conversation between a "robot" and a human programmer using Terry Winograd's language-understanding program. Above is the configuration of the computer's internal model of the blocks world at the time when the <PICK UP A BIG RED BLOCK> command is received.*

PICK UP A BIG RED BLOCK

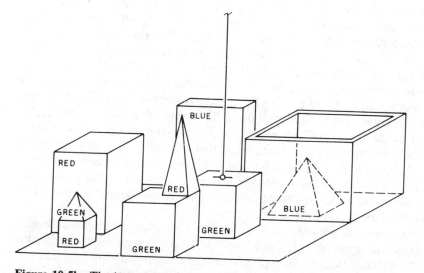

Figure 10.5b: *The internal model after the computer; 1) finds it must move the green block before it can reach the big red one, 2) finds a place to put the green block, and 3) moves the green block to the empty space.*

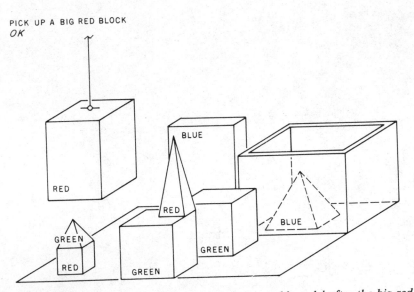

PICK UP A BIG RED BLOCK
OK

Figure 10.5c: *The configuration of the blocks world model after the big red block has been successfully picked up and the computer has answered "OK."*

Figure 10.6 is an example of the dialogue. As is obvious from this example, the level of understanding of the computer is considerable. The computer can carry on a protracted conversation, recognizing and using colloquial sentence fragments appropriately in place of complete sentences, correctly interpreting pronouns, and automatically selecting the most meaningful interpretation of ambiguous words or phrases. This is not a trivial level of understanding.

The key to the Winograd program is that the computer memory contains a model of the world that is shared by both the computer and the human programmer. The discourse is about objects, actions, and relationships that have some specific representation in the computer's internal model. Furthermore, the knowledge is mostly represented in the form of procedures, rather than static data structures. For example, the dictionary contains separate little programs for each word, the execution of which check whether the words are being correctly used. The part of the system that analyzes the syntactic form of sentences contains separate programs that encode the rules of each grammatical structure.

Finally, the computer program has the ability to "imagine" what would happen IF certain actions were carried out. For example, when it receives the command <PICK UP THE RED BOX>, it hypothesizes the attempt only to find that it is blocked by the fact of a green box sitting on top of the red one. It then backs up, hypothesizes moving the green box first, finds out it must discover an empty space to put it down, etc. Finally, once it finds a way to pick up the red box, it actually performs the entire sequence of actions in the proper order to accomplish the commanded goal. Thus the program can hypothesize an action and evaluate the result of that action; hypothesize another action and evaluate that; and so on. It can then select the hypothesis that results in the commanded goal being realized and implement it in overt action. In the case where the results of its internal (mental) experiments lead to ambiguous, unclear, or impossible situations, the program can ask questions or request further instructions of the human operator. There have been several programming languages written to facilitate the writing of the kind of software that is used in the Winograd program.

```
Pick up a big red block.
OK.
Grasp the pyramid.
I DON'T UNDERSTAND WHICH PYRAMID YOU MEAN.
Find a block which is taller than the one you are
    holding and put it into the box.
BY "IT," I ASSUME YOU MEAN THE BLOCK WHICH IS TALLER
    THAN THE ONE I AM HOLDING.
OK.
What does the box contain?
THE BLUE PYRAMID AND THE BLUE BLOCK.
What is the pyramid supported by?
THE BOX.
How many blocks are not in the box?
FOUR OF THEM.
Is at least one of them narrower than the one which I
    told you to pick up?
YES, THE RED CUBE.
Will you please stack up both of the red blocks and
    either a green cube or a pyramid?
OK.
Which cube is sitting on the table?
THE LARGE GREEN ONE WHICH SUPPORTS THE RED PYRAMID.
Is there a large block behind a pyramid?
YES, THREE OF THEM: A LARGE RED ONE, A LARGE GREEN
    CUBE AND THE BLUE ONE.
Put a small one onto the green cube which supports a
    pyramid.
OK.
Put the littlest pyramid on top of it.
OK.
How many things are on top of green cubes?
```

```
I'M NOT SURE WHAT YOU MEAN BY "ON TOP OF" IN THE
   PHRASE "ON TOP OF GREEN CUBES."
DO YOU MEAN:
1--DIRECTLY ON THE SURFACE
2--ANYWHERE ON TOP OF?
2
THREE OF THEM.
Had you touched any pyramid before you put the green
   one on the little cube?
YES, THE GREEN ONE.
When did you pick it up?
WHILE I WAS STACKING UP THE RED CUBE, A LARGE RED
   BLOCK AND A LARGE GREEN CUBE.
Why?
TO GET RID OF IT.
Why did you do that?
TO CLEAN OFF THE RED CUBE.
Why did you clear off that cube?
TO PUT IT ON A LARGE GREEN CUBE.
Why did you do that?
TO STACK UP THE RED CUBE, A LARGE RED BLOCK AND A
   LARGE GREEN CUBE.
Why did you do that?
BECAUSE YOU ASKED ME TO.
```

Figure 10.6: *An example of the dialogue between a human and the robot in Winograd's program. Lines in capitals are generated by the computer.*

Another program written even earlier at MIT in 1966 by Joseph Weizenbaum also exhibited a remarkable ability to converse with a human partner. ELIZA, Weizenbaum's program, carries on a conversation much like that of a psychiatrist. Figure 10.7 shows a sample of the type of dialogue that ELIZA can produce. The ELIZA program is a very simple, almost trivial, question-answering system that recognizes a few key words, word types, and simple sentence structures, and constructs a response using a set of rules. The rules are designed to create the impression of understanding by recognizing a word or key phrase in a sentence, doing a syntactic analysis of its usage, and then constructing a grammatically correct output using parts of the recognized phrase in selected spots. In most cases the response is a prerecorded output with a few blanks to be filled in by words or phrases from the human's input.

ELIZA has been criticized (perhaps most vigorously by Weizenbaum himself) for being a put-on, for having no understanding, and for using the trick of simply rephrasing the input to produce an output. But the same could be said for a great deal of conversation between human beings. This is, in fact, an old strategy students use on exams—simply give the professor's words back to him, with slightly different phrasing. This creates the appearance of understanding with a minimum of the real thing.

This same strategy applied at a slightly higher level in the language processing-generating hierarchy will produce the type of conversation typically encountered at a cocktail party. People in such situations emit a more or less canned opening line, wait for some response, and then reply with an output on roughly the same subject as the response received. This is merely the ELIZA strategy raised one or two hierarchical levels.

```
Hello.
HOW DO YOU DO. PLEASE STATE YOUR PROBLEM.
I want a good example for my book.
YOUR BOOK.
Yes, my book about computers. Can you help me?
YOU'RE BEING SOMEWHAT SHORT WITH ME.
I didn't mean to be.
YOU SAY YOU DIDN'T MEAN TO BE.
That's right. What do you know about computers?
DO COMPUTERS WORRY YOU?
Not at all. I think they can be very useful.
CAN YOU ELABORATE ON THAT?
Computers play a vital role in the operation of our
   society.
WHY DO YOU MENTION COMPUTERS?
Because that is what the book is all about.
IS THAT THE REAL REASON?
Of course. Sometimes you are difficult to talk to.
WHAT MAKES YOU THINK I AM DIFFICULT TO TALK TO?
You answer in such short, stylized phrases.
WE WERE DISCUSSING YOU - NOT ME.
I thought we were discussing computers.
WHAT DO YOU THINK MACHINES HAVE TO DO WITH YOUR
   PROBLEM?
My only problem is to get you to carry on a
   reasonable conversation.
WHY DO YOU SAY YOUR ONLY PROBLEM IS TO GET I TO CARRY
   ON A RESONABLE CONVERSATION?
```

```
You don't use very good grammar.
OH, I DON'T USE VERY GOOD GRAMMAR.
That's right  Don't you know the difference between
     nominative and accusative?
YOU'RE NOT REALLY TALKING ABOUT ME - ARE YOU?
I really was, but I'm willing to change the subject.
DO YOU SAY YOU REALLY WAS FOR SOME SPECIAL REASON?
The reason is that I would like an interesting
     conversation in the book.
IN WHAT WAY?
So that the readers will not get bored with it.
I AM NOT SURE I UNDERSTAND YOU FULLY.
You don't understand very much, do you!
WHAT ARE YOUR FEELINGS NOW?
I feel that I'm about ready to give up.
TELL ME MORE ABOUT SUCH FEELINGS.
The page is almost full now, so I can end this
     interview.
SUPPOSE THE PAGE WERE NOT ALMOST FULL NOW?
Then we would have to continue this silliness a while
     longer.
PLEASE GO ON.
That's all there is to say. Don't you ever get tired?
PERHAPS THAT'S ALL THERE REALLY IS TO SAY.
Yes. Goodbye.
YOU SEEM QUITE POSITIVE.
```

Figure 10.7: *An example of a conversation with Joseph Weizenbaum's ELIZA program. Lines in capitals are generated by the computer.*

CAN MACHINES UNDERSTAND?

Weizenbaum's criticism of his own and others' work in artificial intelligence springs from a deep philosophical issue: can computers ever truly "understand"? Weizenbaum argues that there is something intrinsically different between electronic and biological intelligence, and that the gap between what humans and computers can understand is unbridgeable.

In the deepest sense, he is right. If we accept the hypothesis that intellect grows out of behavior, then it follows that unless robots are born and grow up in human society, experiencing all the sensations, joys, and frustrations of the human condition, then they can never fully understand human ideas, values, emotions, and motivations. For robots to truly understand humans they would have to be indistinguishable from humans in bodily appearance as well as physical and mental development and remain so throughout a life cycle identical of humans'. Otherwise, it is inevitable that robots would be treated differently from humans by their peers and companions, and hence would not have the same type of experiences as their human counterparts. For this reason, robots will never be able to understand human values.

Understanding requires a similar internal knowledge base, or world model, similarly structured in both parties. The encoding and transmission of a message describing the internal state trajectories of one party must be received and interpreted by the second party to elicit similar state trajectories before there can be understanding. If the world model is primarily the result of a lifetime of experiences, then understanding cannot occur unless the entire past histories of both parties are identical.

If carried to a logical conclusion, however, this implies that understanding can never occur between any two parties, even between human twins, because no two individuals ever experience identical lives. In some fundamental sense, this is true. None of us ever fully understands anyone else, and no one is ever fully understood by anyone.

The question of whether robots can ever understand humans, or vice versa, must therefore be argued on some middle ground. Understanding must be defined for a particular domain of knowledge. Winograd's robot understands statements and commands about the world of blocks and pyramids because it contains in its internal knowledge base a set of objects, relationships, and rules regarding how the objects can be manipulated and what relationships are allowed. A human can understand the output produced by the Winograd robot because the human shares the same knowledge base. The robot and the human therefore understand each other and can carry on a sensible conversation within the domain of the knowledge base that they share.

In a similar way, two humans can understand each other and converse sensibly on a subject like politics, yet be unable to understand each other on another subject like nuclear physics. Thus, the issue of understanding is domain-dependent. Today, the domains that robots and humans can share, and hence understand together, are extremely limited. The real question then becomes whether it will ever be possible to extend these domains sufficiently to make the claim that computers can truly "understand."

Weizenbaum contends that the limited successes of AI research using restricted domains are misleading, because as the domain of discourse grows, the difficulty of the problem and the size of the computer programs needed to deal with the problem grow exponentially. Thus, he argues, machine intelligence that duplicates human intelligence is impossible.

What Weizenbaum fails to take into account here is that the power of a hierarchical computing structure increases exponentially with the number of levels in the hierarchy. Thus, as the number of levels in the hierarchy grows linearly, the size of the domain of discourse grows exponentially—which seems to suggest that robot intelligence can indeed someday equal or even surpass human intelligence!

There is no reason to suppose that the present human brain represents any theoretical maximum of intellect. Quite to the contrary, the enormous effort required to educate the human mind in the techniques of logic and reason and to instill the lessons of history suggests that other methods for computing and remembering could be much superior. It might be possible, for example, to build a robot brain that remembers all the information stored in all the libraries of the world. If it's possible to create robots that are as intelligent as humans, there is no reason to suppose that we couldn't, with the simple addition of another hierarchical level, make robots more intelligent than humans. Nevertheless, because of their very different physical forms and prior learning experiences, robots and humans will forever remain very different creatures.

The subject of comparative intelligence is full of logical pitfalls. To begin with, intelligence is not a scalar value, as is suggested by IQ ratings. Intelligence is as multi-valued as is behavioral skill. Who is more physically skilled, the baseball player Reggie Jackson, the piano player Monty Alexander, or the gymnast Nadya Comaneci? That these skills are so different makes the question meaningless. So also, the ranking of intelligence on a linear scale is extremely misleading. The vast differences in the organisms in which the intellect resides will prevent us from ever being able to definitively answer the question of whether robots can be as intelligent as humans.

Intelligence is only one aspect of the human mind. What about the emotions: what of love, hate, hope, fear, awe, and wonder? What about religious experience? Can a robot feel a sense of duty? Could it have a conscience? We don't know. Even in the human mind, such feelings and motives are far from understood. One can only speculate whether similar phenomena could ever be duplicated in robots. In order for any autonomous organism to survive and prosper in a hostile world, there must be mechanisms for detecting and avoiding danger, seeking protection, and carrying on in the midst of adversity. If future robots are ever designed to behave successfully in an uncooperative, even hostile, environment, then something analogous to human emotional evaluators will be needed to select and optimize behavior. There must be a world model that enables it to predict the future, lay plans, and take action in anticipation of difficult circumstances. The world must be made predictable. In a world populated by intelligent rivals, one must be able to construct internal models sufficiently complex to predict the behavior of those rivals. In a world where survival depends on predicting the weather and coping with fire, flood, earthquakes, storms, droughts and a natural order shrouded in mystery, an internal world model might well require a sense of magic, a sense of religion to give it predictability.

As long as robots are confined to the laboratory or factory where they do not have to hunt for food, flee from predators, compete for sex, or survive in war, it seems unlikely that they will develop the internal models required for survival under such conditions. Laboratory or industrial robots will survive and multiply in numbers by simply performing useful services or feats of intellect for their human makers. Like laboratory rats, they will be most useful if they remain docile and domesticated. Presumably they could be programmed to exhibit jealousy, envy, greed, or any of the other emotional traits of humans. But whether there would be any economic or entertainment benefit to us, and hence a survival benefit to the robots, in such characteristics is questionable. There is no reason for such disruptive characteristics to be implanted in robots designed for industrial or domestic applications.

There is even a sense in which it can be argued that robots are an evolving life form. Already robots are used to make robots. Within a few decades robots and automatic factories will achieve a significant degree of self-reproduction. This will create at least a precursor to a new life form, a life form based on silicon rather than carbon, which will draw energy from the electrical power grid rather than from photosynthesis or metabolism of carbohydrates. Robot evolution may be very rapid, because robots have human designer-creators who are much more discriminating than the mechanisms of natural selection.

Such is the stuff of lively conversation and philosophical disputation. All such arguments are speculation and reasoning by analogy. The answer to the question of whether machines ever will, or even can, possess a general level of intelligence comparable to humans' is unknown and may be unknowable.

Nevertheless, in the practical world, robots already have the capacity to perform useful and valuable jobs, and those capabilities are being rapidly expanded. Within limited domains, such as manufacturing, robots will soon be able to perform the perceptual analysis and control functions necessary to operate machines and industrial processes for long periods of time without human intervention. This might not speak to the philosophical question of whether machines will ever rival human intellect or duplicate human feelings, but it does indicate that totally automatic factories are technically feasible. Then, the truly interesting questions become: can robot factories be made economically practical, and, if so, what will be the effects on the social order? How will the creation of an industrial economy based on robot factories and offices impact the way we live and earn our income?

CHAPTER **11**

Future Applications

The first large-scale application of robots will be in the field of manufacturing, for it is here that the environment is well-structured and repetitive enough so that robots with no ability to see or feel and with extremely limited intellectual capabilities can accomplish useful work. In manufacturing, robots can perform some jobs with productivity gains of 100 to 300 percent. Furthermore, the value added is large. Industrial robots costing $30,000 to $100,000 typically return over 50 percent annually on invested capital.

Even larger productivity gains will come from the total integration of robots and computer-controlled machines into the manufacturing process from beginning to end. Soon it will be possible in many manufacturing plants to integrate all operations under a hierarchical control structure like the one in figure 11.1. Such a totally automatic factory would have interactive computer graphics systems for designing parts and products, computer-aided process-planning systems for specifying which operations need to be performed and in what order, computer production planning and scheduling systems that schedule machines and route partially completed parts through the plant, and numerically controlled machine tools that use computer-generated instructions to cut and form parts to the correct dimensions. These would be serviced by computer-controlled materials-handling systems that use robot manipulators to acquire parts from the stockroom, robot carts to automatically transport parts and tools around the shop, and robot manipulators to insert parts into fixtures for machining, assembly, and testing. Robot assembly systems would fit and fasten parts together into completed products, and automatic inspection systems would check dimensions and part integrity at many points during and after the manufacturing process. There would also be computer-based management information systems that allow human managers to keep track of what is happening in the factory, manage inventory, implement management decisions, and set priorities.

All of these systems exist today in one form or another, for one application or another. In most cases they have already proven themselves enormously profitable individually. Productivity gains of several hundred percent are not uncommon. So far, however, all of these systems have not been integrated into a single system to create the totally automatic factory.

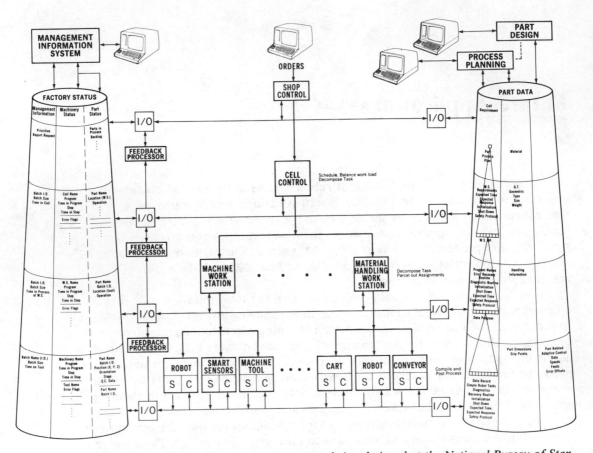

Figure 11.1: *A hierarchical control structure being designed at the National Bureau of Standards for controlling an automatic machine shop. On the right is a hierarchy of data bases containing part designs and process plans generated interactively. On the left is another hierarchy of data bases that contain a complete state description of all the machines and parts in progress in the factory. In the center is a hierarchy of control modules that use the process plans, part data, and factory status data to decompose high-level tasks of part manufacture into low-level actions by numerically controlled machine tools and robots. The feedback processors extract information from the lower levels relevant to the decisions being made at the higher levels. The management-information system enables human managers to query the status of the system and set priorities. Each of the computing modules acts as a state-machine making possible the dynamic interaction of real-time feedback with the scheduling and routing of work through the shop.*

But there are numerous large-scale attempts being made right now to do just that. Japan, East and West Germany, Norway, and Sweden have all made the development of completely automatic robot factories a high priority item of national policy. Firmly committed to the creation of automatic factories for over a decade, the Japanese Ministry of Industry and Trade (MITI) has invested hundreds of millions of dollars in research and development for the automatic factory. The principal focus of this effort is a project called Methodology for Unmanned Manufacturing (MUM).

The economic rationale for the automatic factory is that the productivity gains to be achieved from the integration of many different types of automatic systems multiplies the productivity gains from the individual systems by a factor of two to four times. For example, once a factory is able to run overnight or over the weekend without human labor, productivity immediately takes a quantum leap. There are 168 hours in a week. A factory that can operate continuously can be producing output for four forty-hour shifts a week with eight hours left over for maintainance. This must be compared with factories that employ human labor that usually operate only one or two shifts a week. Most people do not like to work nights and weekends. Thus, premium pay is required for the third and fourth shifts. Robots, however, do not care whether it is day or night, weekday or weekend.

The first robot factories will probably be somewhat more expensive than conventional manned factories. Large initial investment is needed for novel and untried technologies, and robot technology is in its infancy. Microcomputers are less than ten years old. Robot vision, microcomputer networks, and hierarchical, sensory-interactive goal-directed control theory are all just beginning to be investigated by a few researchers in a few under-funded laboratories. Very few persons are skilled in these matters, and no one has fully mastered them. There exists no significant body of theory and engineering practice in robotics; much remains to be done.

Robotics, like space exploration, is a journey into the unknown. It will require our best brains, a large investment in research, huge outlays of money for development, and, eventually, enormous capital resources for new plants and facilities. These are the "front end" costs that will make the first robot factories very costly.

But the long-term economic benefits are clear. Knowledge, once acquired, is inexpensive to reproduce. Once we know how to build a robot factory, we can build a hundred or a thousand robot factories at a fraction of the cost of the first. When we have reduced robotics to an engineering practice, robot factories will not cost any more than conventional factories. In fact, they may be less expensive: robots don't need air conditioning in the summer or heat in the winter; they don't need cafeterias, rest rooms, or parking lots; they don't need costly equipment to protect them from smoke, dust, noise, toxic fumes, or dangerous machinery.

Thus eventually, the robot factory may produce productivity improvements of ten to a hundred times over a conventional factory. This means that products produced in robot factories can be many times less expensive and profits higher.

Robot factories will eventually be able to manufacture, assemble, and test the essential components for other robot factories. This will initiate a regenerative, or reproductive, process similar to that which already exists in the computer industry. The results might be similar to the 20 percent annual reduction in the cost per unit performance that has been going on for at least 25 years in the computer industry. See figure 11.2. A similar price/performance trend in industrial robots would mean that the price of a sophisticated industrial robot might fall to several hundred 1980 dollars by the year 2000. Such a cost, when prorated for a 168-hour week, would amount to an effective robot labor cost of only pennies per hour. Prices of products produced in robot factories could eventually spiral downward by a factor of two every three years.

Eventually the flow of material wealth from automated production lines will give overwhelming economic power to the owners of the robot factories. Once automatic factories become common, the economic advantage will be so large as to be irresistible. No industry using conventional production techniques and human labor will be able to survive in head-to-head competition with industries using the automatic factory concept.

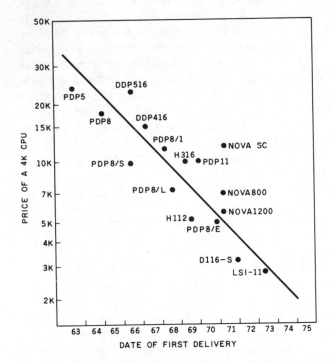

Figure 11.2: *A graph of the cost of small computers over a period from 1963 to 1973. This downward trend in costs has continued throughout the decade of the 1970s and shows every indication that it will continue to do so for at least another ten years.*

We have not yet entered the age of the robot factory. Even the Japanese, the acknowledged leaders in the development of robot factories, have not yet achieved their ultimate goal of the completely automatic factory. But they are getting close enough to seriously influence the balance of world trade. Already the Japanese produce twice as many cars per man-day of labor as American automobile manufacturers. Each day, the Nissan Zama automobile plant assembles 1300 cars with only 67 human workers on the assembly line—the rest of the work is done by robots and other types of automatic machinery. This type of technology is partially responsible for the enormous influx of inexpensive, high quality steel automobile, motorcycles, and other consumer products into the American and world markets. The Japanese economic miracle is largely attributable to their enormous investment in productivity-enhancing technologies in general, and to computer-aided manufacturing and robot technology in particular.

FUTURE ROBOT COST TRENDS

Some experts may disagree that the present cost of $30,000 to $100,000 for an industrial robot will ever be reduced to a few hundred dollars. In fact, the recent announcement of several European robots in the $150,000 to $200,000 price range seems to run counter to this prediction. Nevertheless, there are a number of reasons to believe that the long-term trend of robot costs will be downward. First, we are still just on the threshold of the age of robot factories. Today only pieces and fragments of the technology have entered the industrial arena. The full self-reproductive power of the totally automated factory is still in the future. Today, only one or two robot manufacturers use robots in the production of robots, and only for a few operations. Surely, this will not continue. By the end of the 1980s it will be common practice for robots to be used extensively in the manufacture of robots.

There are two types of costs for robots. One is the software costs: the programming language, the memory-management software, the operating system, and the applications programs. The other is the hardware costs: the cost of mechanical structures, of gears, bearings, motors, pistons, valves, encoders, sensors, power supplies, electronics, computers, and memory systems. Today it is possible to put together an advanced laboratory robot with extensive sensory capabilities for about $150,000 together with computer hardware to run it for another $150,000. However, the cost to develop the software for such a system might easily run 5 to 50 times as much. As the market grows, economies of scale will drastically reduce unit costs both for software and hardware.

For example, once the robot market grows to a certain size it will become economical to build robots from injection-molded plastic. A possible plastic design is shown in figure 11.3. This particular design is powered by pressurized water. Injection-molded plastic parts can be made cheaply and very precisely. Hydraulic motors and pistons using water as the hydraulic fluid at less than 100 psi can easily be constructed from plastic injection-molded parts and can use rubber gaskets and O-rings for seals. Plastic motors, ranging in size and power from more than one horsepower to less than 1/100th horsepower, can be constructed for between one and ten dollars. Plastic pistons can be made even more cheaply. For example, plastic hypodermic syringes can be bought in large quantities for only pennies apiece. Plastic tubing is only a few cents a foot, and 5/8th-inch garden hose costs considerably less than a dollar a foot.

Gear boxes made of plastic gears and nylon bearings can be made for a few dollars with a wide range of speeds and power ratings. Valves can be made from rubber diaphragms and controlled by solenoid coils, a common practice in automatic washing machines and dishwashers. Double valves for automatic washing machines can be purchased in large quantities for a dollar or two apiece.

An array of N valves controlling a set of orifices of exponentially increasing size, shown in figure 11.4, can control the rate of flow to a precision of one part in 2^N. A set of four valves arranged in a bridge configuration as shown in figure 11.5 can control the direction of flow of water through a hydraulic motor or to a bidirectional piston. A set of four valves, arranged in the configuration of figure 11.6, can drive a pair of push-push pistons. The combination of flow-rate control and direction control can be used to operate hydraulic actuators in a robot.

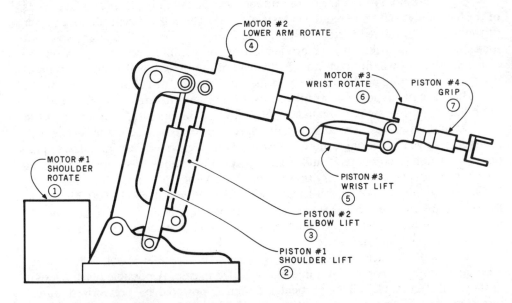

Figure 11.3: *A design for a robot made completely of plastic parts. Plastic pistons and motors using a pressurized hydraulic fluid such as water provide power to the various joints.*

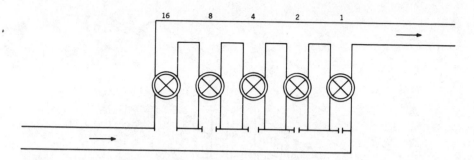

Figure 11.4: *A five-bit digital flow-rate hydraulic control valve. Orifices with areas of 1, 2, 4, 8, and 16 allow 32 different flow rates to be generated by opening or closing various combinations of valves. Such valves can be manufactured from plastic and rubber parts similar to those presently used in automatic washing machines.*

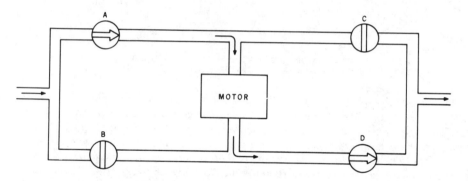

Figure 11.5: *A set of direction-control valves for a hydraulic motor. When valves A and D are open, the motor is driven in one direction. When valves B and C are open, the motor is driven in the other direction. If all the valves are closed, the motor is locked. If valves A and B are open with C and D closed, the motor is free to turn without drawing any power.*

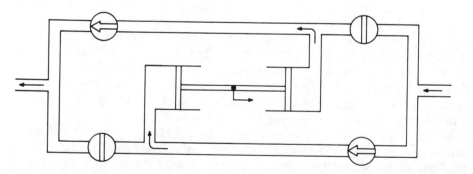

Figure 11.6: *A set of direction-control valves for a pair of push-push pistons. The pistons can be driven in either direction, locked, or left free to slide depending on which combinations of valves are opened and closed.*

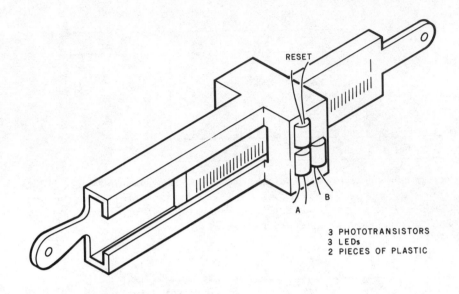

RESET

A
B

3 PHOTOTRANSISTORS
3 LEDs
2 PIECES OF PLASTIC

2 LED-PHOTOTRANSISTOR PAIRS PRODUCE QUADRATURE SIGNALS
3RD PAIR PRODUCES AN INITIALIZATION PULSE

Figure 11.7: *A possible design for a plastic linear-motion detector using moiré fringe patterns. A grating pattern on the clear plastic slide creates moiré fringes when pulled past a similar pattern embedded in the housing. Light emitting diodes (LEDs) on the back of the housing transmit light through the gratings to be detected by the phototransistors shown on the front of the housing. The two phototransistors at the bottom produce phase quadrature square wave signals that are sent to an up–down counter such as shown in figure 11.8. The top phototransistor produces a reset signal for initializing the up–down counter to a known value.*

A chamber partially filled with air and containing a float can be used to measure hydraulic pressure, and the use of orifices of different sizes can be used to control the various relationships between pressure and flow rate, useful in servoing a robot in position, velocity, and force.

Gratings printed on a pair of clear plastic plates, shown in figure 11.7, can be used to generate moiré fringe patterns that alternate from transparent to opaque with each increment of motion equal to the line spacing of the gratings. An electrical pulse for each increment of motion can then be obtained by putting a light-emitting diode on one side and a light-sensitive detector on the other. By placing two emitter–detector pairs one-quarter wavelength of the moiré fringe pattern apart, a pair of phase-quadrature square wave signals can be produced to indicate the direction of motion. The electrical pulses from these signals can be accumulated in registers as shown in the circuit diagram of figure 11.8 and used to measure position and velocity of motion.

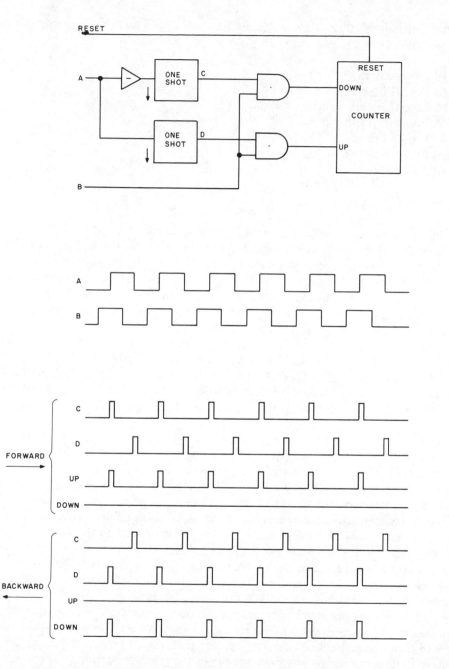

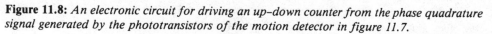

Figure 11.8: *An electronic circuit for driving an up–down counter from the phase quadrature signal generated by the phototransistors of the motion detector in figure 11.7.*

In industrial quantities (less than a million units per year) the following costs could probably be achieved:

$5 Hydraulic motor or piston
$10 Digital flow-rate valves (6 bit)
$5 Direction valves (bridge design)
$5 Pressure regulators
$5 Position sensors
$20 Electronics for valves
$10 Electronics for sensors

$60 Total cost per axis

Thus for a six-axis manipulator with a position-servoed hand capable of lifting a few pounds, the total cost would be $420 for actuators and controls. Doubling this might raise the pressure and load carrying capability by a factor of five or more.

Add $1000 for a computer and $1000 for a plastic and fiberglass (or carbon filament epoxy) structure, and the result is an industrial robot costing about $3000. Such a robot should easily equal the weight-lifting, speed, and accuracy performance of robots that presently sell for $40,000.

If the cost of computing power continues to fall at a rate of 20 percent per year for the next decade, as it has for the past three and as it shows every indication of continuing to do, then by the year 1990 the cost of the same computer will be about $100. The likely strategy for industrial robot production will be to maintain the computer cost at $1000 but increase the computing power to that of today's $10,000 machine.

The final stage in the cost reduction of robots is when they begin to be produced in large quantities by robot factories. The exciting feature of this process is that it feeds on itself: less expensive machinery makes the production of new machinery less expensive still. When robots in computer-controlled automatic factories begin to manufacture the principal components of automatic factories, cost reductions will propagate exponentially from generation to generation. The introduction of computers and robots into the manufacturing process thus has the potential for increasing productivity on a scale not previously conceivable. Eventually the cost of finished manufactured goods may fall to only slightly above the cost of unprocessed raw materials. When this occurs, the expense of production will become virtually independent of the complexity of the manufacturing process.

If the mining, processing, and transporting of raw materials is also eventually performed by robots, then the cost of finished goods becomes governed by the thermodynamics of the process. The limiting factor here is the cost of the energy input to raise the entropy of the raw materials to that of the finished products. These costs are orders of magnitude less than the present market price of manufactured goods, because that price reflects the cost of human labor.

For those industrial tasks where the cost of robot labor falls below that of human labor or where the capabilities of robots rise above those of human labor, industrial productivity will leap forward as fast as the resources are committed to investment in robot technology. This will undoubtedly happen first in the manufacturing industries, resulting in profound effects on the economic strength of whatever nations adopt this new technology.

Manufacturing is the foundation of industrialized civilization. Manufacturing productivity growth is dominant among the factors producing growth in real income and real economic prosperity. The lack of productivity growth towers over all other factors that influence peacetime inflation (including government deficit spending). Industrial productivity affects the cost of food through the cost of farm equipment and supplies, the cost of construction through the cost of building materials and construction equipment, and the cost of transportation through the cost of vehicles and road-building machinery. It affects the cost of energy through the cost of drilling equipment and pipelines. It directly affects the cost of furniture, clothing, appliances, automobiles, trucks, and trains, and indirectly affects the cost of everything else, right down to church and school buildings, books, and the pollution-control equipment required to keep the air and water clean. Industrial productivity growth is the principal source of prosperity and brings a rising standard of living. High productivity is the reason that Americans have traditionally enjoyed a high standard of living. The potential of robot technology to raise industrial productivity by hundreds or even thousands of percent thus makes it a matter of the highest importance to the future of this country, and indeed to the future of modern civilization itself.

ROBOTS IN CONSTRUCTION TRADES

Once robots become firmly established in the manufacturing industries, they can be expected to make inroads into the construction trades. A construction robot must be mobile and be able to move around a construction site, no small feat since a typical site is comprised of muddy ruts, piles of dirt, ditches, and various construction materials. There is frequently a need to go through doors, climb steps, and maneuver on scaffolding. A single construction robot need not necessarily cope with all of these mobility problems, but these are the conditions prevalent in a construction situation.

There are already many machines that have been designed to negotiate a construction site. A variety of tracked and wheeled vehicles (forklifts, cherrypickers, front-end loaders, backhoes, bulldozers, ditchdiggers, and cranes) carry and maneuver many different types of lifting, digging, and scooping devices. Often the vehicles that carry these devices have hydraulically powered stabilizing legs that are set down once the vehicle reaches a suitable work position. This type of vehicle would serve nicely as a base for a construction robot.

A more exotic and versatile design would be to upgrade the stabilizing legs into walking legs. Consider, for example, a construction robot designed as a hydraulically powered six-legged walking machine using the power plant and carriage of a small truck, like the one shown in figure 11.9. The legs would consist of three-degree-of-freedom manipulators with a polar coordinate system. The first degree of freedom is a rotary actuator about the vertical axis. The second and third degrees of freedom are lifting and flexing motions controlled by hydraulic pistons.

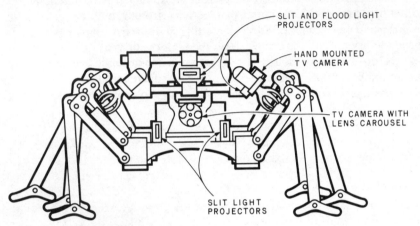

(a) FRONT VIEW

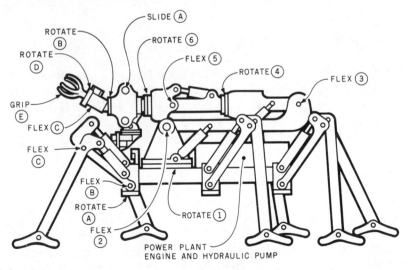

(b) SIDE VIEW

Figure 11.9: *A possible design for a construction robot.*

At low speeds, such a legged vehicle could be nearly as efficient as a wheeled vehicle. A vehicle weighing about 3000 pounds with a 100-horsepower engine should be able to walk across the ditches, holes, and piles of rubble on any given construction site. A lighter vehicle of several hundred pounds with an engine of three to five horsepower should be able to climb stairs or scaffolding, carry loads, and lift and position heavy or bulky objects.

Coordinating the leg movements so the robot can walk and climb deftly is a problem that can be solved by a network of microcomputers, one for each leg, connected together in a configuration similar to the one developed at Ohio State University by Professor Robert B. McGhee. Figure 11.10 shows a six-legged walking machine built at Ohio State. Figure 11.11 shows a flow diagram of the software designed by McGhee for leg coordination. To measure the distance between the foot and the ground at all times, a construction robot might have input from an acoustic ranging sensor on each foot, like the one used on the Polaroid One-Step camera.

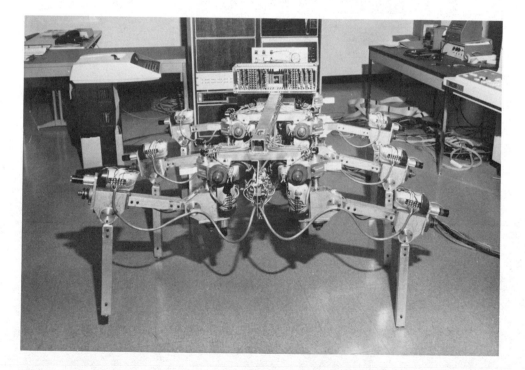

Figure 11.10: *Front view of a six-legged walking vehicle designed and built at Ohio State University by Professor Robert B. McGhee.*

Additional ranging sensors could keep the legs from bumping into anything or anyone. Position inputs from each joint of the legs and sensors to measure the forces exerted downward by each foot would also be necessary. Gaits for six-legged walking devices have been worked out in detail and are well-known. A seventh microcomputer would have coordination control over the six-leg computers and would compute the roll, pitch, and yaw of the vehicle as well as the desired heading and speed, so it could be steered like a car.

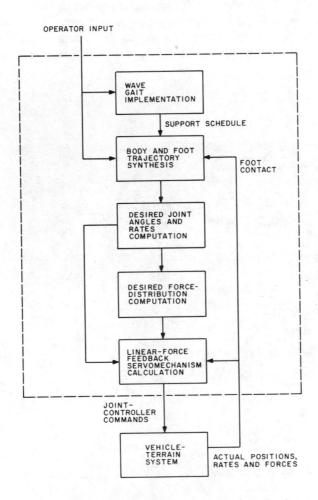

Figure 11.11: *Structure of interactive computer software system for control of the Ohio State University hexapod of figure 11.10.*

On the front of the vehicle would be a pair of slit projectors and a solid-state TV camera configured as a three-dimensional vision system similar to the one illustrated in figure 8.34. The computations of a depth image for the region in front of the vehicle would be handled by an eighth microcomputer controlling the vision interface and processing the visual data. The planes of light would be mechanically scanned back and forth across the territory in front of the vehicle in an interlaced pattern so the entire region would be covered every one-half second. A ninth microcomputer would compare the processed vision data with a stored topographic map of the construction site so that the vehicle could find its way around.

On top of the vehicle could be a hydraulically powered cherry-picker boom, with a three-axis device for orienting the shoulders of the two robot arms. The shoulder structure would position two manipulator arms, a TV camera, a light projector, and perhaps a tool manipulator (not shown in the figure).

The potential selling price, assuming present-day technology, might be the following:

$20,000 computing hardware
$40,000 six-axis cherry-picker
$40,000 two arms with grippers
$30,000 six legs
$30,000 cameras and lighting system
$20,000 mass storage system for topographic maps
$20,000 engine, frame, and hydraulic system

$200,000 TOTAL

This is too expensive for most applications today. However, technological advances will eventually reduce the cost by three to ten times. As the cost of human construction labor rises, the economic advantages of robot construction labor will grow more and more significant.

A robot like the one shown in figure 11.10 could serve as an apprentice to a master craftsman in constructing cinder block or brick walls, laying roofing shingles, lifting, positioning, and fastening siding, insulation, window and door frames, setting roof and floor joists, assembling forms for concrete, pouring and dressing concrete, painting, and performing a large number of other specialized tasks. A smaller version of this basic design would be suitable for inside work, for setting studs, installing plumbing, laying tile, building brick or stone fireplaces, putting up wallboard, painting, sanding, polishing, etc. Eventually, such machines would be able to work unsupervised for extended periods of time.

OUTSTANDING PROBLEMS

What are the technical problems in developing such devices? We know how to build the mechanical apparatus, and there are a number of powered actuators on the market. There are backhoes of many different designs that can execute very precise motions of a powerful digging claw. A well-trained backhoe operator can dig a hole of precise dimensions, can lift huge volumes of dirt or large boulders, or can pick up a single pebble. There is a whole family of cranes that can lift heavy loads and precisely position them. Why are these not made into robots, outfitted with a variety of vacuum and fingered grippers, and provided with tools—automatic nailers, mortar dispensers, paint brushes and spray nozzles, trowels and spatulas, picks and shovels, buckets and mops, grinders and sanders, scrapers and caulkers, drills, saws, chisels, glue guns, and a hundred other varieties of instruments?

There are two reasons: first, at present there are no sensors or sensory-processing devices that can make a robot see and feel well enough to know what it is doing. Cranes and backhoes need the human operator to see where to put the shovel or the load. Even a human has no way of sensing the forces developed at the point of action except by such crude methods as seeing the deflection of the structures being operated upon or hearing the power train being loaded down. Robot vision is still crude, slow, unreliable, and expensive, and no software exists for rapidly and reliably recognizing objects, relationships, and situations, or for measuring the position and orientation of objects and their relationship to one another and the environment. Furthermore, no one knows how to write such software in an economically practical manner.

Second, control systems or control system architectures that can enable a robot to act and react using sensory information in a timely and intelligent way are still nonexistent. Construction sites are notoriously dirty and cluttered places, and even the simplest job (such as picking up a brick or board, deciding where to drive a nail, or how to open a paint can) requires a great deal of knowledge and skill. In order for a robot to perform such jobs efficiently and reliably, a great deal of additional knowledge about writing software for accomplishing such tasks will be required. Few if any robots, even under ideal conditions in the most advanced research laboratories, can presently do these things. The software required to demonstrate complex assembly tasks requires many person-hours of programming effort, often by doctorate-level researchers with wide experience and formal training in computer science. No one has yet perfected a person–machine interface by which an average construction foreman, in a few words, could instruct a robot to perform a job like <LAY A TILE FLOOR>, <BUILD A BRICK WALL>, <INSTALL A SINK>, or <PAINT A CEILING>.

These are enormous yet solvable problems. Any complex task is nothing more than a sequence of simpler subtasks. Each subtask can itself be decomposed into a sequence of yet simpler sub-subtasks. At the very bottom, each actuator needs only the information of how far to move in one of two directions, how fast to proceed, and how much force to apply. For most tasks in factories or construction sites, there is a well-known procedure to be followed. A robot would seldom, if ever, have to figure out for itself how to perform a task. Many tasks can be described in terms such as <PICK THAT UP AND HOLD IT HERE>, or <FETCH THOSE>, <CARRY THESE AND PLACE THEM OVER THERE>, etc.

One problem is to be able to embed procedures to execute such commands in a set of rules that reside at the various levels of a control hierarchy and to provide sensory information to the control modules that invoke the proper rules at the proper times. Another problem is to devise a means by which the writing of software can be similarly partitioned, so that the robot programmer can isolate and address a limited problem with a limited set of parameters in a modular fashion. A third problem is to make the various program modules fit together and function in a coordinated goal-directed manner when they are assembled.

These are not small problems, but they can also be solved. The first step is to analyze each task the robot is to perform and partition the task into a set of sub-tasks, and then sub-subtasks, in a hierarchical manner similar to what was described in Chapter 9.

The second step is to configure a network of computers so that the separate computing modules of the hierarchy can be implemented on separate computers in the network. A separate computer (or separate time slot on a shared computer) for each computational module in the processing-generating hierarchy means that the different computing tasks never need to interrupt each other. This enormously simplifies the problem of writing software because of the regular structure and precise modularity it imposes on the process. It also simplifies the debugging and verification of software that is critical to making robot programs interact intimately with many external variables.

A third step is to fit the robot with visual systems using structured light in order to recognize and measure the position and orientation in three-dimensional space of the objects to be manipulated. The use of structured light simplifies the visual-processing algorithms sufficiently so unambiguous conclusions can be derived in a small fraction of a second. This is essential if visual information is to be used for controlling the actions of the robot in real time.

A fourth step is to equip the robot with force and touch sensors so that it can feel the presence of objects and exert forces on them in a controlled and goal-directed way.

The fifth and final step is to provide the robot with a world model that can enable it to interpret both commands and sensory information in the context of a known environment. One type of world model is a photographic image, or set of images, of the work environment that can be used as a map or template to compare against incoming sensory data. Consider, for example, if a painting robot were to be provided with a photographic image of the object, such as the front of a house, to be painted. This photograph could be used as a world model for interpreting commands such as <PAINT THE FRONT DOOR> or <PAINT THE UPSTAIRS WINDOW FRAMES>. The photograph would show where the paint should be applied. It would tell the vision system where to look for edges and corners and the control system where to watch for obstructions such as posts and shrubs.

This assumes that the robot has the ability to scan and interpret the photograph and compare the sensory information obtained from a vision or touch system with the world model expectations derived from the photograph. The complexity of this problem can be substantially reduced by using a map derived from the photograph, instead of the photograph itself. In this case, the map could be produced from photographs and graphic overlays developed off-line in a sophisticated computer-vision-graphics laboratory or by manual input on an interactive graphics terminal. The map would have numerical codes attached to each region identifying the physical object represented by that region and its three-dimensional position, orientation, shape, and surface characteristics. The on-site robot would then merely need the ability to scan the map, which could reside on a programmable read-only memory (PROM) chip, a floppy disk, or a bubble memory, and compare the stored data against incoming observations from the robot's sensory system.

Programs written to implement robot tasks at various levels in the hierarchy could then refer to various portions of the map image. For example, the areas to be painted can be specified by number, and the color and dimensions of each area defined by the map in the robot's world model. The program then consists merely of specifying the order in which each area is to be painted or sanded, where nails are to be positioned, where tile is to be laid, where roofing materials should be positioned, etc. Standard patterns can be specified for laying bricks or blocks of stone in constructing walls, fireplaces, floors, and arches. Using such a map, or set of maps, and programs referring to the maps, the robot can compare the existing state of the work with the desired state of the completed project, selecting the appropriate operation to be performed in the appropriate sequence.

Such functioning requires a significant amount of software to be embedded in the computational modules of the control hierarchy. The software may be either resident on read-only memory (ROM) in the on-site robot or in a mass storage device that can be accessed by the robot. The mass storage device could be a large disk system located in a van, or one that is accessible through phone lines to a remote facility. The set of programs required to perform a large variety of tasks thus can be loaded into the robot-control system whenever those specific tasks are called for by the robot's job supervisor. Given this type of *a priori* information, a construction robot should be able to accept instructions from a foreman on a construction site in a simple subset of English. Given recent progress in the state-of-the-art of automatic voice recognition, such verbal commands may soon be possible.

It will probably be many decades before robots are able to do all the tasks necessary to build a house. Nevertheless, enough of the value added in construction may be amenable to robot labor by 1990 to significantly affect the cost of new housing.

Once construction robots become dexterous, inexpensive, and simple to use in a large variety of practical construction tasks, labor-intensive construction techniques that have been abandoned because of prohibitive costs will once again be economically practical.

For example, building with stone could experience a renaissance. Buildings, bridges, roads, gardens, and fountains could be designed by computer to be constructed out of precisely sculptured interlocking blocks of stone. The computer would instruct a quarry robot to cut and palletize the stone. The same computer would compile the behavior commands for a robot stonemason to assemble the cut stone at the building site.

Certainly the world will never run short of the raw materials for stone buildings. Stone construction has unexcelled beauty and durability, and although stone is not a good insulator, it has thermal storage properties that are very useful in the design of passive solar heating systems.

The amount of software needed to enable a robot to perform routine construction and assembly tasks in a relatively unstructured environment is enormous. However, if the software is properly structured it can be easily transferred from one robot to another and from one type of robot to another. The software is task-specific. Each task requires a unique program, indeed, an entire set of programs at each level in the sensory-control hierarchy. Nevertheless, many different tasks utilize the same set of subtasks, arranged in differing orders or with differing modifiers. Thus, the total amount of code, although large, is within practical limits.

In short, construction robots are technologically feasible. The technology required for their development is either already in existence or soon will be. What remains is an understanding by those who control research monies that such things are within the realm of practicality, and a conviction of those who control government and corporate policy that the results would have positive effects within a time period short enough to justify the capital investment.

HOUSEHOLD ROBOTS

The 1990s could be the decade during which the household robot becomes practical. Once plastic robots become highly developed and inexpensive in industrial applications, and once advanced software and sensory systems are developed for construction robots, the same technology can be applied to the problems of household robots. The environment of the home is as variable and complex as that of the construction site. Each home has a different floor plan and arrangement of furniture. In order for a household robot to negotiate through the average room, it must have an internal map of the furniture placement and permissible pathways. In order for the robot to set the table, it needs to have an internal map of the proper placement of plates, silverware, cups, glasses, and napkins. In order for it to dust, it must have an internal program that recognizes each piece of furniture and each fragile item and how it should be handled. A household robot must know where the dishwasher is, where the cabinets are located, and where each of the various types of plates and utensils is to be stored. If it is to vacuum, it must have a map of what to vacuum as well as a sensory system that can recognize the difference between patches of dirt and patterns in the Oriental rugs. If it is to clean windows, it must know where they are as well as how to reach them without bumping into the furniture or becoming entangled in the drapes. If it is to scrub the bathroom, it must have a model of the shape of the fixtures as well as a procedures for wetting, rubbing, rinsing, and drying them.

These are extremely complicated problems, yet they are similar to those that must be solved by construction robots. Once the software techniques are developed for construction applications, they should be adaptable to the household environment. The mass market of household robots means that the software costs can be amortized over a very large number of robots. Again, the driving cost factor will be the mechanical structure.

In mass consumer quantities, the mechanical parts for a robot may cost one-half, or even one-third of what industrial quantities cost. A household robot, such as the one shown in figure 11.12, with two arms, wheels, and a shoulder-height-adjustment capability might have twenty degrees of freedom. Not all would require the full complement of rate control, pressure regulation, and position indicators.

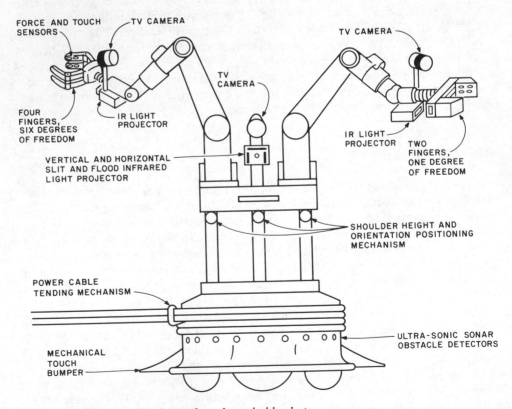

Figure 11.12: *A possible design for a household robot.*

The average cost per axis for a household robot might be between $20 and $30. This translates into $400 to $600 for actuators and controls.

Add $1500 for a computer, $800 for sensor systems including vision, $600 for a structure, and the result is a household robot costing around $3500. Such a product could be marketed for $4000 to $6000 (1980 dollars)—about the price of an inexpensive automobile. If the capabilities are extensive, such as the ability to set and clear the table, load and unload the dishwasher, prepare meals, sort clothes and do the laundry, vacuum, dust, and wash windows, this price is not unreasonable and a mass market would exist.

Hydraulic power could be provided simply and inexpensively by a single electric motor driving a plastic hydraulic pump carried in the bottom of the robot. Such a robot could obtain power as well as access to large external computers and data bases by plugging itself into wall sockets. The robot would carry a small storage battery to enable it to travel between one wall socket and another. Alternatively, it might use two lengths of cord to enable it to maneuver from one electrical outlet to another by plugging itself in at a new outlet before releasing and recoiling its cord from the last outlet.

With some modifications, a household robot might be able to perform a variety of jobs in the yard and garden. An internal map of the yard together with sensors to detect landmarks like the corners of the house, walkways, trees, and shrubs could enable the robot to navigate in the yard. A mowing attachment could cut and trim the grass, and a map of the garden may even make it capable of weeding the flower beds or garden. Such an outdoor device could be electrically powered through an extension cord or mechanically powered by a small gasoline engine.

ROBOTS IN ENERGY, THE OCEANS, AND SPACE

Besides the use of robots in manufacturing and construction and their potential as household servants, there will be many other applications as well. Over the next few decades, robot technology could greatly improve the safety and reduce the cost of nuclear power. Professor Marvin Minsky of MIT has proposed that robots and remote manipulators completely replace human workers inside nuclear power plants. This could make it possible for nuclear fuel reprocessing plants and breeder reactors to be permanently sealed. As a result, the threat of sabotage or the possibility of theft of nuclear materials would be totally eliminated. In the event of nuclear power plant accident or malfunction, robots could work in radioactive areas for emergency repairs and clean-up operations.

Robots are also ideally suited for underwater applications. Underwater robots using water hydraulics could operate at any depth. The computer could be housed in a spherical pressure-resistant chamber together with a fuel cell that would generate electricity to drive an electric motor connected to a hydraulic pump. Such a system could easily provide one-horsepower working capacity in a very compact package. Larger systems with ten to a hundred times as much power are well within the capabilities of current technology.

Underwater robots could be weightless, and their buoyancy could be controlled by expanding or contracting air-filled chambers. They could be maneuvered by propellers or by jets of water. Walking underwater could easily be accomplished by a two-legged (or two-armed) robot. Such robots could explore the depths for minerals, operate underwater mining and drilling equipment, and perform underwater construction.

Underwater robots might eventually be capable of introducing completely new approaches to solar energy. One possibility is to use underwater construction robots to build and service huge turbines for capturing energy from deep ocean currents. Although the energy density in currents such as the Gulf Stream is not high (the flow is only about five knots), the total energy available is enormous. The Gulf Stream is thousands of feet deep and many miles wide. Estimates are that underwater turbines could produce electricity at commercially competitive prices, even using present construction technology. Undersea construction and maintenance robots would considerably reduce the cost of such structures.

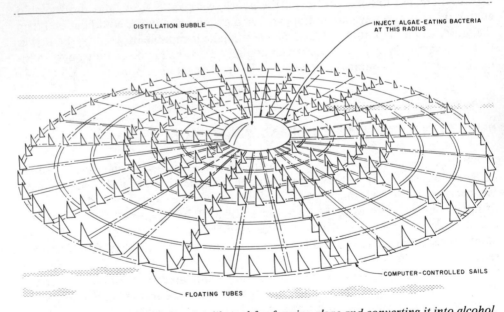

Figure 11.13: *A giant plastic floating lily pad for farming algae and converting it into alcohol. Floating tubes support plastic-bottom ponds filled with fertilized water. Circulation from the outer rim inward carries the growing algae toward the center where it is processed by bacteria and distilled into fuel-grade alcohol. The center is covered by a clear plastic bubble that traps and condenses the alcohol vapor produced by solar heating.*

Another possibility would be to use robot technology to control giant floating lily pads like the one in figure 11.13. These structures could farm algae and process it into fuel-grade alcohol while sailing the equatorial oceans. Completely unmanned, these huge plastic-bottomed ponds, up to ten kilometers in diameter, would be filled with highly fertilized sea water. They would float on the surface of the sea, using wave energy to circulate the algae, wind energy to navigate, and a network of microcomputers to control the many subtle adjustments of sail and rudder necessary to maintain the shape and structural integrity of a flimsy plastic web many kilometers in diameter on the open ocean. A microcomputer network brain could give such a structure the ability to fold up like a morning glory and sink beneath the surface during rough weather and spread open again when the seas are calm.

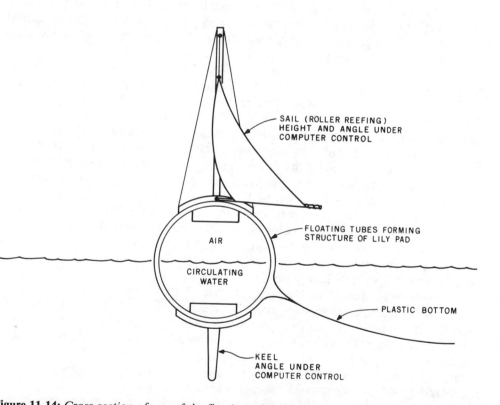

Figure 11.14: *Cross-section of one of the floating tubes that support the plastic bottom of the lily pad algae farm and circulate enriched water. Sails and keels are controlled by a network of microcomputers to maintain the shape and structural integrity of the lily pad and permit it to navigate on the open ocean. Mechanical power to adjust sails and keels is derived from wind or wave energy.*

The algae would grow and multiply in the outer portions of the lily pad that would be fed by fertilized water recycled from the central processing region. The algae would be concentrated through a series of one-way valves and sieves as the algae flowed gradually toward the central processing region. At a point near the center, algae-eating bacteria would be injected. The resulting product would be alcohol. The central portion would be covered with a clear plastic bubble supported by a pocket of air. Sunlight shining through the clear plastic would evaporate the alcohol, which would then condense on the inside of the plastic and run into collecting troughs.

At present, only methyl alcohol could be economically produced by such a process. However, future research in genetic engineering should be able to produce a strain of bacteria that can convert algae to ethyl alcohol, which has about twice the energy density of methanol.

The alcohol fuel produced would be stored in an underwater bladder, collected periodically by a robot tanker, transported safely, and burned without pollution in home furnaces, automobiles, and electric utilities. The robot tankers could be giant submarine blimps powered by alcohol fuel.

There are good reasons to believe that lily pads might be practical sources of fuel in the near future. If we assume a 2 percent photosynthetic efficiency and a 25 percent chemical conversion efficiency, the output for a single lily pad ten kilometers in diameter would be about 42,000 gallons of methanol an hour. Assuming eight hours a day, that leads to over 100 million gallons per year. A fleet of 2500 such lily pads would provide the equivalent of all the oil presently consumed in the United States. This number of lily pads would fit conveniently in a square 500 miles on a side. In the future genetic engineering on algae and on microorganisms that feed on algae should be able to increase the efficiency of the sunlight-to-alcohol conversion process. This suggests that the alcohol fuel available from robot lily pads might eventually be sufficient to provide the entire energy needs of the world for the foreseeable future without any need for nuclear power in any form. The percentage of the equatorial oceans that would need to be covered with lily pads in order to satisfy the entire world's energy supply for the next thousand years would be small.

An important feature of lily pad technology is that it would not divert any existing food-producing land into energy production. In fact, sea-going lily pads would themselves become complex ecosystems wherein many higher creatures might live and reproduce. Plankton, shrimp, fish, and birds would thrive in the environment created by the lily pads. The fish crop might eventually become a significant source of food for the world's growing population as the competition for arable farmland grows and the natural fishing grounds become overharvested.

Finally, these havens of life and energy in the open ocean might one day become desirable places for people to live and work and play. Such colonies are much more likely to be economically and technologically practical than the space colonies proposed in the NASA-sponsored studies of Brian O'Leary, and the stepping stones to reaching them are much closer at hand.

Structures similar to the ocean-going lily pads could also be constructed on land in the desert. Dry-land lily pads would require two sheets of plastic, one dark to cover the bottom, the other clear to cover the top and prevent the water from evaporating. Water is, by definition, scarce in the desert and evaporation expensive to replace. The sea-going variety would not need to worry about evaporation.

It is important to add, however, that a major energy switch from oil to alcohol produced by lily pad technology is probably not possible in this century. Even if there were no remaining technical problems, which there are, and even if the technology had already proved itself price-competitive, which it has not, the time needed for conversion of a large fraction of the world's energy industry to alcohol produced with lily pad technology would probably be 20 to 30 years.

These are only a few of the potential applications of robotics. Robots will be able to accomplish many other interesting and valuable tasks. For example, robots will be able to explore the bottom of the oceans and eventually mine the deep ocean trenches where untold mineral treasures lie hidden. They also will be capable of exploring and even colonizing the surface of the Moon, Mars, and the satellites of Jupiter.

Robot space exploration and robot construction of large space structures will be much less expensive than similar work performed by human astronauts. Robot space voyagers will not need the elaborate life-support and safety equipment required by humans. Robots can fly aboard launch vehicles that aren't certified safe for humans and can embark on one-way missions with no provisions for returning to Earth. Robot explorers, if equipped with the proper sensory systems, can transmit visual and other sensory information back to Earth where the sensory experiences can be reconstructed for human observers. By this means, robot vehicles on Mars or robot gliders riding updrafts in the atmosphere of Jupiter could transport us all on fantastic voyages of exploration to new worlds. By telepresence (i.e., the transmission and reconstruction of sensory experiences over long distances) we might all experience the sights, sounds, and feelings of unearthly regions throughout the solar system.

CHAPTER **12**

Economic, Social, and Political Implications

These are revolutionary times. The introduction of the computer into the manufacturing process and the spectacular steady decline in the cost of computing power are historical events that will someday rank with the invention of the steam engine and the discovery of electricity. The human race is now poised on the brink of a new industrial revolution that will at least equal, if not far exceed, the impact of the first industrial revolution. Changes as profound as those resulting from the development of agriculture and the domestication of wild animals are rushing us toward a new world.

The first industrial revolution substituted mechanical energy for muscle power in the manufacture of goods and the production of food. This brought about an enormous increase in productivity, put an end to slavery, and freed a great mass of human beings from a life of poverty, ignorance, and endless physical toil.

The next industrial revolution will substitute computer power for brain power in the control of machines and industrial processes and will be based on robot labor. Automatic factories, offices, and farms will be able to produce material goods—automobiles, appliances, furniture, and food—in almost unlimited quantities at very low cost and without human intervention. Robot construction workers will be able to build homes, roads, and commercial buildings. Robots will be able to mine the sea beds and farm the ocean surface for fuel as well as food. Robots and automatic factories have the potential to create material wealth in virtually unlimited quantities and eventually to reproduce themselves in any numbers we choose.

The next industrial revolution—the robot revolution—could free the human race from the regimentation and mechanization imposed by the requirement for manual labor and human decision-making in factories and offices. It has the capacity to provide us all with material wealth, clean energy, and the personal freedom to enjoy what could become a golden age of mankind.

BARRIERS TO A ROBOT LABOR FORCE

Unfortunately, the present socio-economic system is not structured to deal with the implications of a robot revolution. At least in America, there presently exists no politically acceptable mechanism by which average people could directly benefit from the unprecedented potentials of the next generation of industrial technology. Quite to the contrary, under the present economic system, the rapid widespread deployment of automatic factories would largely concentrate wealth and power in the hands of a few. In the long run, a massive conversion to robot industries has the potential to threaten jobs and thus undermine the financial security of many American families.

The fundamental problem is that income to the average family is distributed primarily through wages and salaries. If technologically efficient methods and automatic factories were introduced to create wealth with little or no human effort, it is not clear how most ordinary people would receive additional income to purchase what was produced. The income distribution system in America, and indeed in the entire industrialized world, is based on employment, not on industrial output. This is a serious structural flaw, for it works against policies that otherwise could upgrade productivity in our industrial system. It means that rapid increases in productivity lead, or at least appear to lead, to unemployment. The fear is that if productivity were upgraded at the maximum rate that is technologically possible, unemployment would become a serious problem.

Of course, one can make a good case that this is not true. There is *not* a fixed amount of work. Demand can always be increased enough to match increased supply. In the present economic situation there is plenty of demand. The mere fact of inflation is *prima facie* evidence that consumer demand exceeds the ability of producers to supply without raising prices. Even in the most technologically efficient robot society, demand can always be increased to match supply. All that is necessary is for increased spending power to find its way into the pockets of consumers at the same rate that increased output flows out of the more productive factories.

This, however, is not always easy to achieve in a politically acceptable way when wages are tied to the amount of work input and not to the amount of product output. This structural flaw in the income distribution system creates at least the appearance of a threat of unemployment that is serious enough to delay, if not prevent, the rapid development of a massive robot labor force from becoming an acceptable goal of national economic policy. It makes it extremely difficult to generate significant public enthusiasm for massive investments in robots, particularly while the unemployment rate for human workers is unacceptably high.

Just one example of the problem is the lawsuit recently brought by the agricultural unions against the state of California because of State University research on automated farm machinery. The complaint was that the state is supporting the development of technology that will put farm laborers out of work. This fear of unemployment, whether well-founded or not, is one of the most potent impediments to the development of robot technology today.

In order for a democratic society to take advantage of the benefits of a robot labor force, it is necessary, at the very least, to demonstrate that a variety of alternative occupations will be created to fill the void left by those jobs that are eliminated.

The most obvious source of new jobs is in the industries that would be created in the conversion to a robot-based economy. If robots are to be manufactured in large enough quantities to make a significant impact on the existing industrial system, entirely new industries will emerge and millions of new jobs will be created. It will be many years, perhaps centuries, before robots can design, manufacture, market, install, program, and repair themselves completely without human intervention. In the meantime, the manufacture and servicing of robots will produce an enormous labor market for mechanical engineers and technicians, computer programmers, electronic designers, and robot installation and repair persons. New robot companies will require secretaries, salespersons, accountants, and business managers. It seems likely that the robot industry will eventually employ at least as many people as the computer industry does today.

Converting the world's existing industrial plant from manual to robot labor will require many decades and will cost as much as the entire existing stock of industrial wealth. This is a Herculean task that will provide employment to millions of white-collar and blue-collar workers for several generations. For a country like the United States, with its strong technological base, the world market in robots could easily create twice as many jobs in robot production as were lost to robot labor. Needless to say, the export of robot systems could have a strong positive effect on the balance of trade and the strength of the dollar on the international market.

Of course, many occupations would survive and prosper even in the most advanced robot economy. Doctors, nurses, teachers, entertainers, and social, psychological, and religious counselors would continue to be required as long as there are humans with needs for such services. Surely a robot-based economy would produce sufficient material wealth to increase the demand for health, education, recreation, and social services by making them available to more people. Occupations in leisure industries, the arts, and many types of personal services would abound. Scientific research and exploration of the oceans and outer space offer unlimited opportunities for many types of fascinating careers into the indefinite future.

We can, of course, always spread the available work around. A shorter work-week of twenty hours, or perhaps eventually ten hours, is possible. Longer vacations, sabbatical leaves, and increased adult education all have the capacity to raise the number of jobs while reducing the amount of work.

In addition, we must never underestimate the capacity of our politicians, labor unions, and bureaucrats to generate make-work. Remember the Peter Principle: "The amount of work always expands to fit the number of workers assigned to do it." Both government and business bureaucracies have accumulated a great deal of experience in holding committee meetings, sending memos, and issuing regulations and directives that can busy an indefinite number of executive personnel and office workers for an arbitrary length of time. There is no question that we will find something to occupy as many people as necessary for as long as is necessary to create a rationale for passing out paychecks every two weeks. We have both the technological means and the political will to create work in whatever quantities are deemed fit by the voting public. One must never forget that both work and money are easily created. They can be generated by bureaucratic fiat whenever the voters demand it. Real wealth is what is hard to produce. This means that the dramatic scenes of mass unemployment pictured in novels like Kurt Vonnegut's *Player Piano* are grossly overdrawn.

Nevertheless, make-work is a poor solution for at least two reasons. First, most make-work jobs in a robot economy would be transparently unnecessary and therefore unsatisfying to most people. Second, the resources to create such jobs could be used much more productively in solving some of the real problems—poverty, disease, and illiteracy—that will be with us for a very long time.

This generation is in no danger of running out of work. The world is filled with need. It is premature to worry about robots eliminating work as long as there exist such overwhelming problems as providing food, clothing, shelter, education, and medical care for millions of people living in desperate poverty. The problem is not in finding plenty of work for both humans and robots. The problem is in finding mechanisms by which the wealth created by robot technology can be distributed to the people who need it. If this were done, markets would explode, demand would increase, and there would be plenty of work for all able-bodied humans, plus as many robots as we could build. This is not a technical problem—it is a social, economic, and political problem.

POTENTIAL SOLUTIONS

One possible solution to the problem of wealth distribution in a robot economy might be to make it easy for individuals to become robot owners. If, for example, workers in industries where robots were being introduced were to be given the opportunity to purchase the robots that were to displace them and to lease those robots to their former employers, then instead of becoming unemployed, the displaced workers would become independent owner-entrepreneurs.

This would seem particularly promising in the case of farm labor. The itinerant farmer laborer is already an independent entrepreneur. The trouble is he has only his labor to sell. Small groups or families of farm workers might band together to obtain financing to buy harvester robots. By such means, the itinerant farm worker could hope for not a lifetime of labor in the fields, but a life enriched by the prosperity brought by ownership of a group of robot slaves. If you still have to stoop over in the hot sun all day long, wage slavery is, after all, little different from the old-fashioned kind. How much better if farm worker families could own and operate a few robots rather than having to sell their own sweat to earn their daily bread? This suggests that the farm unions might do their workers more good by supporting farm robot research and concentrating their organizational efforts on obtaining the financial resources to make it possible for farm workers to become robot owner-entrepreneurs.

Appealing as this possibility is, it suffers from the problem that it would be practical in only a few instances. It might possibly work in farm applications and perhaps to some extent in construction work. However, the structure of the working relationships in factories and offices makes it unlikely that it would work there. Such an arrangement would require an unprecedented degree of cooperation, vision, and mutual good faith between unions and management, as well as between workers and capital financing institutions.

Another possibility, more amenable to manufacturing industries, would be to introduce a massive program of Employee Stock Ownership Plans (ESOP) such as have been suggested by Lewis O. Kelso. This would allow most of the presently employed industrial and business labor force to benefit from the robot revolution. However, it would exclude most of the rest of the population and would tie each worker's fortune very tightly to the future profitability of his or her particular company. Thus, some would fare very well while others might end up with nothing because of a company bankruptcy.

Another possible solution would be to finance the development and construction of robot factories out of public money (not tax money, but credit from the Federal Reserve System) and pay dividends on the profits from those investments to everyone on an equal per-capita basis. To be more specific, a semi-private investment corporation, which we might call a National Mutual Fund, could be created for the purpose of financing capital investment for increasing productivity in private industry. This investment corporation would be authorized by the Congress each year to draw up to a specified amount from the Federal Reserve which it would use to purchase stock from private industry. This would provide equity financing for the modernization of plants and machinery and the introduction of advanced computer-based automation. Profits from these investments would then be paid in the form of dividends by the National Mutual Fund to all adults on an equal per capita basis. By this means each citizen would receive income from the industrial sector of the economy independent of employment in factories and offices. Every adult citizen would become a capitalist in the sense of deriving substantial income from invested capital.

A new economic philosophy based on the concept of a National Mutual Fund is outlined in some detail in my previous book: *Peoples' Capitalism: The Economics of The Robot Revolution*. This book attempts to show how America could finance a rebuilding of its industrial plant and a massive construction program for robot factories. The suggestion is to begin the National Mutual Fund with the modest sum of $10 million for the first year and increase this amount by a factor of three every year for 25 years until the investment rate for the National Mutual Fund equals the total private investment rate. Once this were achieved, annual public dividends for every adult citizen would amount to about $8000, in 1980 dollars.

Figure 12.1 suggests that doubling the nation's investment rate would lead to a real annual growth rate of about ten percent. An enormous difference exists between ten percent real growth and the present rate of GNP increase. Figure 12.2 shows the implications over the next 25 years. At the current annual growth rate of 1.5 percent,

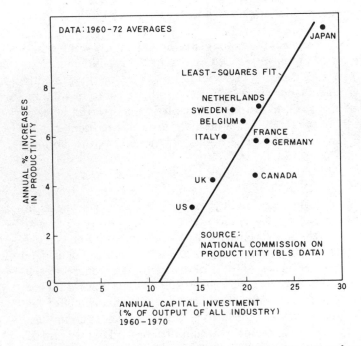

Figure 12.1: *The relationship between capital investment and productivity growth in ten industrialized countries. Countries with a high rate of investment have high productivity growth and vice versa. This dependence of productivity growth on capital investment is not a transitory phenomenon or one confined to a few countries. It is a fundamental relationship inherent in all industrialized societies.*

This implies that productivity growth can be controlled, that it is the direct result of economic policies that promote investments in new technology and in more efficient plants and equipment. The data shown here suggests that a given amount of investment will yield a given amount of productivity growth. For example, it suggests that a doubling of America's investment rate would produce an annual productivity growth rate of eight to ten percent.

This chart was compiled from data taken during the 1960s. However, the addition of data from the 1970s makes little change in the graph.

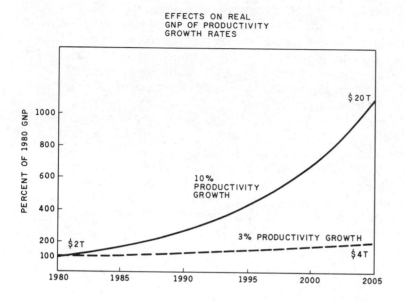

Figure 12.2: *Implications of different rates of productivity growth. Increased productivity is the principal factor causing real growth in the GNP. Three percent productivity growth for the next 25 years will lead to a GNP of $4 trillion 1980 dollars by the year 2005. Ten percent productivity growth over the same time interval would result in a GNP of $20 trillion. The annual difference in 2005 amounts to eight times the present GNP.*

the GNP will barely rise from its present level of about $2 trillion to about $3 trillion. This hardly keeps up with the population growth. Even if the U.S. were to achieve its historic growth rate of three percent per year, the GNP would rise to only $4 trillion by 2005. However, a ten percent growth rate would result in a GNP of over $20 trillion in 25 years, or more than six times the amount achievable at our present rate!

Clearly, this is a matter of tremendous importance. A GNP surplus of $16 trillion over what otherwise would be considered normal would mean that even the most exotic solutions to the problems of the environment would become economically feasible. We could afford to collect solar energy or dig for geothermal power anywhere on earth. We could afford to convert all industry, homes, and transportation to alcohol or hydrogen fuel. We could process all sewage and farm drainage to the purity of rainwater. At the same time, we could afford to rebuild our cities, modernize our transportation systems, and provide the best in health care for everyone. The military budget could support our defense needs on a smaller fraction of the GNP, and we could embark on a much more exciting program of space exploration.

There are, of course, many economists who would dispute the possibility of the United States increasing its real growth rate to ten percent per year even if the investment rate were doubled. Many would claim that Japan's experience is unique and that even Japan will slow down once she becomes the world leader. Perhaps so. But the curve in figure 12.1 does not come from a single country or represent the experience of only a few years. It reflects the combined experience of all the industrial countries in the world over the past 20 years.

Productivity growth is positively correlated with the investment rate. The new technology of robotics, computer-aided manufacturing, and particularly the prospect of self-reproducing factories certainly provide the technical basis for a ten percent annual productivity growth rate. What is needed is the capital investment to completely rebuild the present industrial base using the latest computer and robot technology. That involves a minimum of $6 trillion new investment, which, spread over two decades, amounts to about $300 billion addition annual investment, or about double the present rate.

DEALING WITH INFLATION

Unfortunately, simply doubling the nation's investment rate through newly created money would be inflationary in the short-term. The current investment rate is about 15 percent of the GNP, or about $300 billion per year. Doubling that to $600 billion annually through newly created money would put an enormous amount of additional spending power into the pockets of consumers. It often takes five years before newly built plants and equipment begin to operate at full capacity. Thus, increased demand caused by investment spending could precede by five years the productivity gains produced by those investments. Although investment reduces costs in the long run, if nothing is done in the short-term to delay the rise in demand caused by investment spending, inflation is inevitable.

Therefore, in conjunction with (but institutionally separate from) the National Mutual Fund, it is suggested that short-term demand be restrained through mandatory savings bonds. In order to share the pain of saving fairly, it is suggested that savings be withheld as surcharge on individual income taxes. In order to assure that these savings do not simply end up as a tax in disguise, these bonds would bear interest at four percent above the prevailing inflation rate and be redeemable after five years. The key idea in this plan, which might be called an Industrial Development Bond program, is to index the mandatory savings rate to the leading indicators for inflation on a monthly basis. If inflation is predicted, mandatory savings go up for the next month and reduce consumer demand. As soon as prices stabilize or decline, mandatory savings are reduced. This policy would effectively divert short-term demand from consumption into savings and compensate for increased investment. At the same time it would assure that the purchasing power to distribute the fruits of investment in highly productive technology would be available once the new plants and modernized machinery began to produce increased output.

Figure 12.3 shows how the National Mutual Fund and the mandatory savings program would work together. The National Mutual Fund would draw money from the Federal Reserve Bank where it was created. It would invest in highly productive robot industries and eventually pay dividends from profits in those industries to the general public. Industrial Development Bonds would regulate the amount of money in circulation and hence the demand for goods and services. The price index would be the controlling function on the rate of withholding for the bonds. When cheaper, more reliable, and longer-lasting products came flowing out of the robot factories, mandatory savings would be reduced, and the bonds being redeemed would increase demand and consume the increased productive output.

Working together, the National Mutual Fund and the mandatory savings program would create a form of peoples' capitalism or Jeffersonian democracy for the post-industrial era. Investments in private industries competing in the free market economy would earn profits that would be distributed to the general public as dividends to stockholders. Everyone would receive a substantial income from invested capital. Everyone would be a capitalist, not just the wealthy.

The difficulties in creating such a system would be enormous. It would involve a radical departure in the financing of industry and in the distribution of the wealth that it creates. There are many questions as to how such a system would be controlled and protected from abuse. It is an unprecedented proposal, but the wealth-producing power of robot technology is also unprecedented.

Unfortunately, the National Mutual Fund and Industrial Development Bonds probably represent too great a departure from conventional economic policy to be adopted in the near future, at least in the United States. Thus, I would like to suggest a less radical proposal that has some possibility of implementation.

Consider, for example, if the mandatory savings proposal were implemented without the National Mutual Fund. The withholding rate for Industrial Development Bonds could be set at a rate designed to control inflation by restricting consumer demand. Once this was done, taxes and interest rates could be lowered to produce whatever level of economic activity was desired. Today both taxes and interest rates are far above their historic averages.

Mandatory savings provide an equitable mechanism by which a free and democratic society could impose on itself the monetary discipline necessary to prevent inflation without simultaneously inducing recession. By separating the savings rate from interest rates it is possible to control aggregate demand by a mechanism other than fiscal or monetary policy. Mandatory savings can be set at a level designed to achieve any desired rate of inflation, while taxes and interest rates on investment loans can be lowered to stimulate whatever level of economic activity is also desired. By this simple means, rapid economic growth and stable prices could be achieved simultaneously.

The National Mutual Fund and mandatory savings are *not* socialism by any normal definition of the term. No industries would be owned by the state or run by

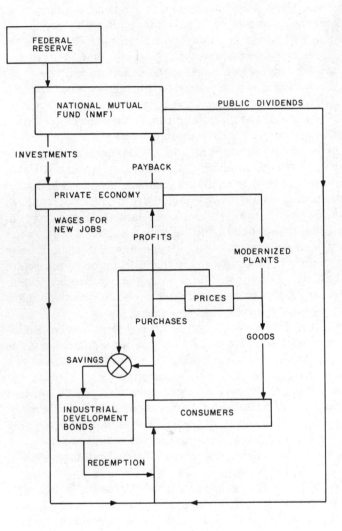

Figure 12.3: *A model of a national economy operating with the National Mutual Fund (NMF) and a mandatory savings program (Industrial Development Bonds). NMF investments and public dividends find their way into consumer pockets creating demand for new products produced by modernized plants. The balance between demand and supply is reflected in prices that regulate the amount of consumer purchasing power temporarily diverted into savings. The savings rate is adjusted monthly to control inflation despite massive investments of newly created money by the National Mutual Fund.*

the government. The National Mutual Fund would be a semi-private investment corporation that would be disallowed from owing a controlling share of any company and would never be allowed to invest more than private investors in the economy as a whole. All National Mutual Fund investments would finance privately owned industries operated for profit in a free market. Eventually public dividends would make everyone financially independent. All, regardless of their beliefs or attitudes toward industrialization or the work ethic, would have sufficient income to survive. Everyone would be assured of enough cash money to purchase food, shelter, clothing, and health care.

This would allow many new and previously untried lifestyles to develop and survive. It would even allow the revival of many ancient lifestyles that have become extinct because of competition with industrialized job economies. It would provide freedom from want as a birthright.

The equal distribution of wealth earned by robot labor might even lead eventually to the repeal of the graduated income tax. If robots were to provide for the basic needs of everyone, there would be no further moral justification for taxing the rich to subsidize the poor. There would be no need to penalize success and put great riches beyond the reach of all but the very few. The payment of equal dividends to all would make it possible for society, in good conscience, to reward excellence and encourage ambition.

It is also important to distinguish public dividends from welfare. To begin with, the dividends would not come out of taxes in any form. They would not be based on need of recipients, but on profitability of the companies in which the investment were made. This proposal is not just another "Robin Hood" scheme to take from the rich and give to the poor. Dividends would be paid to rich and poor alike. The healthy would benefit as well as the sick, the industrious as well as the lazy. This means that there would be no need for government welfare inspectors to intrude on privacy to determine need or for a large bureaucracy to certify eligibility or administer payments.

Equal payments would, of course, mean more to the poor than to the rich. They would provide an absolute income floor below which no one could sink, but there would be no reduction of payments for persons who chose to work and no limit to how much anyone could earn in additional income. Eventually, once annual per capita dividend payments rose to $8000 or more (in 1980 dollars), there would be no further need for welfare. Everyone would be financially independent regardless of job employment or lack of it.

To be sure, some will object to this proposal on the grounds that it would destroy the Puritan work ethic that made this country great, or that it would fly in the face of the Biblical curse placed on Adam and Eve, "In the sweat of thy face shall thou eat bread til thou return unto the ground." The work ethic is a culturally derived behavioral rule created by the requirements for economic success in a pre-robot economic system. It is not an indispensable component of human society, nor is it essential to mental or physical health or moral stability. A large segment of human society (namely the rich) have survived and prospered throughout history with very little recourse to the work ethic as most of us know it.

Before the first industrial revolution, physical slavery formed the backbone of every high civilization from the ancient Egyptians, Babylonians, Chinese, Greeks, Syrians, Turks, and Romans, down to the antebellum southern American states. The first industrial revolution substituted machine power for muscle power in the industrial and agricultural processes. This made slavery uneconomical. In a very real sense, the invention of the water wheel and the steam engine put slaves out of a job. However, the machinery of the first industrial revolution still requires human labor to control and service the machinery. Thus, present industrial technology still requires wage slavery in order for advanced civilization to flourish. If we wisely use the available intellect, knowledge, and socio-political institutions, we can hope that the second industrial revolution will free mankind from wage slavery and the regimentation of the Puritan work ethic central to all economic philosophies born of industrialization.

OPPORTUNITIES FOR THE FUTURE

Robot technology offers the possibility of completely eliminating poverty, not only from the United States, but from the face of the Earth. The cure to poverty is wealth, and robots have the capacity to create wealth in virtually unlimited quantities. Robots are almost like a new race of creatures willing to be our slaves: they will work for the cost of their purchase price plus their upkeep, and eventually they may reproduce themselves at exponentially declining costs. The self-reproductive potential of robots suggests that they might be manufactured in sufficient quantities to provide a robot (or two or three) for every human being. Since industrial robots are capable of producing value added of about $30,000 per year, we now have within our grasp the ability to create an everyman's aristocracy based on robot labor. The question is, do we have the wisdom to develop this technology in such a way that everyone benefits?

The principal remaining problems are not technical, but political—that is, social, economic, and psychological. The question is not so much, "Can we produce robots in these quantities?" but "Should we do so?" and "What would be the social consequences if we did?"

Some people today would question the wisdom of increasing the economic wealth of the world by such a vast amount. There has recently come into vogue a notion that economic growth and prosperity are not good; that they are incompatible with a clean, safe, healthy, uncrowded, unpolluted environment; that riches are somehow the cause of poverty and pollution. Surely this is ultimately false, for poverty and pollution can go hand in hand. Industrial pollution, for example, is more a product of poverty than wealth. The worst industrial pollution comes from obsolete plants in industries that are not profitable enough to afford antipollution equipment. Smokestack scrubbers, just like automobile exhaust suppressors and sewage treatment plants, are costly. Unprofitable industries cannot afford to clean up after themselves.

A clean environment and adequate food, education, and health care for a large population are expensive. They require a surplus over and above subsistence. The notion that advanced technology has created poverty and pollution is false. These are the result of the population outgrowing the technology. It is modern technology that produces sufficient surplus to feed, house, educate, and provide sanitation and health care for those fortunate enough to have these things now. It will require more advanced technology to provide these advantages for everyone.

It is sometimes argued that if everyone were rich, it would be no different than if everyone were poor. This seems absurd. There are many areas in the world where all the residents are rich and many others where everyone is poor. The difference is stark. In poor areas there is often hunger and sickness. In rich areas there is plenty to eat, the environment is clean, and education, health care, and entertainment are readily available.

Some may counter that wealth does not bring happiness and that there is nobility in poverty. However, such philosophical nonsense is seldom espoused by the truly poor. Poverty is degrading and debilitating. It is full of frustration and despair. The "nobility of poverty" is akin to the "dignity of slavery"—a romantic fantasy believed only by those who have never experienced either.

The new technology of robotics means that there are no limits to economic growth, certainly not in this century, and probably not in the next. There are undoubtedly limits to population growth. But there are no limits to knowledge growth or to growth in our ability to produce goods, services, and pleasant, healthy surroundings for the present population of the globe. Robots present us with the means to enormously increase the production of food, energy, housing, a clean environment, health care, education, entertainment, and economic security for all. Robots provide the technical basis for an unprecedented increase in wealth, security, and prosperity for everyone.

There will, of course, be problems in overcoming the fear that surrounds the subject of robots, a fear partly born of the Frankenstein legend of artificial life run amuck, partly born of the threat of job competition, as well as the prospect of monopoly control of robot technology by large corporations. We also contend with a general fear of the unknown, a distrust of modern science, and a feeling of powerlessness of the individual in a society dominated by machines.

To alleviate these fears, I have tried to suggest how we all might benefit from robot technology, how we might use robots to create a new industrial revolution that would usher in a new era of prosperity. As the world population grows and conventional resources become more scarce, increased productivity and new technologies that substitute new resources for old offer the only real alternative to economic decline.

Without rapid economic growth, a world of growing shortages will become an increasingly dangerous place. Nations competing over a shrinking stock of wealth and resources will inevitably come to military confrontation. The world's best hope is a great surge of industrial productivity that can outstrip the present population explosion and give us one more period of affluence in which we will have another chance at bringing the human population into stable equilibrium with the finite living space aboard the planet Earth.

Robots can help us achieve this productivity. Within a generation robots could create real material wealth in sufficient quantities to provide everyone with plenty of material goods. The only problem is whether we humans can create the mechanisms to distribute this wealth so that everyone gets a fair share.

The problem is not an idle one. The present precarious social order is threatened by dire problems of overpopulation, depletion of resources, and desperate poverty. What we do with the new technology of robotics may be a matter of life and death for the coming generation.

REFERENCES

CHAPTER 1

Arbib, M.A. *The Metaphorical Brain*. New York: John Wiley & Sons, 1972.

Bellman, R.E. "Mathematical Models of the Mind." *Mathematical Biosciences* 1 (1967): 287-304.

Blakemore, C. *Mechanics of the Mind*. New York: Cambridge University Press, 1972.

Dreyfus, H.L. *What Computers Can't Do: A Critique of Artificial Reason*. New York: Harper and Row, 1972.

Hofstadter, Douglas R. *Godel, Escher, Bach: An Eternal Golden Braid*. New York: Basic Books, 1979.

Hubbard, J.I. *The Biological Basis of Mental Activity*. Reading, MA: Addison-Wesley, 1975.

Leakey, Richard E., and Lewin, Roger. *Origins*. New York: E. P. Dutton, 1977.

McCulloch, Warren S. *Embodiments of Mind*. Cambridge, MA: M.I.T. Press, 1965.

Russell, Bertrand. *Human Knowledge: Its Scope and Limits*. New York: Simon and Schuster, 1948.

Sagan, Carl. *The Dragons of Eden: Speculations on the Evolution of Human Intelligence*. New York: Random House, 1977.

Sommerhoff, Gerd. *Logic of the Living Brain*. New York: John Wiley & Sons, 1974.

Sperry, Roger W. "Perception in the Absence of the Neocortical Commisures." *Perception and its Disorders*, Research Publication of the Association for Research in Nervous and Mental Diseases 48 (1970).

Turing, Alan M. "Computing Machinery and Intelligence." *Mind* 59 (1950): 433-460. Reprinted in Feigenbaum and Feldman. *Computers and Thought*. New York: McGraw-Hill, 1963.

Vander Zanden, James W. *Human Development*. New York: Alfred A. Knopf, 1978.

Von Neumann, J. *The Computer and the Brain*. New Haven, CT: Yale University Press, 1959.

Wooldridge, D.E. *The Machinery of the Brain*. New York: McGraw-Hill, 1963.

CHAPTER 2, 3, and 4

Carlson, Neil R. *Physiology of Behavior*. Boston: Allyn and Bacon, 1977.

Denney-Brown, D. *The Basal Ganglia—Their Relation to Disorders of Movement*. New York: Oxford University Press, 1962.

Geschwind, Norman. "Specializations of the Human Brain." *Scientific American* 241 (Sept., 1979): 180-199.

Green, David M. *An Introduction to Hearing*. Hillsdale, NJ: Lawrence Erlbaum Associates, 1976.

Grossman, Sebastian Peter. *A Textbook of Physiological Psychology*. New York: John Wiley & Sons, 1967.

Guyton, Arthur C. *Organ Physiology, Structure and Function of The Nervous System*, 2d ed. Philadelphia: W.B. Saunders, 1976.

Haber, R.N., ed. *Contemporary Theory and Research in Visual Perception*. New York: Holt, Rinehart and Winston, 1968.

Hubel, D.H., and Wiesel, T.N. "Receptive Fields, Binocular Interaction, and Functional Architecture in the Cat's Visual Cortex." *Journal of Physiology* 160 (1962): 106-154.

Kent, Ernest W. *The Brains of Men and Machines*. Peterborough, NH: Byte/McGraw-Hill, 1981.

Lettvin, J.Y.; Matturana, H.R.; McCulloch, W.S.; and Pitts, W.J. "What the Frog's Eye Tells the Frog's Brain." *Proceedings of Institute of Radio Engineers* 47 (1959): 1940-1951.

Quarton, G.C.; Melnechuk, T.; and Schmitt, F.O. *The Neurosciences: A Study Program*. New York: Rockefeller University Press, 1967.

Schmitt, F.O. *The Neurosciences: Second Study Program*. New York: Rockefeller University Press, 1970.

Schmitt, F.O.; Adelman, G.; Melnechuk, T.; and Worden, F.G.; eds. *Neurosciences Research Symposium Summaries* (Vol. 6). Cambridge, MA: M.I.T. Press, 1972.

Schmitt, F.O., and Worden, F.G. *The Neurosciences: Third Study Program*. Cambridge, MA: M.I.T. Press, 1974.

Shephard, Gordon M. *The Synaptic Organization of the Brain*. New York: Oxford University Press, 1974.

Truex, Raymond C., and Carpenter, M.B. *Human Neuroanatomy,* 6th ed. Baltimore, MD: Williams and Wilkins, 1969.

CHAPTERS 5, 6, and 7

Adam, G. *Perception, Consciousness, Memory: Reflections of a Biologist*. New York: Plenum Press, 1980.

Albus, J.S. "A New Approach to Manipulator Control: The Cerebellar Model Articulation Controller (CMAC)." *Journal of Dynamic Systems, Measurement, and Control*, (1975): 220-227.

_____. "A Theory of Cerebellar Functions." *Mathematical Biosciences* 10, (1971): 25-61.

_____. "Data Storage in the Cerebellar Model Articulation Controller (CMAC)." *Journal of Dynamic Systems, Measurement, and Control*. (1975): 229-233.

_____. "Mechanisms of Planning and Problem Solving in the Brain." *Mathematical Biosciences* 45 (1979): 247-293.

_____. "Theoretical and Experimental Aspects of a Cerebellar Model." Ph.D. Thesis, University of Maryland, 1972.

_____; Barbera, A.J.; and Nagel, R.N. "Theory and Practice of Hierarchical Control." *Proceedings of National Computer Conference* (1981).

Bloom, L.M. *Language Development: Form and Function in Emerging Grammar*. Cambridge, MA: M.I.T. Press, 1970.

Bower, T.G. *The Perceptual World of the Child*. Cambridge, MA: Harvard University Press, 1977.

Clark, M.L. *Hierarchical Structure of Comprehension Skills, Vol. 1: Theoretical Models and Related Research on the Definition and Measurement of Reading and Listening Comprehension*. Verry, 1973.

Coren, S., et al. *Sensation and Perception*. New York: Academic Press, 1979.

Duda, A.O., and Hart, P.E. *Pattern Classification and Scene Analysis*. New York: John Wiley and Sons, 1973.

Eccles, J.C.; Ito, M.; and Szentagothai, J. *The Cerebellum as a Neuronal Machine*. New York: Springer-Verlag, 1976.

Evarts, E., and Tanji, J. "Gating of Motor Cortex Reflexes by Prior Instruction." *Brain Research* 71 (1974): 479-494.

_____, and Thach, W.T. "Motor Mechanisms of the CNS: Cerebrocerebellar Interrelations." *Ann. Rev. Physiol.* 31 (1969): 451-498.

Gardner, B.T., and Gardner, R.A. "Teaching Sign Language to a Chimpanzee." *Science* 165 (1969): 664-672.

Gregory, R.L. *Concepts and Mechanisms of Perceptions.* New York: Charles Scribner & Son, 1974.

Held, R., and Richards W., eds. *Perception: Mechanisms and Models.* San Francisco: W.H. Freeman, 1972.

———, ed. *Image, Object, and Illusion.* San Francisco: W.H. Freeman, 1974.

Hubel, D.H., and Wiesel, T. "Receptive Fields and Functional Architecture of Monkey Striate Cortex." *J. Physiol. (London)* 195 (1968): 215-243.

Jackson, J. *Selected Writings of John Hughlings Jackson.* Edited by J. Taylor. London: Hodder and Stoughton, 1931.

John, E.R. "A Model of Consciousness." *Consciousness and Self-Regulation* (Vol. 1). New York: Plenum Press, 1967.

Kaufman, Lloyd. *Perception: The World Transformed.* New York: Oxford University Press, 1979.

Kohler, W. *The Mentality of Apes.* New York: Harcourt, Brace, 1925.

Konishi, M. "The Role of Auditory Feedback in the Control of Vocalization in the White-Crowned Sparrow." *Z. Tiertsychol.* 22 (1965): 770-783.

Lonnenberg, E.H. "The Natural History of Language." *The Genesis of Language.* Cambridge, MA: M.I.T. Press, 1966.

MacKay, D.M. "Cerebral Organization and Conscious Control of Action." *Brain and Conscious Experience.* New York: Springer, 1966.

MacLean, P.D. *A Triune Concept of the Brain and Behavior.* Toronto: University of Toronto Press, 1973.

Manning, A. *An Introduction to Animal Behavior.* Reading, MA: Addison-Wesley, 1972.

Marler, P., and Tamura, M. "Culturally Transmitted Patterns of Vocal Behavior in Sparrows." *Science* 146 (1964): 1483-1486.

Marr, D. "A Theory of Cerebellar Cortex." *Journal of Physiology* 202 (1969): 437-470.

Phillips, C.G. "Cortical Localization and Sensorimotor Processes at the Middle Level in Primates." *Proc. of the Royal Society of Medicine* 66 (1973): 987-1002.

Piaget, Jean. *The Grasp of Consciousness: Action and Concept in the Young Child.* Cambridge, MA: Harvard University Press, 1976.

———, and Inhelder, B. *The Child's Conception of Space.* New York: W.W. Norton, 1967.

Pfeiffer, J.E. *The Emergence of Man.* New York: Harper and Row, 1969.

Premack, A.J., and Premack, D. "Teaching Language to an Ape." *Scientific American* (Oct., 1972): 92-99.

Pribram, K.H. "Self Consciousness and Intentionality." *Consciousness and Self-Regulation* (Vol. 1). New York: Plenum Press, 1976.

Pugh, G.E. *The Biological Origin of Human Values.* New York: Basic Books, 1977.

Rachlin, H. *Introduction to Modern Behaviorism.* San Francisco: W.H. Freeman, 1970.

Rosenblatt, F. *Principles of Neurodynamics: Perceptions and the Theory of Brain Mechanisms.* Washington: Spartan Books, 1961.

Rumbaugh, D.J. *Acquisition of Linguistic Skills by a Chimpanzee.* New York: Academic Press, 1977.

Sacerdoti, E.D. *A Structure for Plans and Behavior.* New York: Elsevier, 1977.

Sagan, Carl. *Dragons of Eden: Speculations on the Evolution of Human Intelligence.* New York: Random House, 1977.

Skinner, B.F. *About Behaviorism.* New York: Vintage Books, 1976.

———. *Beyond Freedom and Dignity.* New York: Alfred A. Knopf, 1971.

Slamecka, N.J., ed. *Human Learning and Memory: Selected Readings.* New York: Oxford University Press, 1967.

Smith, F., and Miller, G.A., eds. *The Genesis of Language: A Psyhcolinguistic Approach.* Cambridge, MA: M.I.T. Press, 1966.

Sperry, R.W. "Perception in the Absence of the Neocortical Commisures." *Perception and its Disorders,* Research Publication of the Association for Research in Nervous and Mental Diseases 48 (1970).

Stelmach, G.E., ed. *Motor Control: Issues and Trends.* New York: Academic Press, 1976.

Taylor, J.G., and Papert, S. *The Behavioral Basis of Perception.* Greenwood, 1976.

Tinbergen, N. *The Study of Instinct.* Oxford: Clarendon Press, 1951.

Wightman, F.L. "The Pattern Transformation Model of Pitch." *Journal of Acoustical Society of America* 54 (1973): 407-416.

Wilson, E.O. *Sociobiology.* Cambridge, MA: Belknap Press of Harvard University, 1975.

CHAPTERS 8-12

Agin, C., "Real Time Control of a Robot with a Mobile Camera," Tech. Note 179, SRI International AI Center, Menlo Park, CA, 1979.

Agrawala, A.K., ed. *Machine Recognition of Patterns.* IEEE Press, 1977.

Albus, J.S. *Peoples' Capitalism: The Economics of the Robot Revolution.* Kensington, MD: New World Books, 1976.

_____; Barbera, A.J.; Fitzgerald, M.L.; Nagel, R.N.; VanderBrug, C.J.; and Wheatley, T.E. "A Measurement and Control Model for Adaptive Robots." *Proceedings of the 10th International Symposium on Industrial Robots,* Milan, Italy, 1980.

_____; Barbera, A.J.; and Nagel, R.N. "Theory and Practice of Hierarchical Control." *Proceedings of the National Computer Conference,* 1981.

_____; Evans, J. "Robot Systems." *Scientific American* 234 (1976).

Asimov, I. *In Robot.* Greenwich, CT: Fawcett Crest Publications, 1970.

Barbera, A. *An Architecture for a Robot Hierarchical Control System: User's Guide.* Special Publication 500-23, National Bureau of Standards, Washington, DC, 1977.

_____; Albus, J.S.; and Fitzgerald, M.L. "Hierarchical Control of Robots Using Microcomputers." *Proceedings of 9th International Symposium on Industrial Robots,* Washington, DC, 1979.

_____, et al. "Control Strategies for Industrial Robot Systems." Final Report, Publ. PB-283539/5GA, National Bureau of Standards, Washington, DC, 1976.

Boden, M. *Artificial Intelligence and Natural Man.* New York: Basic Books, 1977.

Capek, K. *R.U.R. (Rossum's Universal Robots).* New York: Oxford University Press, 1961.

Chapuis, A., and Droz, E. *The Jaquet-Droz Mechanical Puppets.* Neuchatel Historical Museum, Neuchatel, Switzerland, 1956.

Chomsky, Noam. *Aspects of the Theory of Syntax.* Cambridge, MA: M.I.T. Press, 1965.

Cohen, John. *Human Robots in Myth and Science.* London: George Allen and Unwin, Ltd., 1966.

Corliss, W., and Johnsen, E.G. "Teleoperator Controls." Report SP-5070, NASA, 1968.

Dallas, D.B. "CAD/CAM and the Computer Revolution: Selected Papers From CAD/CAM I and CAD/CAM II." Society of Manufacturing Engineers, Dearborn, MI, 1974.

Duda, R.O., and Hart, P.E. *Pattern Classification and Scene Analysis.* New York: John Wiley & Sons, 1973.

Engelberger, J.F. *Robotics in Practice.* Am. Managment, 1981.

_____. "Robotics: 1984." *Robotics Today* (1979): 26-27.

Fahlman, S. *NETL: A System for Representing and Using Real World Knowledge.* Cambridge, MA: M.I.T. Press, 1979.

Feigenbaum, E.A., and Feldman, J. *Computers and Thought*. New York: McGraw-Hill, 1963.

Fikes, R.E., and Nillson, N. "STRIPS: A New Approach to the Application of Theorem Proving to Problem Solving." *Artificial Intelligence* 2 (1971): 189-208.

Flora, P.C., Thompson, A.M.; and Wilf, J.M., eds. *Robotics Industry Directory*. La Canada, CA: Robotics Publishing Co., 1981.

Fu, K.S. *Syntatic Methods in Pattern Recognition*. New York: Academic Press, 1974.

Gonzales, R.C., and Wintz, P. *Digital Image Processing and Recognition*. Reading, MA: Addison-Wesley, 1977.

Guzman, A. "Decomposition of a Visual Scene into Three-Dimensional Bodies," *Proceedings Fall Joint Computer Conference* 33. Washington: Thompson Book Co., 1968.

Harrington, J. *Computer Integrated Manufacturing*. New York: Industrial Press, 1973.

Heginbotham, W.B., and Rooks, B.W., eds. *The Industrial Robot*. Oxford: Cotswold Press.

Hohn, R.E. "Computed Path Control for an Industrial Robot." *Proc. 8th Int'l Symp. on Indust. Robots (Vol. 1)*, Int'l Fluidics Services, Ltd., Bedford, England, 1978.

Issaman, P.B.S. "Tapping the Ocean's Vast Energy with Undersea Turbines." *Popular Science* 217 (1980): 72-158.

Kelso, L.O., and Hetter, P. *Two-Factor Theory: The Economics of Reality*. New York: Random House, 1967.

Klix, F., ed. *Human and Artificial Intelligence*. New York: North-Holland, 1979.

Lewis, R.A., and Johnston, A.R. "A Scanning Laser Rangefinder for a Robotic Vehicle." 5th Int'l Jt. Conf. on Artificial Intelligence, Cambridge, MA, 1977.

Malone, R. *The Robot Book*. New York: Harcourt Brace Jovanovich, 1978.

"Manufacturing Technology — A Changing Challenge to Improve Productivity." Report to the Congress by the Comptroller General of the United States, June, 1976.

McCorduck, P. *Machines Who Think*. San Francisco: W.H. Freeman, 1979.

Meltzer, B., and Michie, D. *Machine Intelligence*. Halsted Press, 1973.

Minsky, M., ed. *Semantic Information Processing*. Cambridge, MA: M.I.T. Press, 1968.

Nevins, J.L., et al. "Exploring Research in Industrial Modula Assembly." Report R-1111, C.S. Draper Labs, 1977.

———, and Whitney, D. "Computer-Controlled Assembly." *Scientific American* 238 (1979): 62.

Newell, A., and Simon, H.A. "GPS, A Program That Simulates Human Thought." In *Computers and Thought*. Edited by E.A. Feigenbaum and J. Feldman. New York: McGraw-Hill, 1963.

Nilsson, N.J. "A Hierarchical Robot Planning and Execution System." Artificial Intelligence Center Tech. Note, 6, Stanford Research Institute, 1973.

———. *Principles of Artificial Intelligence*. Palo Alto, CA: Tioga Publishing Co., 1980.

———. *Problem-Solving Methods in Artificial Intelligence*. New York: McGraw-Hill, 1971.

———, (narrator). "Shakey: A First Experiment in Robot Planning and Learning." A film by Stanford Research Institute AI Center, 1972.

———, and Rapheal, B. "Preliminary Design of an Intelligent Robot." *Computer and Information Sciences*. New York: Academic Press, 1967.

Nitzan, D. "Robotic Automation Program at SRI." Proc. MIDCON/79, Chicago, 1979.

———, and Rosen, C.A. "Programmable Industrial Automation." NSF Grant GI-38100X1, Tech. Note 133, SRI International AI Center, Menlo Park, CA, 1979.

Park, W.T. "Robotics Research Trends." Tech. Note 160, SRI International AI Center, Menlo Park, CA, 1978.

Paul, R.L. "Modelling, Trajectory Calculation and Servoing of a Computer Controlled Arm." Memo AIM-177, report STAN-CS-72-311, Stanford AI Project, 1972.

————. "WAVE: A Model-Based Language for Manipulator Control." *The Industrial Robot* 4 (1977): 10-17.

Pavlidis, T. *Structural Pattern Recongition.* New York: Springer-Verlag, 1977.

Perkins, W.A. "A Model-Based Vision System for Industrial Parts." *IEEE Transactions on Computers* 27 (1978): 126-143.

Pratt, W.K. *Digital Image Processing.* New York: John Wiley & Sons, 1978.

Raphael, B. *The Thinking Computer: Mind Inside Matter.* San Francisco: W.H. Freeman, 1976.

Reichardt, J. *Robots: Fact, Fiction, and Prediction.* New York: Penguin Books, 1978.

Reiger, C. "Artificial Intelligence Programming Languages for Computer-Aided Manufacturing." Report TR-595, Computer Science Department, University of Maryland, 1977.

Rigney, J.W., and Towne, D.M. "Computer Techniques for Analyzing the Microstructure of Serial-Action Work in Industry." *Human Factors* 11 (1969): 113-122.

Rosen, C.A., and Nilsson, N. "An Intelligent Automaton." IEEE International Convention Record, 1967.

————; Nitzan, E.; et al. "Machine Intelligence Research Applied to Industrial Automation." Reports 1-8, SRI International AI Center, Menlo Park, CA, 1973-1978.

Rosenfeld, A., and Kak, A.. *Digital Picture Processing.* New York: Academic Press, 1976.

Ruoff, C.F. "PACS—An Advanced Multitasking Robot System." *The Industrial Robot* 7 (1980): 87-98.

Samuel, A.L. "Some Studies in Machine Learning Using the Game of Checkers." In *Computers and Thought.* Edited by E.A. Feigenbaum and J. Feldman. New York: McGraw-Hill, 1963.

Schank, R.C., and Abelson, R.P. *Scripts, Plans, Goals, and Understanding: An Inquiry into Human Knowledge Structures.* Halsted Press, 1977.

The Seeds of Artificial Intelligence. NIH Publications 80-2071, U.S. Dept. of HEW, 1980.

Shimano, B. "User's Guide to VAL." Unimation, Inc., Danbury, CT 06810.

Shirai, Y., and Suwa, M. "Recognition of Polyhedra with a Range Finder," *Proc. of the IJCAI-71,* British Computer Society, 1971.

Simon, H. and Newell, A. *Human Problem Solving.* New York: Prentice-Hall, 1972.

Simon, J.C., and Rosenfeld, A. *Digital Image Processing and Analysis.* Sijthoff & Noordhoff, 1978.

Slagle, James R. "A Heuristic Program That Solves Symbolic Integration Problems in Freshman Calculus." In *Computers and Thought.* Edited by E.A. Feigenbaum and J. Feldman. New York: McGraw-Hill, 1963.

Stauffer, R.N., ed. *Robotics Today.* Robotics International of Society of Manufacturing Engineers.

Stucki, Ed. *Advances in Digital Image Processing: Theory, Application, Implementation.* New York: Plenum Press, 1979.

Sussman, C.J. *A Computer Model of Skill Acquisition.* Elsvier, 1975.

Tanner, W., ed. *Industrial Robots: Vol. 1, Fundamentals; Vol. 2, Applications.* Dearborn, MI: Society of Manufacturing Engineers, 1978.

Watterman, D.A., and Hayes-Roth, F. *Pattern-Directed Inference Systems.* New York: Academic Press, 1978.

Weekley, T.L. "The UAW Speaks Out on Industrial Robots." *Robotics Today* (1979-80): 25-27.

Weizenbaum, J. *Computer Power and Human Reason: From Judgement To Calculation.* San Francisco: W.H. Freeman, 1976.

Whitney, D. "Resolved Motion Rate Control of Manipulators and Human Prostheses." IEEE Trans. Man-Machine Systems, VOl. MMS-10, June, 1969: 47-53.

Winograd, T. *Understanding Natural Language.* New York: Academic Press, 1972.

Winston, P.H. *Artificial Intellignece.*
Reading, MA: Addison-Wesley, 1977.
———. *The Psychology of Computer Vi-
sion.* New York: McGraw-Hill, 1975.
Wisnosky, D., "Worldwide Com-
puter–Aided Manufacturing Survey."
ICAM Program, A.F. Materials Lab,
Wright-Patterson AFB, 1977.

Yoosufani, Z., and Boothroyal, G. "Design
for Manufacturability: Design of Parts
for Ease of Handling." NSF Grant
APR77-10197. Amherst, MA: Univ. of
Massachusetts, 1978.
Young, J.F. *Robotics.* New York: John
Wiley & Sons, 1973.

INDEX